Frontiers in Metabolism 1

Series Editor:
Keith Snell

FRONTIERS IN METABOLISM

Metabolic Regulation

A Human Perspective

by Keith N. Frayn

PORTLAND PRESS

Published by Portland Press Ltd, 59 Portland Place,
London W1N 3AJ, U.K.

In North America orders should be sent to Ashgate Publishing Co.,
Old Post Road, Brookfield, VT 05036-9704, U.S.A.

Copyright © **1996 Portland Press Ltd, London**

ISBN 1 85578 048 8   ISSN 1353 6516

British Library Cataloguing-in-Publication Data
A catalogue record for this book is available from the British Library

Typeset by Portland Press Ltd.
Printed in Great Britain by Henry Ling Ltd. Dorchester

Contents

3   Metabolic characteristics of the organs and tissues

4 Some important endocrine organs and hormones

5 Integration of carbohydrate, fat and protein metabolism in the whole body

6   The nervous system and metabolism

7 Coping with some extreme situations

8 Lipoprotein metabolism

9　Diabetes mellitus

10　Energy balance and body weight regulation

Editor's preface

Frontiers in Metabolism is a new series of books aimed at university or college students of biochemistry, medical and life sciences. In general such students are well served by excellent textbooks of molecular cell biology. But when it comes to the biochemical transformations for harnessing and utilizing chemical energy and for synthesizing macromolecules for cell replication and self-preservation — i.e. metabolism — the available textbooks are dated, dry or both.

Small wonder then that to some *Frontiers in Metabolism* may sound like a contradictory statement. After all, the majority of biochemical pathways, which form the structure of cellular metabolism, have already been discovered and described. However, having defined the structural framework of metabolism, the real frontiers now lie in determining its functional operation and the controlling mechanisms involved. It is the control of function which determines the specialization of biochemical behaviour which marks one tissue from another in a multicellular organism. It is in these respects that current textbooks fail to deliver.

Control systems and metabolic specialization operate at multiple levels and this series will explore these various levels. This first volume in the series deals with the integrative control mechanisms which govern the physiology of the human organism as a whole. It explores the sociological mechanisms which ensure the co-operation and integration of pathways in different tissues to promote the harmonious well-being of the whole animal and enable it to adapt to changing internal and external circumstances. The primary aim of this book, as with the others in the series, is to convey a modern picture of metabolism which emphasizes the dynamics of the subject — a picture which shows that there is more to understanding metabolism than regurgitating pathway sequences!

Keith Snell
Institute of Cancer Research
University of London

January 1996

Author's preface

The great triumph of modern biochemistry has been the reductionist approach. For instance, in the field of lipid metabolism, the 1960s was the era of incubating isolated fat pads to look at the control of fat mobilization. In the 1970s it became possible to isolate individual fat cells to study their metabolism. During the last decade, we have developed the ability to look at fat cell metabolism in molecular terms. Within a few years we may know the entire sequence of the human genome. These are powerful tools and will undoubtedly lead to great advances in our understanding of biochemistry at a fundamental level. However, there is a danger that we shall forget that, for most of us, the purpose of studying biochemistry is to do something useful for people or animals. The human body is more than just a collection of molecules or even cells: it is an extremely organized collection of cells capable of responding in a highly coordinated manner. Some very important situations for humans, such as starvation, stress or physical exercise, can only be understood at the level of the whole body. Most cells are very susceptible to starvation, but most people can survive a month of starvation with few ill effects. This is because of the coordinated interplay between the different tissues and organs of the body — something which cannot be studied at the cellular or molecular level. This book is an attempt to rebuild an integrated view of metabolism and metabolic regulation. It is set firmly in a human context, since I think many of us find humans among the most interesting of species. I hope you find it useful. Even more, I hope you will find it interesting.

Keith Frayn
Oxford Lipid Metabolism Group
Nuffield Department of Clinical Medicine
University of Oxford

November 1995

Abbreviations

ACTH	adrenocorticotropic hormone
ADH	antidiuretic hormone
AGE	advanced glycosylation end-product
AIB	α-amino-isobutyric acid
BMI	body mass index
BMR	basal metabolic rate
CCK	cholecystokinin
CE	cholesteryl ester
CETP	cholesteryl ester-transfer protein
CNS	central nervous system
CoASH	coenzyme A
CPT-1	carnitine O-palmitoyltransferase-1
DAG	diacylglycerol
DIT	diet-induced thermogenesis
FBPase	fructose 1,6-bisphosphatase
FH	familial hypercholesterolaemia
F 6-P	fructose 6-phosphate
F 1,6-P_2	fructose 1,6-bisphosphate
FQ	food quotient
FSH	follicle-stimulating hormone
GH	growth hormone
Gly-K	glycerol kinase
GK	glucokinase
GLUT	glucose transporter
G 6-P	glucose 6-phosphate
G 6-Pase	glucose-6-phosphatase
glycerol 3-P	glycerol 3-phosphate
HDL	high-density lipoprotein
HMG-CoA reductase	hydroxymethylglutaryl-CoA reductase
HSL	hormone-sensitive lipase
IDDM	insulin-dependent diabetes mellitus
IGF	insulin-like growth factor
IMP	inositol monophosphate
IP$_3$	inositol 1,4,5-trisphosphate
LCAT	lecithin–cholesterol acyltransferase
LDH	lactate dehydrogenase
LDL	low-density lipoprotein
LH	luteinizing hormone

LPL	lipoprotein lipase
MAG	monoacylglycerol
M_r	relative molecular mass
NEFA	non-esterified fatty acid
NIDDM	non-insulin-dependent diabetes mellitus
PCr	phosphocreatine
PDH	pyruvate dehydrogenase
PFK	phosphofructokinase
P_i	inorganic phosphate
PL	phospholipid
RER	respiratory exchange ratio
RQ	respiratory quotient
SGLT	sodium–glucose co-transporter
T_3	tri-iodothyronine
T_4	thyroxine
TAG	triacylglycerol
TCA cycle	tricarboxylic acid cycle
TSH	thyroid-stimulating hormone
VLDL	very-low-density lipoprotein

Some important concepts

1.1   Metabolic regulation in perspective

To many students, metabolism sounds a dull subject. It involves learning pathways with intermediates with difficult names and even more difficult formulae. Metabolic regulation may sound even worse. It involves not just remembering the pathways, but remembering what the enzymes are called, what affects them and how. This book is not simply a repetition of the molecular details of metabolic pathways; rather, it is an attempt to put metabolism and metabolic regulation into a physiological context, to help the reader to see the relevance of these subjects. Once their relevance to everyday life becomes apparent, then the details will become easier, and more interesting, to grasp.

This book is written from a human perspective because, as humans, it is natural for us to find our own metabolism interesting — and it is very important for understanding human health and disease. Nevertheless, many of the principal regulatory mechanisms to be discussed are common to other mammals. Some mammals, such as ruminants, have rather specialized patterns of digestion and absorption of energy; such aspects will not be covered in this book.

A consideration of metabolic regulation might begin with the question: why is it necessary? An analogy is with mechanical devices, which require an input of energy, and convert this energy to a different and more useful form. The waterwheel is a simple example: this device takes the potential energy of water in a reservoir — the mill-pond — and converts it into mechanical energy which can be used for turning machinery, for instance, to grind corn. As long as the water flows, its energy is extracted, and useful work is done. If the water stops, the wheel stops. A motor vehicle has a different pattern of energy intake and output (Figure 1.1). Energy is taken in very spasmodically — only when the driver stops at a filling station — and is converted into useful work (acceleration and motion) with an entirely different pattern. A long journey might

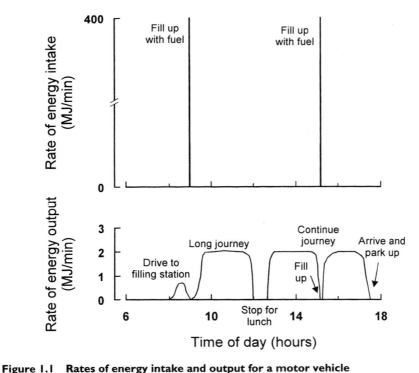

Figure 1.1   Rates of energy intake and output for a motor vehicle
The rate of intake (top panel) is zero except for periods in a filling station, when it is suddenly very high. The rate of output (bottom panel) is zero while the car is parked with the engine off; it increases as the car is driven to the filling station, and is relatively high during a journey. Note that when totalled up over a long period, the areas under the two curves must be equal (energy intake = energy output), except for any difference in the amounts of fuel in the tank before and after. (Notice that the scales are different for intake and output.)

be undertaken without any energy intake. Clearly, the difference from the water-wheel lies in the presence of a storage device, the fuel tank. But the fuel tank alone is not sufficient: there must also be a control mechanism to regulate the flow of energy from the store to the device which produces useful work, i.e. the engine. In this case, the regulator is in part a human brain, deciding when to move, and in part a mechanical system controlling the flow of fuel.

What does this have to do with metabolism? The human body is also a device for taking in energy (chemical energy, in the form of food) and converting it to other forms. Most obviously, this is in the form of physical work, such as lifting heavy objects. However, it can also be in more subtle forms, such as producing and nurturing offspring. Every activity requires energy. Again, this is most obvious if we think about performing mechanical work: lifting a heavy object from the floor onto a shelf requires conversion of chemical energy (ultimately derived from food) into potential energy of the object. But even maintaining life involves work: breathing, pumping blood around the vascular system, chewing food and digesting it or replacing cells

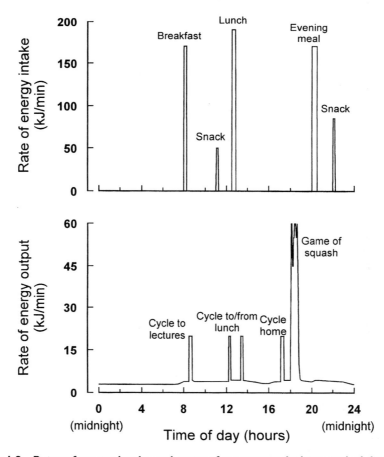

Figure 1.2   Rates of energy intake and output for a person during a typical day
The rate of energy intake (top panel) is zero except when eating or drinking, when it may be very high. The rate of energy output (heat + physical work; bottom panel) is at its lowest during sleep; it increases on waking and increases even more during physical exertion, e.g. cycling to and from lectures, or playing games. As with the car, the pattern of energy intake may not resemble that of energy expenditure, but over a long period the areas under the curves will roughly balance, except for any difference in the amounts of energy stored (mainly as body fat) before and after.

which have become damaged. At a cellular level, there is constant work performed in the pumping of ions across membranes, and the synthesis and breakdown of the chemical constituents of cells.

What is your pattern of energy intake in relation to energy output? For most of us, the majority of energy intake occurs in three relatively short periods during each 24 hours, whereas energy expenditure is largely continuous (the *resting metabolism*) with occasional extra bursts of external work (Figure 1.2). It is clear that we, like the motor vehicle, must have some way of storing food energy and releasing it when required. As with the motor vehicle, the human brain may also be at the beginning of the regulatory mechanism, although it may not be the conscious part of the brain that is involved: we do not have to think when we need to release some energy from our fat stores, for instance. Some of the important regulatory systems that will be covered in this book lie outside the brain, in organs that secrete hormones, particularly the pancreas. But whatever the internal means used to achieve this regulation, we manage to store our excess food energy and to release it just as we need.

This applies to the normal 24 hour period in which we eat meals and go about our daily life. However, the body also has to cope with less-well-organized situations. In many parts of the world, there are times when food is not that easily available, and yet people are able to maintain relatively normal lives. Clearly, the body's regulatory mechanisms must recognize that food is not coming in and allow an appropriate rate of release of energy from the internal stores. In other situations, the need for energy may be suddenly increased. Strenuous physical exercise may increase the total rate of metabolism in the body to twenty times its resting level: something must recognize the fact that there is a sudden need to release energy at a high rate from the body's stores. During severe illness, such as that associated with infection, the rate of metabolism may also be increased; this is manifested in part by the rise in body temperature. Often the sufferer will not feel like eating normally. Once again, the body must have a way of recognizing the situation, and regulating the necessary release of stored energy.

What we are now discussing is, indeed, *metabolic regulation*. Metabolic regulation in human terms covers the means by which we take in nutrients in discrete meals, and deliver energy as required, varying from moment to moment and from tissue to tissue in a pattern which may have no relationship at all to the pattern of intake. Metabolic regulation works ultimately at a molecular level, mainly by modulation of the activities of enzymes. But one should not lose sight of the fact that these molecular mechanisms are there to enable us to lead normal lives despite fluctuations in our intake and expenditure of energy. In this book, the emphasis will be on the systems within the human body that sense the balance between energy coming in and energy required, particularly the *endocrine* (hormonal) and the *nervous* systems. These systems regulate the distribution and storage of nutrients after meals and their release from stores and delivery to individual tissues as required.

The intention of this preamble is to illustrate that, underlying our everyday lives, there are very precise and beautifully coordinated regulatory systems which control the flow of energy within our bodies. Metabolic regulation is not a dry, academic subject thought up just to make biochemistry examinations difficult, it is at the heart of human life and affects each one of us at every moment.

1.2   The chemistry of food (and of bodies)

Energy is taken into the body in the form of food. The components of food may be classified as *macronutrients* and *micronutrients*. Macronutrients are those components present in a typical serving, in amounts of grams rather than milligrams or less. They are the well-known carbohydrates, fats and proteins. Water is another important constituent of many foods, although it is not usually considered to be a nutrient. Micronutrients are vitamins, minerals and nucleic acids. Although these micronutrients play vital roles in the metabolism of macronutrients, they will not be discussed in any detail in this book, which is concerned with the broader aspects of what is often called *energy metabolism*.

The links between nutrition and energy metabolism are very close: we eat carbohydrates, fats and proteins; within the body these are broken down to smaller components, rearranged, stored, released from stores and further metabolized. But essentially, whether we are discussing food or metabolism, the same categories of carbohydrate, fat and protein can be distinguished. This is not surprising since our food itself is of organic origin, whether plant or animal.

To understand metabolism and metabolic regulation, it is useful to have a clear idea of some of the major chemical properties of these components. This is not intended as a treatise in physical or organic chemistry, but the discussion assumes a basic understanding of the meaning of the terms atom and molecule, and of chemical reactions and catalysis, and some understanding of chemical bonds (particularly the distinction between ionic and covalent bonding).

1.2.1   Some important chemical concepts

1.2.1.1   Polarity

Some aspects of metabolism are more easily understood through an appreciation of the nature of *polarity* of molecules. Polarity refers to the distribution of electrical charge over the molecule. A *non-polar* molecule has a very even distribution of electrical charge over its surface and is electrically neutral overall (the negative charge on the electrons is balanced by the positive charge of the nucleus). A *polar* molecule has an overall charge, or at least an uneven distribution of charge. The most polar small particles are ions, i.e. atoms or molecules which have entirely lost or gained one or more electrons. However, even completely covalently bonded organic molecules may have a sufficiently uneven distribution of electrical charge to affect their behaviour. Polarity is not an all-or-none phenomenon: there are gradations, from the strongly polar to the completely non-polar.

Polarity is not difficult to predict in the molecules that are important in biochemistry. We will contrast two simple examples: the water molecule and that of methane, another simple molecule. Their relative molecular masses are similar — 18 for water, 16 for methane — and yet their physical properties are very different. Water is a liquid at room temperatures and does not boil until it is heated to a temperature of 100 °C, whereas methane is a gas ('natural gas') which only liquifies when cooled to −161 °C. We might imagine that similar molecules of similar size would have the same tendency to move from the liquid to the gas phase, and that they would have similar boiling points. The reason for their different behaviours lies in their relative polarity. The molecule of methane has the three-dimensional structure shown in Figure 1.3(a). The outer electron 'cloud' has a very even distribution over the four hydrogen atoms, each of which has an equal tendency to pull electrons its way. The molecule has no distinct electrical poles — it is non-polar. Because of the very even distribution of electrons, molecules near each other have very little tendency to interact. In contrast, in the water molecule (Figure 1.3b) the oxygen atom has a very distinct tendency to pull electrons its way, shifting the distribution of the outer electron cloud so that it is more dense over the oxygen atom, and correspondingly less dense elsewhere. Therefore, the molecule has a rather negatively charged region around the central oxygen

Figure 1.3 (a) Three-dimensional structure of the methane molecule and (b) the molecular structure of water
(a) The hydrogen atoms of methane (CH_4) are arranged symmetrically in space, at the corners of a tetrahedron. (b) Top, view of the 'electron cloud' surrounding the molecule; bottom, interactions between water molecules. The molecule has a degree of *polarity*, and this leads to electrical interactions between neighbouring molecules by the formation of *hydrogen bonds* (dotted lines). These bonds are not strong compared with covalent bonds, and are constantly being formed and broken. Nevertheless, they provide sufficient attraction between the molecules to account for the fact that water is a liquid at room temperature whereas the non-polar methane is a gas.

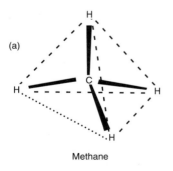

(a)

Methane

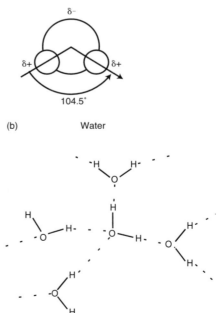

(b)   Water

atom, and correspondingly positively charged regions around the hydrogen atoms. Thus it has distinct electrical poles — it is a relatively polar molecule. Now, it is easy to imagine that water molecules near to each other will interact in some way: like electrical charges repel each other, unlike ones attract. This gives water molecules a tendency to line up so that the positive regions of one molecule attract the negative region of an adjacent molecule (Figure 1.3b). So water molecules, unlike those of methane, tend to 'stick together': the energy needed to break them apart and form a gas is much greater than for methane. Hence at room temperature and pressure water is a liquid whereas methane is a gas. The latent heat of evaporation of water is 2.5 kJ/g, whereas that of methane is 0.6 kJ/g. Note that the polarity of the water molecule is not as extreme as that of an ion — it is merely a rather uneven distribution of electrons, but this is enough to affect its properties considerably.

The contrast between water and methane may be extended to larger molecules. Organic compounds composed solely of carbon and hydrogen — for instance, the alkanes or 'paraffins' — all have the property of extreme non-polarity: the chemical (covalent) bond between carbon and hydrogen atoms leads to a very even distribution of electrons, and the molecules have little interaction with each other. A result of this is that polar molecules, such as those of water, and non-polar molecules, such as those of alkanes, do not mix well: the water molecules tend to bond to each other and to exclude the non-polar molecules, which can themselves pack together very closely because of the lack of interaction between them. In fact, there is an additional form of direct attraction between non-polar molecules, the *van der Waals* forces. Random fluctuations in the density of the electron cloud surrounding a molecule lead to minor, transient degrees of polarity; these induce an opposite charge in a neighbouring molecule, with the result that there is a transient attraction between them. These are very weak attractions, however, and the effect of the exclusion by water is considerably stronger. The non-polar molecules are said to be *hydrophobic* (water-fearing or water-hating).

A strong contrast is provided by an inorganic ionic compound such as sodium chloride. The sodium and chlorine atoms in sodium chloride are completely ionized under almost all conditions. They pack very regularly in crystals in a cubic form. The strength of their attraction for each other means that considerable energy is needed to disrupt this regular packing — sodium chloride does not melt until it is heated to temperatures above 800 °C. However, it dissolves very readily in water, i.e. the individual ions become separated from their close-packing arrangement rather as they would on melting. This is because the water molecules, by virtue of their polarity, are able to come between the ions and reduce their attraction for one another. In fact, each of the charged sodium and chloride ions will become surrounded by a 'shell' of water molecules, shielding it from the attraction or repulsion of other ions. Sodium chloride is said to be *hydrophilic* (water loving). The terms polar and hydrophilic are for the most part interchangeable. Similarly, the terms non-polar and hydrophobic are virtually synonymous.

Ionic compounds, the extreme examples of polarity, are not confined to inorganic chemistry. Organic molecules may include ionized groups. These may be almost entirely ionized under normal conditions: e.g. the esters of orthophosphoric acid ('phosphate groups') in the compounds AMP, ADP and ATP, in metabolites such as glucose 6-phosphate, and in phospholipids. Most of the organic acids involved in intermediary metabolism, such as lactic acid, pyruvic acid and the long-chain carboxylic acids (fatty acids), are also largely ionized at physiological hydrogen ion concentrations (Box 1.1). Thus generation of lactic acid during exercise raises the hydrogen ion concentration (the acidity) both within the cells where it is produced and generally within the body, since it is released into the bloodstream.

As stated earlier, polarity is not difficult to predict in organic molecules. It relies upon the fact that certain atoms always have *electronegative* (electron-withdrawing) properties in comparison with hydrogen. The most important such atoms biochemically are those of oxygen, phosphorus and nitrogen. Therefore, certain functional groups based on these atoms have polar properties. These include the hydroxyl group (-OH), the amino group ($-NH_2$), and the orthophosphate group ($-OPO_3^{2-}$). Compounds that contain these groups will have polar properties, whereas those containing just carbon and hydrogen will have much less polarity. The presence of an electronegative atom does not always give polarity to a molecule — if it is part of a chain and balanced by a similar atom this property may be lost: for instance, the ester link in a triacylglycerol molecule (discussed below) contains two oxygen atoms but has no polar properties.

Examples of relatively polar, and thus water-soluble, compounds are sugars (with many -OH groups), organic acids such as lactic acid (with a $-COO^-$ group) and most other small metabolites. Most amino acids also fall into this category (with their amino and carboxyl groups), although some fall into the *amphipathic* ('mixed') category discussed below.

Another important point about polarity in organic molecules is that within one molecule there may be both polar and non-polar regions. These molecules are called amphipathic compounds, and this category includes phospholipids and long-chain fatty acids (Figure 1.4). Cell membranes are made up of a double-layer of phospholipids, interspersed with specific proteins such as transport molecules and hormone receptors, and molecules of cholesterol (Figure 1.5). The phospholipid bilayer presents its polar faces — the polar 'heads' of the phospholipid molecules — to the aqueous external and internal environments; within the thickness of the membrane is a non-polar, hydrophobic region. Molecules crossing this membrane must pass through both the hydrophilic, polar faces and the hydrophobic interior. In general, this presents less of a problem for non-polar hydrophobic molecules; thus many hydrophobic drugs are able to enter cells readily. It has long been assumed that

Box 1.1 Ionization state of some acids at normal hydrogen ion concentrations

The normal pH in blood plasma is around 7.4. (It may be somewhat lower within cells). This corresponds to a hydrogen ion concentration of 3.98×10^{-8} mol/l (since $-\log_{10}$ of 3.98×10^{-8} is 7.4).

The ionization of an acid HA is described by the equation:

$$HA <===> H^+ + A^-$$

$$\frac{[H^+][A^-]}{[HA]} = K_i$$

where K_i is the dissociation or ionization constant, and is a measure of the strength of the acid: the higher the value of K_i the stronger (i.e. the more dissociated) the acid.

K_i in the equation above relates the concentrations expressed in molar terms (e.g. mol/l). (Strictly, it is not the concentrations but the 'effective ion concentrations' or ion activities which are related; these are not quite the same as concentrations because of inter-ion attractions. In most biological systems, however, in which the concentrations are relatively low, it is a close approximation to use concentrations. If activities are used, then the symbol K_a is used for the dissociation constant of an acid.)

Some biological acids and their K_a values are listed in the table below, together with a calculation of the proportion ionized at typical pH (7.4).

The calculation is done as follows (using acetic acid as an example).

$$K_a = 1.75 \times 10^{-5} = \frac{[H^+][Ac^-]}{[HAc]}$$

(where HAc represents undissociated acetic acid, Ac^- represents the acetate ion).

At pH 7.4, $[H^+] = 3.98 \times 10^{-8}$ mol/l. Therefore,

$$\frac{[Ac^-]}{[HAc]} = \frac{[1.75 \times 10^{-5}]}{[3.98 \times 10^{-8}]} = 440$$

(i.e. the ratio of ionized to undissociated acid is 440:1; it is almost entirely ionized).

The percentage in the ionized form $= \dfrac{440}{441} \times 100\% = 99.8\%$.

Acid	K_a	% ionized at pH 7.4
Acetic acid, CH_3COOH	1.75×10^{-5}	99.8
Lactic acid, $CH_3CHOHCOOH$	1.38×10^{-4}	99.9
Palmitic acid, $CH_3(CH_2)_{14}COOH$	1.58×10^{-5}	99.8
Glycine, CH_2NH_2COOH (carboxyl group)	3.98×10^{-3}	100

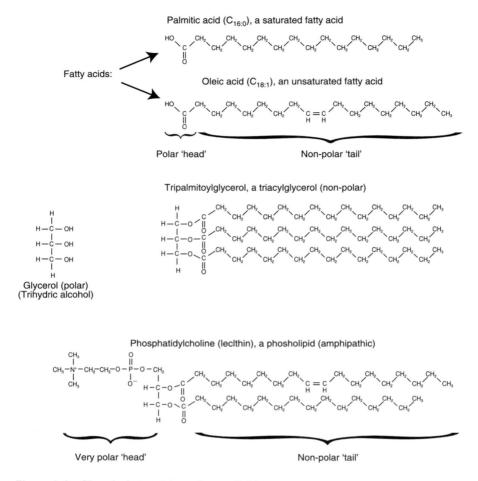

Figure 1.4   Chemical structures of some lipids
A typical saturated fatty acid (palmitic acid) is shown with its polar carboxylic group and non-polar hydrocarbon tail. *Glycerol* is a hydrophilic alcohol. However, it is a component of many lipids, as its hydroxyl groups may form ester links with up to three fatty acids, as shown. The resultant *triacylglycerol* has almost no polar qualities. The *phospholipids* are diacylglycerols with an additional polar group, usually a nitrogen-containing base such as choline (as shown) or a polyalcohol derivative such as phosphoinositol. The fatty acids in phospholipids are commonly long-chain unsaturated on the 2-position: oleic acid ($C_{18:1}$) is shown.

all hydrophobic molecules can enter cells by simple diffusion, but this is now increasingly under question as more and more specific transporter proteins are described. One example which will be common in this book is that of long-chain fatty acids entering cells: for many years this process was thought to occur by diffusion, but within the last few years specific *fatty-acid transport proteins* have been described. It should not surprise us, since it is difficult to imagine how the largely non-polar fatty acid might cross the extremely polar outer layers of a phospholipid bilayer. Furthermore, it makes good physio-

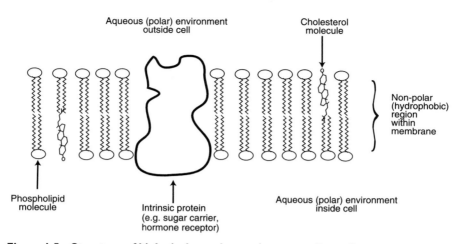

Figure 1.5   Structure of biological membranes in mammalian cells
Cell membranes and intracellular membranes, such as the endoplasmic reticulum, are composed of bilayers of phospholipid molecules with their polar head-groups facing the aqueous environ-ment on either side and their non-polar 'tails' facing inwards, forming a hydrophobic centre to the membrane. The membrane also contains *intrinsic proteins*, such as hormone receptors and sugar transport proteins, and molecules of cholesterol, which stabilize the membrane and regulate its fluidity.

logical sense because the movement of molecules in and out of cells by simple diffusion is, by its very nature, not a process over which any active control can be exerted. On the other hand, if the movement occurs more by a carrier-mediated process, then immediately there are possibilities for regulation: some cells may have more carriers than others, or the number or activity of the carriers may be altered by hormones. General characteristics of the movement of substances across membranes are discussed in Box 1.2.

The long-chain fatty acids fall into the amphipathic category — they have a long, non-polar hydrocarbon tail but a more-polar carboxylic group head (-COO⁻). Another compound with mixed properties is cholesterol (Figure 1.6); its ring system is very non-polar, but its hydroxyl group gives it some polar properties. However, the long-chain fatty acids and cholesterol may lose their polar aspects completely when they join in ester links. An ester is a compound formed by the condensation (elimination of a molecule of water) of an alcohol (-OH) and an acid (e.g. a carboxylic acid, -COO⁻).

Cholesterol, through its -OH group, may become esterified to a long-chain fatty acid, forming a *cholesteryl ester* (e.g. cholesteryl oleate; see Figure 1.6). The cholesteryl esters are extremely non-polar compounds. This fact will be important when we consider the metabolism of cholesterol in Chapter 8.

The long-chain fatty acids may also become esterified with glycerol to form triacylglycerols (Figure 1.4). Again, the polar properties of both partners are lost, and a very non-polar molecule is formed. This fact underlies one of the most fundamental aspects of mammalian metabolism: the use of triacyl-glycerol as the major form for storage of excess energy.

Box 1.2 Movement of molecules across membranes

The cell membrane, and membranes within cells, are formed from a phospholipid bilayer (see Figure 1.6). Most biological molecules, especially polar molecules and ions, do not diffuse freely across such a membrane. Instead, there are specific proteins embedded in the membranes which 'transport' molecules and ions from one side to the other. This box describes some general properties of the movement of molecules across membranes. (More details of the specific transport proteins for glucose are given in Box 3.1, Chapter 3.)

A substance will cross a membrane to move from one solution to another if (i) the membrane is permeable to the substance, and (ii) there is a *concentration gradient* in the appropriate direction: i.e. it will move from a region of high concentration to one of lower concentration. (In reality, there will be movement in both directions because of random molecular movements, but the *net movement* will be *down* the concentration gradient.)

There are two major means by which such movement may occur: *free diffusion*, i.e. unassisted movement by diffusion, brought about simply by the overall effect of random molecular motions, and *facilitated diffusion (carrier-mediated diffusion)*, i.e. movement assisted by a specific transport protein. A third means of movement, is *active transport*, in which substances may move *up* a concentration gradient, i.e. from a lower concentration to a higher one. This can only be brought about by the supply of energy, either electrical (charge on the membrane) or chemical; for instance, the enzyme *Na^+/K^+-exchanging ATPase* (EC 3.6.1.37) is a membrane protein which hydrolyses ATP and pumps sodium ions out of cells, against a strong concentration gradient, and potassium ions in, also against a strong concentration gradient.

The two forms of movement down concentration gradients, free diffusion and facilitated diffusion, can be distinguished by their kinetic characteristics. Since the movement of substances by a transport protein is similar in many ways to enzyme catalysis, it has ☞

Among amino acids, the branched-chain amino acids, leucine, isoleucine and valine, have non-polar side-chains and are thus amphipathic. The aromatic amino acids phenylalanine and tyrosine are relatively hydrophobic, and the amino acid tryptophan is so non-polar that it is not carried free in solution in the plasma.

The concept of the polarity or non-polarity of molecules thus has a number of direct consequences for the aspects of metabolism to be considered in later chapters. It is worth listing some of these consequences here.

1. Lipid fuels — fatty acids and triacylglycerols — are largely hydrophobic and are not soluble in the blood plasma. There are specific routes for their absorption from the intestine and specific mechanisms by which they are transported in blood.

☞ **Box 1.2 (continued)**

similar characteristics: there is a characteristic *affinity* of the transport protein for the molecule, and a maximum rate of transfer of the molecule which will depend, in turn, on the intrinsic 'rate of action' of the protein, and the number of transport proteins available in the membrane. Thus if we measure the rate of transport at differing concentrations of the substrate to be transported, we will find a hyperbolic curve similar to a 'Michaelis–Menten' plot of enzyme action. On the other hand, if transport occurs by free diffusion, there is no limitation to the rate, and it will be simply proportional to the concentration of substrate (strictly, to the magnitude of the concentration gradient across the membrane). These are illustrated here.

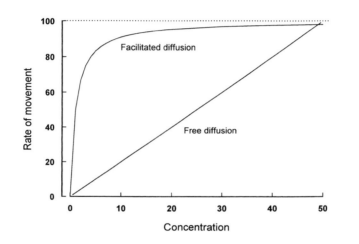

The presence of active transport will usually be identified by its need for energy: blocking of ATP synthesis (for instance, by inhibition of oxidative phosphorylation) will reduce or abolish such transport.

2. Carbohydrates are hydrophilic. When carbohydrate is stored in cells it is stored in a hydrated form, in association with water. In contrast, fat is stored as a lipid droplet from which water is excluded. Mainly because of this lack of water, fat stores contain considerably more energy per unit weight of store than do carbohydrate stores.

3. The entry of fats into the circulation must be co-ordinated with the availability of the specific carrier mechanisms. In the rare situations in which it arises, uncomplexed fat in the bloodstream may have very adverse consequences.

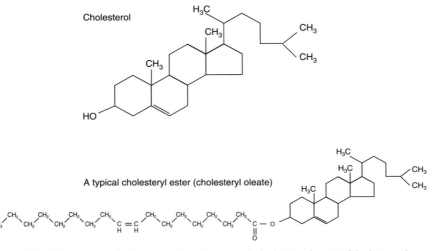

Figure 1.6 Structures of cholesterol and a typical cholesteryl ester (cholesteryl oleate)
In the structure of cholesterol, not all atoms are shown (for simplicity): each 'corner' represents a carbon atom, or else -CH or -CH$_2$. Cholesterol itself has amphipathic properties because of its hydroxyl group, but when esterified to a long-chain fatty acid the molecule is very non-polar.

1.2.1.2 Osmosis

The phenomenon of *osmosis* underlies some aspects of metabolic strategy — it can be seen as one reason why certain aspects of metabolism and metabolic regulation have evolved in the way that they have. It is outlined only briefly here to highlight its relevance.

Osmosis is the way in which solutions of different concentrations tend to even out when they are in contact with one another via a *semi-permeable membrane*. In solutions, the *solvent* is the medium in which substances dissolve (e.g. water) and the *solute* the substance that dissolves. A semi-permeable membrane allows molecules of solvent to pass through, but not those of solute. Thus it may allow molecules of water but not those of sugar to pass through. Cell membranes are close approximations to semi-permeable membranes when water is the solvent. Although the relatively polar water molecules do not diffuse freely through a phospholipid bilayer, cell membranes contain specific protein 'channels' through which water molecules pass, apparently as though by simple diffusion.

If solutions of unequal concentration, e.g. a dilute and a concentrated solution of sugar, are separated by a semi-permeable membrane, then molecules of solvent (in this case water) will tend to pass through the membrane until the concentrations of the solutions have become equal on either side of the membrane. To understand this intuitively, it is necessary to remember that the particles (molecules or ions) of solute are not just moving about freely in the solvent: each is surrounded by molecules of solvent, attracted by virtue of the polarity of the solute particles. (In the case of a non-polar solute in a non-polar solvent, we would have to say that the attraction is by virtue of the non-polarity: it occurs through weaker forces such as the van der Waals.) In the more concentrated solution, the proportion of solvent molecules engaged in such attachment to the solute particles is larger, and there is a net attraction for further solvent molecules to join them, in comparison with the more dilute solution; solvent molecules will tend to move from one solution to the other until the proportion involved in such interactions with the solute particles is equal.

The consequence of this in real situations may not be simply the dilution of a more concentrated solution, and the concentration of a more dilute one, until their concentrations are equal. Usually there are physical constraints. This is simply seen if we imagine a single cell, which has accumulated within it, for example, amino acid molecules taken up from the outside fluid by a transport mechanism which has made them more concentrated inside than outside. Water will then tend to move into the cell to even out this concentration difference. If water moves into the cell, the cell will increase in volume. Cells can swell so much that they burst under some conditions (fortunately not usually encountered in the body). For instance, red blood cells placed in water will burst (*lyse*) from just this effect: the relatively concentrated mixture of dissolved organic molecules within the cell will attract water from outside the cell, increasing the volume of the cell until its membrane can stretch no further and ruptures.

In the laboratory, we can avoid this by handling cells in solutions that contain solute — usually sodium chloride — at a total concentration of solute particles which matches that found within cells. This total concentration of particles is usually measured in mmol per kg of water, and is referred to as the *osmolality*. Solutions which match this osmolality are referred to as *isotonic*; a common laboratory example is *isotonic saline* solution which contains 9 g of NaCl per litre of water, with a molar concentration of 154 mmol/l. Remember that, since this will be fully ionized into Na^+ and Cl^- ions, the particle concentration is 308 'milliparticles' (sometimes called milliosmoles) per litre. We refer to this as an osmolarity of 308 mmol/l, but it is not 308 mmol of NaCl per litre. (The conversion between concentration of particles in mmol per litre of solution, strictly called *osmolarity*, and osmolality, in mmol per kg solvent, is not significant here, and the difference need not concern us.)

The phenomenon of osmosis has a number of repercussions in metabolism. Most cells have a number of different 'pumps' or active transporters in their cell membranes which can be used to regulate intracellular osmolality, and hence cell size. This process requires energy and is one of the components of basal energy expenditure. It may also be important in metabolic regulation; there is increasing evidence that changes in cell volume are part of a signalling mechanism that brings about changes in the activity of intracellular metabolic pathways. The osmolality of the plasma is maintained within narrow limits by specific mechanisms within the kidney, regulating the loss of water from the body via changes in the concentration of urine. Most importantly, potential problems posed by osmosis can be seen to underlie the metabolic strategy of fuel storage, as will become apparent in later sections.

1.2.2   The chemical characteristics of macronutrients

1.2.2.1   Carbohydrates

Simple carbohydrates have the empirical formula $C_n(H_2O)_n$; complex carbohydrates have an empirical formula which is similar to this (e.g. $C_n(H_2O)_{0.8n}$). The name carbohydrate reflects the idea, based on this empirical formula, that these compounds are hydrates of carbon. It is not strictly correct, but illustrates an important point about this group of compounds: the relative abundance of hydrogen and oxygen in carbohydrate molecules, in proportions similar to those in water. From the discussion above, it will be apparent that carbohydrates are mostly relatively polar molecules, miscible with, or soluble in, water. Carbohydrates in nature include the plant products starch and cellulose and the mammalian storage carbohydrate glycogen, as well as various simple sugars, of which glucose is the most important from the point of view of human metabolism. The main source of carbohydrate we eat is the starch in vegetables, such as potatoes, rice and other grains.

The chemical definition of a sugar is that its molecules consist of carbon atoms, each bearing one hydroxyl group (-OH), except for one carbon atom which bears a carbonyl group (=O) instead. In solution, the molecule exists in an equilibrium between a 'straight-chain' form and a ring structure; however, as the ring structure predominates, sugars are usually shown in this form.

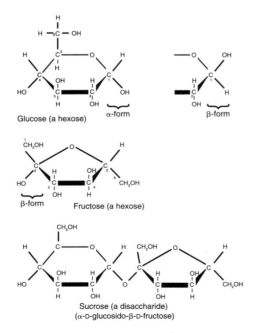

Glucose (a hexose)

α-form

β-form

β-form

Fructose (a hexose)

Sucrose (a disaccharide)
(α-D-glucosido-β-D-fructose)

Figure 1.7 Some simple sugars and disaccharides

Glucose and fructose are shown in their 'ring' form. Even this representation ignores the true three-dimensional structure, which is 'chair' shaped. Imagine that the middle part of the glucose ring is flat; the left-hand end slopes down and the right-hand end slopes up. Glucose forms a six-membered ring and is described as a pyranose; fructose forms a five-membered ring and is described as a furanose. In solution, the α- and β-forms are in equilibrium with each other and with a smaller amount of the straight-chain form. The orientation of the oxygen on carbon atom 1 becomes fixed when glucose forms links via this carbon to another sugar, as in sucrose: α- and β-links then have quite different properties (e.g. compare cellulose with starch or glycogen).

Nevertheless, some of the chemical properties of sugars can only be understood by remembering that the straight-chain form exists. The basic carbohydrate unit is known as a monosaccharide. Monosaccharides may have different numbers of carbon atoms, and the terminology reflects this: a hexose molecule has six carbon atoms, a pentose has five, etc. Pentoses and hexoses are the most important monosaccharides in terms of mammalian metabolism. These sugars also have 'common names' which often reflect their natural occurrence. The most abundant in our diet and in our bodies are the hexoses *glucose* (grape sugar; named from the Greek *glykys*, meaning sweet), *fructose* (fruit sugar; from the Latin *fructus* for fruit) and *galactose* (derived from lactose, milk sugar; from the Greek *galaktos* meaning milk), and the pentose *ribose*, a constituent of nucleic acids (the name comes from the related sugar arabinose; named after Gum arabic).

Complex carbohydrates are built up from the monosaccharides by covalent links between sugar molecules. The term *disaccharide* is

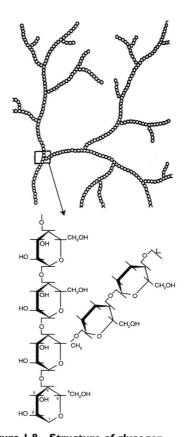

Figure 1.8 Structure of glycogen
Each circle in the upper diagram represents a glucosyl residue. Most of the links are of the α-1,4 variety. One of the branch points, an α-1,6 link, is enlarged below. Amylopectin, a component of starch, has a similar structure. Amylose, the other component of starch, has a linear α-1,4 structure.

used for a molecule composed of two monosaccharides (which may or may not be the same); *oligosaccharide* is used for a short chain of sugar units and *polysaccharide* for longer chains (>10 units), as found in starch and glycogen. Disaccharides are abundant in the diet and, again, their common names often denote their origin: *sucrose* (table sugar, named from the French sucre) which contains glucose and fructose (Figure 1.7); *maltose* (from malt) contains two glucose molecules; *lactose* (from milk) contains galactose and glucose. The bonds between individual sugar units are relatively strong at normal hydrogen ion concentrations, and sucrose (for instance) does not break down when it is boiled, although it is steadily broken down in acidic solutions such as cola drinks; however, there are specific enzymes in the intestine (described in

Chapter 2) which hydrolyse these bonds to liberate the individual monosaccharides.

Polysaccharides differ from one another in a number of respects: their chain length, and the nature (α- or β-) and position (e.g. ring carbons 1-4, 1-6) of the links between individual sugar units. Cellulose consists mostly of β-1,4-linked glucosyl units; these links give the compound a close-packed structure which is not attacked by mammalian enzymes. In humans, therefore, cellulose largely passes intact through the small intestine where other carbohydrates are digested and absorbed. It is broken down by some bacterial enzymes. Ruminants have complex alimentary tracts in which large quantities of bacteria reside, enabling the host to obtain energy from cellulose, the main constituent of the ruminant's diet of grass. In humans there may be some bacterial digestion in the large intestine (see Chapter 2). Starch and the small amount of glycogen in the diet are readily digested (Chapter 2).

The structure of glycogen is illustrated in Figure 1.8. It is a branched polysaccharide; most of the links between sugar units are of the α-1,4 variety but, after every 9–10 residues, there is an α-1,6 link, which creates a branch. Glycogen is stored within cells, in organized structures which can be seen as granules on electron microscopy. The enzymes of glycogen metabolism appear to be intimately linked with these granules.

The carbohydrates share the property of relatively high polarity. Cellulose is not strictly water soluble, because of the tight packing between its chains, but even cellulose can be made to mix with water (e.g. paper pulp and wallpaper paste). The polysaccharides tend to make 'pasty' mixtures with water, whereas the small oligo-, di- and monosaccharides are completely soluble. These characteristics have important consequences for the metabolism of carbohydrates, some of which are as follows:

1. Glucose and other monosaccharides circulate freely in the blood and interstitial fluid, but their entry into cells is facilitated by specific transport proteins.

2. Perhaps because of the need for a specific transporter for glucose to cross cell membranes (thus making its entry into cells susceptible to regulation), glucose is an important fuel for many tissues, and an obligatory fuel for some. Carbohydrate cannot be synthesized from the more abundant store of fat within the body. The body must, therefore, maintain a store of carbohydrate.

3. Because of the water-soluble nature of sugars, this store will be liable to osmotic influences. It cannot, therefore, be in the form of simple sugars or even oligosaccharides because of the osmotic problem this would cause to the cells. This is overcome by the synthesis of the macromolecule glycogen, so that the osmotic effect is reduced by a factor of many thousand compared with monosaccharides. The synthesis of such a

polymer from glucose, and its breakdown, are brought about by enzyme systems which are themselves open to regulation, thus giving the opportunity for precise control of the availability of glucose.

4. Glycogen in an aqueous environment (as in cells) is highly hydrated; in fact, it is always associated with about three times its own weight of water. Thus storage of energy in the form of glycogen carries a large weight penalty (this will be discussed further in Chapter 7).

1.2.2.2 Fats

Just as there are many different sugars, and carbohydrates built from them, so there are a variety of types of fat. The term *fat* comes from Anglo-Saxon times and is related to the filling of a container or vat. The term *lipid*, from Greek, is more useful in chemical discussions since fat can have so many shades of meaning. Lipid materials are those substances which can be extracted from tissues in organic solvents such as petroleum or chloroform. This immediately distinguishes them from the largely water-soluble carbohydrates.

Among lipids there are a number of groups (Figure 1.4). The most prevalent, in terms of amount, are the *triacylglycerols* (or *triglycerides*; referred to in older literature as 'neutral fat' since they have no acidic or basic properties). These compounds consist of three individual fatty acids, each linked by an ester bond to a molecule of glycerol. As discussed above, the triacylglycerols are very non-polar, hydrophobic compounds. The *phospholipids* are another important group of lipids: constituents of membranes and also of the lipoprotein particles, which will be discussed in Chapter 8. *Steroids*, which are compounds with the same nucleus as cholesterol (see Figure 1.6), form yet another important group and will be considered in later chapters: steroid hormones in Chapter 4 and cholesterol metabolism in Chapter 8.

Fatty acids are the building blocks of lipids, analogous to the monosaccharides. Those important in metabolism are mostly unbranched, long-chain (12 carbon atoms or more) carboxylic acids with an even number of carbon atoms. They may contain no double bonds (*saturated fatty acids*); one double bond (*mono-unsaturated fatty acids*); or several double bonds (*polyunsaturated fatty acids*). Many individual fatty acids are named, like monosaccharides, according to the source from which they were first isolated. Thus *lauric acid* (C_{12}, saturated) comes from the laurel tree; *myristic acid* (C_{14}, saturated) from the *Myristica* or nutmeg genus; *palmitic acid* (C_{16}, saturated) from palm oil; and *stearic acid* (C_{18}, saturated) from suet (Greek *steatos*). *Oleic acid* (C_{18}, mono-unsaturated) comes from the olive (Latin *olea* for olive or *oleum* for oil). *Linoleic acid*, C_{18} with two double bonds, is a polyunsaturated acid common in certain vegetable oils; it is obtained from linseed (Latin *linum* for flax and *oleum* for oil).

The fatty acids mostly found in the diet have some common characteristics. They are composed of even numbers of carbon atoms, and the most abundant have 16 or 18 carbon atoms. There are three major series or families of fatty acid, grouped according to the distribution of their double-bonds (Box 1.3).

Differences in the metabolism of the different fatty acids are not very important from the point of view of their roles as fuels for energy metabolism; in fact, it has been extremely difficult to show that there are specificities for the major fatty acids in the provision and storage of energy. When considering the release, transport and uptake of fatty acids the term *non-esterified fatty acids* will, therefore, be used without reference to particular molecular species. In a later section (Section 8.4.2.2) some differences in their effects on the serum cholesterol concentration and propensity to heart disease will be discussed.

It will be seen from Figure 1.4 that saturated fatty acids, such as palmitic acid ($C_{16:0}$), have a natural tendency to fit together in nice orderly arrays. The unsaturated fatty acids, on the other hand, have less regular shapes. This is reflected in the melting points of the corresponding triacylglycerols: saturated fats, such as beef suet (with a high content of stearic acid, $C_{18:0}$), tend to be solid at room temperature, whereas unsaturated fats, such as olive oil, are liquid. This feature may have an important role in metabolic regulation, although its exact significance is not yet clear. We know that cell membranes with a high content of unsaturated fatty acids in their phospholipids are more 'fluid' than those with more saturated fatty acids. This may make them better able to regulate metabolic processes; for instance, muscle cells with a higher content of unsaturated fatty acids in their membranes respond better to the hormone insulin, probably because the response involves the movement of proteins (insulin receptors, glucose transporters) within the plane of the membrane and this occurs faster if the membrane is more fluid.

An important feature of the fatty acids is that, as their name implies, they have within one molecule both a hydrophobic tail and a polar carboxylic acid group. Fatty acids are almost insoluble in water; they are carried in the plasma loosely bound to the plasma protein albumin. Nevertheless, they are more water-miscible than triacylglycerols, which are carried in plasma in the complex structures known as lipoproteins. The simpler transport of non-esterified fatty acids is perhaps why they serve within the body as the immediate carriers of lipid energy from the stores to the sites of utilization and oxidation; they can be released very rapidly from stores when required and their delivery to tissues is regulated on a minute-to-minute basis.

But non-esterified fatty acids would not be a good form in which to store lipid fuels in any quantity. Their amphipathic nature means that they aggregate in micelles (small groups of molecules, formed with their tails together and their heads facing the aqueous environment); they would not aggregate easily in a very condensed form for storage. Triacylglycerols, on the other hand, do so readily; the hydrophobic molecules form uniform lipid droplets, from which water is completely excluded, which are an extremely efficient form in which to store energy (in terms of kJ stored per g). Thus, in brief, triacyl-

---

Box 1.3 The structures and inter-relationships of fatty acids

In the orthodox nomenclature, the position of double bonds is counted from the carboxyl end. Thus α-linolenic acid (C_{18}, polyunsaturated) may be represented as cis-9,12,15-18:3, and its structure is:

$$CH_3-CH_2-CH=C^{15}H-CH_2-CH=C^{12}H-CH_2-CH=C^9H-(CH_2)_7-C^1OOH$$

(where the superscripts denote the numbering of carbon atoms from the carboxyl end). However, this is also known as an *n*-3 (or sometimes as an ω3) fatty acid, since its first double bond, counting from the non-carboxyl (ω) end, is after the third carbon atom. On this basis, unsaturated fatty acids can be split into three main families: *n*-3, *n*-6 and *n*-9.

The saturated fatty acids can be synthesized within the body. In addition, many tissues possess the *desaturase* enzymes to form *cis*-6 or *cis*-9 double bonds, and to elongate the fatty acid chain by addition of 2-carbon units at the carboxyl end. But these processes do not alter the position of the double bonds relative to the ω end, so fatty acids cannot be converted from one family to another. Thus *cis*-9-18:1 (oleic acid) (*n*-9 family) can be synthesized, but the body cannot form *n*-6 or *n*-3 fatty acids. Since the body has a need for fatty acids of these families, they must be supplied in the diet (in small quantities). Some patients receiving all their nutrition intravenously have become deficient in these fatty acids. The problem is easily cured by rubbing sunflower oil into the skin!

Family	Source	Typical member	Simplified structure
Saturated	Diet or synthesis	Myristic acid	14:0
		Palmitic acid	16:0
		Stearic acid	18:0
n−9	Diet or synthesis	Oleic acid	9-18:1
n−6	Diet	Linoleic acid	9,12-18:2
n−3	Diet	α-Linolenic acid	9,12,15-18:3
Based on Gurr (1988).			

glycerols are the form in which most fat is stored in the human body — and in the bodies of other organisms; hence they are the major form of fat in food. Non-esterified fatty acids, on the other hand, are the form in which lipid energy is transported in a highly regulated manner from storage depots to sites of utilization and oxidation.

1.2.2.3 Proteins

Proteins are polymers of amino acids linked through peptide bonds. Individual proteins are distinguished by the number and order of amino acids in the chain — the sequence, or primary structure. Within its normal environment, the chain of amino acids will assume a folded, three-dimensional shape, represent-ing the secondary structure (local folding into α-helix and β-sheet) and tertiary structure (folding of the complete chain on itself). Two or more such folded peptide chains may then aggregate (quaternary structure) to form a complete enzyme or other functional protein.

In terms of energy metabolism, the first aspect we shall consider is not how this beautiful and complex arrangement is brought about but rather how it is destroyed. Protein in food is usually *denatured* (its higher-order structures disrupted) by cooking or other treatment; then, within the intestinal tract, the disrupted chains are broken down to short lengths of amino acids before absorption into the bloodstream. Within the bloodstream and within tissues we shall be concerned with the transport and distribution of individual amino acids. These are mostly sufficiently water-soluble to circulate freely in the aqueous environment of the plasma. Only tryptophan is sufficiently hydrophobic to require a transporter — it is bound loosely, like the non-esterified fatty acids, to albumin. Amino acids, not surprisingly, do not cross cell membranes by simple diffusion; there are specific transport proteins, which carry particular groups of amino acids. Many of these await detailed characterization.

Protein is often considered to be the structural material of the body, although it should not be thought of as the only structural material; it can only assume this function because of the complex arrangements of other cellular constituents, especially phospholipids which form cell membranes. Nevertheless, apart from water, protein is the largest single component in terms of mass of most tissues.[1] Within the body, the bulk of protein is present in the skeletal muscles, mainly because of their sheer weight (usually around 40% of the body weight) but also because each muscle cell is well packed with the proteins (actin and myosin) that constitute the contractile apparatus. But it is important to remember that most proteins act in an aqueous environment and are, therefore, associated with water. This is relevant if we consider the body's protein reserves as a form of stored chemical energy. Since protein is associated with water, it suffers the same drawback as a form of energy storage as does glycogen: with every gram of protein is associated about 3 g of water. It is not an energy-dense storage medium. Further, although protein undoubtedly represents a large source of energy which is drawn upon during starvation, it should be remembered that there is, in animals, no specific storage form of protein; all proteins have some function other than storage of energy. Thus utilization of protein as an energy source involves loss of the substance of the body. In evolutionary terms we might expect this to be minimized (i.e. the use of the specific storage compounds glycogen and triacylglycerol to be favoured) and, as we shall see in later chapters, this is exactly the case.

---

[1] *One important exception is mature white adipose tissue, in which triacylglycerol is the major constituent by weight.*

1.3 Some physiological concepts

The emphasis of this book on the integration of metabolism in different tissues and organs is akin to physiology rather than to molecular biology. This short section is intended to provide some physiological concepts for those from more biochemical backgrounds.

1.3.1 Circulation, capillaries and interstitial fluid

Blood is pumped around the body by the heart (Figure 1.9). Strictly speaking, it is pumped by the left ventricle, out into the aorta — the main artery — and its various branches, which supply blood to all tissues. Within tissues, the arterial vessels supplying blood divide into smaller and smaller vessels, and eventually into the capillaries — small vessels whose interior lumen is approximately 0.01 mm diameter, just large enough for red blood cells to pass through in single file.

The density of capillaries, in terms of number per unit area when the tissue is examined in cross-section under the microscope, varies between different tissues; however, in most tissues, at least one capillary is in close proximity to each cell. The inner walls of the capillaries are lined with flat endothelial cells, but in most tissues there are gaps between the endothelial cells and/or 'fenestrations' (passages) through the endothelial cells; these gaps are not large enough to let red blood cells through, but they are large enough for proteins and other molecules, such as metabolites and hormones, to pass. Outside the capillaries, surrounding the cells of the tissue, is an aqueous medium known as the interstitial fluid. For the most part, it is believed that substances diffuse from cells through the interstitial fluid into the capillaries, and from the capillaries through the interstitial fluid to cells, following concentration gradients

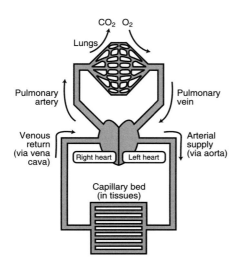

Figure 1.9 The circulatory system
Oxygenated blood from the lungs returns in the pulmonary veins to the left heart, from where it is pumped through the aorta and its various branches (arteries) to the tissues and organs. It returns from the tissues and is pumped to the lungs for re-oxygenation and expiration of CO_2. The key feature from the point of view of integration of metabolism is that blood returning from all tissues (and from endocrine glands) is mixed within the heart and lungs, and then redistributed to tissues. Thus the bloodstream (the circulation) acts as an efficient means of interchange of nutrients, metabolites and hormones between tissues.

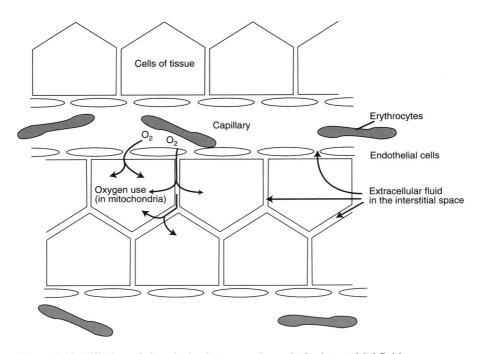

Figure 1.10 Diffusion of chemical substances through the interstitial fluid
A typical tissue is shown (schematically) in cross-section. The diffusion of oxygen from erythrocytes to cells in the tissue is shown as an example. It diffuses down a concentration gradient, from the erythrocytes, via the plasma and the interstitial fluid, into the cells where its concentration is depleted as it is used in mitochondrial oxidation. Note that the interstitial fluid occupies the space between cells known as the *extracellular space*; this is not a true empty space, but in reality is occupied by glycoproteins and other molecules joining the cells. Nevertheless, it offers a path for diffusion of substances.

(Figure 1.10). Thus oxygen, at its highest concentration in the blood supply at the arterial end of the capillary, will diffuse towards cells which are using it and thus depleting its local concentration in interstitial fluid; carbon dioxide will diffuse from cells which are generating it and thus creating a high local concentration, into the capillaries where the concentration is lower because it is continuously being removed by the flow of blood. There are some substances for which this cannot be entirely true, especially the non-esterified fatty acids; this will be discussed in more detail later.

There are different types of capillary; those with abundant fenestrations in the endothelial cells occur in tissues where there are high rates of exchange of molecules with the cells, for instance in the mucosa (absorptive lining) of the small intestine, where substances are absorbed, and in endocrine tissues where there is rapid secretion of hormones. In the brain the endothelial cells are tightly joined to one another, and this is believed to be the structural basis of the 'blood–brain barrier'; a number of substances, including non-esterified fatty acids and many drugs, are thus denied access to the cells of the brain.

The capillaries in turn lead to larger and larger vessels, which merge to form the major veins, through which blood returns to the heart. The returning blood enters the right ventricle, from where it is pumped through the lungs, collecting O_2 and losing CO_2; it then returns to the left heart and starts its journey anew.

The bloodstream is the major means of carrying substances from one tissue to another. For instance, it carries non-esterified fatty acids liberated from adipose tissue to other tissues where they will be oxidized, and it carries hormones from endocrine organs to their target tissues. The term *the circulation* is often used to mean the bloodstream; we speak of a substance being carried in the circulation, or even of *circulating glucose* (for example), meaning glucose in the bloodstream. In the metabolic diagrams, used extensively later in this book, the clear area in which different organs and tissues sit is meant to represent the bloodstream, and it may be assumed that substances will be efficiently carried across these blank spaces from one tissue to another.

1.3.2   Blood, plasma and serum

The blood itself is an aqueous environment, consisting of the liquid *plasma* — a solution of salts, small organic molecules such as glucose and amino acids, and a variety of peptides and proteins — and the blood cells, mostly red blood cells (*erythrocytes*). The erythrocyte membrane is permeable to, or has transport proteins for, some molecules but not others. Glucose, for instance, partially equilibrates across the erythrocyte membrane. Its concentration is somewhat lower inside the cell than outside, since the erythrocyte uses some for glycolysis and the transport must be somewhat limiting for this process. Nevertheless, glucose and some amino acids are carried around both in blood cells and in the plasma. On the other hand, lipid molecules are excluded from red blood cells and carried in the plasma. On the whole, the term 'in the plasma' will be used for those substances confined to that compartment, and 'in the blood' or 'in the bloodstream' for those which are carried in both compartments.

If blood is allowed to clot and then centrifuged, a yellow fluid can be removed: this is *serum*. It is like plasma but lacks the protein *fibrinogen*, which is used in the clotting process. Serum is often collected from patients for measurement of the concentration of cholesterol or triacylglycerol, mainly because it is convenient to let the blood clot. Thus 'serum cholesterol' simply refers to the concentration of cholesterol in the serum; it would be almost exactly the same as the plasma cholesterol concentration.

1.3.3   Lymph and lymphatics

The interstitial fluid is formed by 'filtration' of the blood plasma through the endothelium (vessel lining), as described earlier. Some of the fluid which leaves the bloodstream in this way will naturally find its way back to the blood vessels, but some is drained away from tissues in another series of vessels, the lymphatics. These are, for the most part, smaller than blood vessels. The fluid within them, the lymph, resembles an ultrafiltrate of plasma — i.e. it is like plasma but without red blood cells and without some of the larger proteins of plasma. The lymphatic vessels merge and form larger vessels and eventually discharge their contents into the bloodstream. We shall be concerned with one particular branch of the lymphatic system — that which drains the walls of the small intestine. The products of fat digestion enter these lymphatic vessels, which collect together and form a duct running up the back of the chest, known as the *thoracic duct*. The thoracic duct discharges its contents into the bloodstream in the upper chest. The lymphatic system also plays an important role in defence against infection, but this immunological role is beyond the scope of this book.

Suggestions for further reading

General metabolic biochemistry and metabolic regulation and other useful textbooks

Newsholme, E.A. & Leech, A.R. (1983) *Biochemistry for the Medical Sciences*, John Wiley, Chichester

Salway, J.G. (1994) *Metabolism at a Glance*, Blackwell Scientific Publications, Oxford

White, D.A. & Baxter, M. (1994) *Hormones and Metabolic Control (2nd edn)*, Edward Arnold, London

More detail on physiological and nutritional aspects

Bender, D.A. (1993) *Introduction to Nutrition and Metabolism*, UCL Press, London

Hunt, S.M. & Groff, J.L. (1990) *Advanced Nutrition and Human Metabolism*, West Publishing Co, St Paul, MN

Marieb, E.N. (1989) *Human Anatomy and Physiology*, Benjamin/ Cummings, Redwood City, CA. (Any textbook of physiology will provide more detail on the physiological and anatomical aspects. I like this one as it has exceptionally clear figures.)

Digestion and intestinal absorption

In a book which describes the events that connect the eating of food and the utilization of nutrients within the body it is necessary to look at the processes that come between food entering the mouth and its components appearing in the bloodstream. These are the processes of digestion and intestinal absorption. The aim of this chapter is to show the relationships between food and the substrates whose metabolism will be considered in later chapters. In addition, the process of digestion illustrates some interesting examples of integration by hormones and by the nervous system. The general layout of the digestive tract is shown in Figure 2.1 and typical amounts of the major nutrients eaten each day on a Western diet are given in Table 2.1. We shall deal here only with the macronutrients. Vitamins and minerals are also taken in with the diet, of course, but their handling is outside the scope of this book.

2.1　The strategy of digestion

2.1.1　Carbohydrate

Dietary carbohydrate may take a number of forms. In most real meals (as opposed to the pure glucose loads studied in many experimental situations) there is a mixture of simple sugars, oligosaccharides and complex carbohydrates. Of the complex carbohydrates, some will be readily digestible, i.e. *starch*, which is composed of the straight-chain *amylose* and the branched-chain *amylopectin*, and very small amounts of glycogen in animal tissues. Amylose consists of long chains of glucosyl units joined by α-1,4 links; amylopectin consists of chains of α-1,4-linked glucosyl units, with α-1,6-linked branches very like glycogen (see Figure 1.8). There are other types of starch which are resistant to digestion in the small intestine but fully digested in the large intestine; they are referred to as *resistant starch*. Their chemical structure is identical to that of starch, which is more easily digested, but the polysaccharide chains are in a semi-crystalline state, which makes the bonds

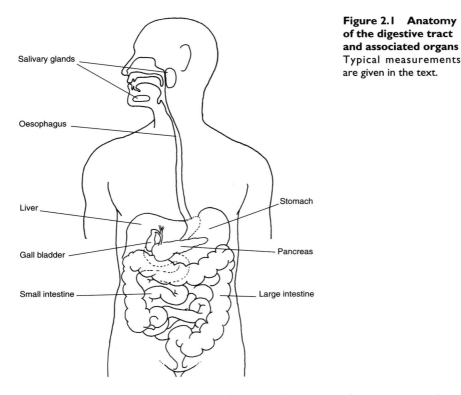

Figure 2.1 Anatomy of the digestive tract and associated organs Typical measurements are given in the text.

Salivary glands

Oesophagus

Liver

Gall bladder

Small intestine

Stomach

Pancreas

Large intestine

inaccessible to the usual enzymes of starch digestion. The remaining, less-digestible, carbohydrate is referred to as *non-starch polysaccharide*, or, more generally, as *dietary fibre*. Cellulose, one of the main components of the non-starch polysaccharide fraction, consists of long, β-1,4-linked chains of glucosyl units.

The digestible carbohydrates are, for the most part, absorbed from the small intestine in the form of monosaccharides. The strategy of the digestive process, therefore, is to have them in that form as they reach the small intestine. Digestion of dietary carbohydrate to monosaccharide units takes place in two stages: *luminal digestion*, digestion which occurs in the intestinal lumen, and *membrane digestion*, the hydrolysis of certain small oligosaccharides by enzymes that form part of the microvillus membrane, the absorptive surface of the cells lining the small intestine.

2.1.2 Fats

The majority of dietary fat is in the form of triacylglycerol, with some cholesterol and small amounts of other lipids, such as phospholipids (Table 2.1). Fat-soluble vitamins are ingested with other foods. Some are taken in as relatively water-soluble precursors or *provitamins*, such as carotene in carrots and other vegetables. Others, such as vitamin D, are taken in with fatty foods and absorbed along with the fat.

Table 2.1 Average daily intake of macronutrients

Nutrient	Amount per day	Constituents		Percentage by weight
Carbohydrate	300 g	Polysaccharides		
		Starch		65
		Glycogen		0.5
		Disaccharides		
		Sucrose		25
		Lactose		6
		Monosaccharides		
		Fructose	}	3
		Glucose		
Fats	100 g	Triacylglycerols		94
		Phospholipids		5
		Cholesterol		1
Protein	100 g			100

The figures apply to a typical Western diet. Not shown is a very variable amount of non-digestible carbohydrate (fibre), typically 10–20 g per day.

The digestion and absorption of fat necessitates that the fat is made accessible to the enzymes which break it down for digestion. This is achieved by emulsification — formation of microscopic droplets in which the ratio of surface area (where enzymes can act) to mass is very large. Thus, in considering the digestion and absorption of fat, we are concerned both with physico-chemical changes and with enzymic processes.

2.1.3 Protein and amino acids
Protein in the diet may take many forms. For the most part, this makes little difference to its handling in the digestive process; proteins are hydrolysed to free amino acids and dipeptides for absorption.

2.2 Stages of digestion

2.2.1 The mouth
The process of digestion and preparation for the absorption of food may begin even before food enters the mouth. The *cephalic phase* represents the brain's anticipation of food, through the sight or smell or even thought of food; it is reinforced by the taste of food in the mouth. Cephalic stimulation of the flow of saliva occurs through activation of the parasympathetic nervous supply to

the salivary glands. (The parasympathetic nervous system will be discussed in detail in Section 6.2.2.2.) Stimulation of gastric juice secretion also occurs, and there is evidence for cephalic-phase secretion of insulin, showing the control of insulin secretion by the nervous system (to be discussed in more detail later; see Section 6.4). The presence of food in the mouth stimulates nerve receptors both mechanically and chemically through taste receptors to reinforce the cephalic stimulus to saliva production.

Saliva is produced in pairs of glands which are located along the line of the jaw: the parotid, submandibular and sublingual glands. It is slightly buffered by its content of bicarbonate and phosphate ions, and contains a number of enzymes as well as the glycoprotein *mucin*, which gives it its lubricating properties. The major enzyme in saliva is an α-*amylase* (EC 3.2.1.1), which hydrolyses α-1,4 links to begin the process of carbohydrate digestion; this is probably not extensive unless the food is chewed for an abnormal length of time before swallowing. The most important process occurring in the mouth is mechanical breakdown of the food and its hydration with saliva.

A lipase, *lingual lipase*, is also secreted into the mouth from glands in the tongue and soft palate. It is not thought to produce much hydrolysis of lipids in adults; however, it may have a more important role in neonates which consume milk in which a large proportion of the energy is in the form of tria-cylglycerol. Its pH optimum is low (around 5) and it may produce some lipid hydrolysis in the stomach.

2.2.2   The stomach
2.2.2.1   General description
After swallowing, the chewed food is propelled rapidly, in a matter of seconds, through the oesophagus to enter the stomach. The stomach is a distensible muscular sac, about 25 cm long, with a volume of around 50 ml when empty, but it can expand to hold up to 1.5 litres or more. Its walls are made of three layers of smooth muscle running in different directions, giving the stomach the ability to churn food around and physically break it up further and mix it with the stomach's own digestive juices.

The cells of the *epithelium* (inner lining) of the stomach produce both mucus and an alkaline bicarbonate-containing fluid, which protect them from attack by the stomach's own acidic digestive juices. Interspersed with these cells are many millions of small holes, visible microscopically: these are the openings of the *gastric pits* or *gastric glands*. The gastric pits are lined with further epithelial, mucus-secreting cells, but also contain specialized cells which secrete different substances: the *parietal* or *oxyntic cells* secrete HCl (hydrochloric acid), and the *chief cells*, also known as zymogenic or peptic cells, which secrete proteins, particularly the pro-enzyme *pepsinogen*. The oxyntic cells also secrete the glycoprotein known as *intrinsic factor*, which is necessary for absorption of vitamin B_{12}.

2.2.2.2 Regulation of digestive processes in the stomach

The secretion of these various substances is not continuous in time; it is co-ordinated with the ingestion of food and its arrival in the stomach.

The control of acid secretion is summarized in Figure 2.2. Secretion of HCl is stimulated by three factors which act at specific receptors on the oxyntic cells: *acetylcholine*, the parasympathetic neurotransmitter (discussed in

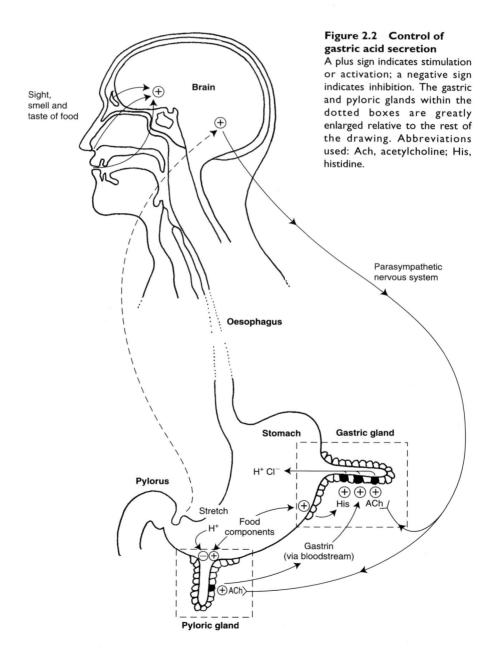

Figure 2.2 Control of gastric acid secretion
A plus sign indicates stimulation or activation; a negative sign indicates inhibition. The gastric and pyloric glands within the dotted boxes are greatly enlarged relative to the rest of the drawing. Abbreviations used: Ach, acetylcholine; His, histidine.

Section 6.1.1); *histamine*; and the peptide hormone *gastrin*. Maximal acid production is only achieved when all three signals are present; any one of the three will only give weak stimulation of acid production.

Histamine is released from cells in the stomach wall in response to food in the stomach. It acts locally, and thus it is not a true hormone but acts in a *paracrine* manner. It acts at specific receptors, known as H_2-receptors, on the oxyntic cells; drugs which block binding at these receptors, the H_2-antagonists (e.g. cimetidine, ranitidine), have found widespread use as anti-ulcer agents, since they reduce acid secretion. The parasympathetic nervous system is activated during digestion, as noted earlier, by the taste, smell and sight of food; when food enters the stomach, distension of its walls activates *stretch receptors* which send signals to the brain, which in turn cause further activation of the parasympathetic nervous system (the *vagus nerve*), and enhance acid secretion. A traditional surgical treatment for gastric ulcers (now out of fashion) was to sever the vagus nerve, thus removing one stimulus for acid secretion. When we consider other effects of the vagus nerve (e.g. the modulation of insulin secretion), we shall see that this could have widespread, unwanted effects. In recent years, so-called *highly selective vagotomy* was introduced, in which only those branches innervating the stomach were cut, but even this treatment has now been superseded by the use of H_2-antagonists.

Gastrin, the third regulator of acid secretion, is a 17 amino acid peptide produced by *enteroendocrine cells*, which are found in gastric pits in the region of the *pylorus* — the exit from the stomach in to the first part of the small intestine (the *duodenum*). Gastrin is a true hormone: it is released from the enteroendocrine cells into the bloodstream and circulates in the bloodstream. There is no apparent short-cut for it, although the cells it affects are near to those that secrete it. The release of gastrin is stimulated by a number of factors arising from the food in the stomach: some amino acids and peptides released from partially digested protein in the stomach, caffeine, calcium and alcohol. In addition, stimulation of gastrin secretion is reinforced by the parasympathetic nervous system, activated during the digestive process. Gastrin acts directly on the oxyntic cells to stimulate acid secretion. It also has other actions in the small intestine, which will be considered below.

The secretion of gastrin is inhibited by too high an acidity in the stomach: when the pH falls below about 2 (the optimum for the action of pepsin) gastrin secretion declines. This seems to be brought about by release from adjacent cells of the 14 amino acid peptide *somatostatin*. Somatostatin is a widespread inhibitor of peptide hormone secretion: it is found throughout the intestine, in the brain and in the pancreas, and, when given intravenously, will inhibit the secretion of many peptide hormones — including growth hormone, gastrin, insulin and glucagon. [Its name comes from the inhibition of growth hormone (or somatotropin) secretion.] Clearly, it could have very non-specific effects if released in sufficient quantities into the circulation. Somatostatin appears, like histamine, to act locally on adjacent or nearby cells; it is a paracrine regulator of hormone secretion. Excess acidity appears to act directly to stimulate somatostatin secretion and thus inhibit gastrin release.

The inhibition of gastrin release by excess acidity is a good example of feedback inhibition brought about by a hormonal regulator. Large amounts of protein in the stomach act as a buffer, 'soaking up' excess acid, so the pH will rise and more gastrin will be released; as the pH falls below the optimum for pepsin action, gastrin release — and thus acid production — is diminished. The system maintains a relatively constant and optimum hydrogen ion concentration for digestion.

2.2.2.3 Digestive processes in the stomach

The acidic environment in the stomach stops the action of the salivary amylase as it reaches the interior of the boluses of food that arrive from the oesophagus. Nevertheless, the contractile activity of the stomach is greatest near the pylorus, and, after a large meal, boluses of food may remain relatively undisturbed and salivary amylase may continue to act for up to an hour in the upper part of the stomach. It has been estimated that up to 50% of dietary starch (but usually less) may be digested by the time food leaves the stomach.

Beyond that, in the stomach the digestion of carbohydrate and fat is confined to mechanical disruption and liquefaction of the food. The acidity of the stomach also has an antibacterial action. Therefore, the main digestive action in the stomach is on protein, although it should be said that it is quite possible to live without a stomach (except for the need for injections of vitamin B_{12}, which cannot be absorbed because of the lack of intrinsic factor).

Most proteins are denatured in an acidic environment, i.e. their quaternary, tertiary and secondary structures are lost. (Adding lemon juice to milk or egg white will 'curdle' it.) Denaturation makes the peptide chains more accessible to proteolytic enzymes, which break the peptide bonds linking the amino acids. The proteolytic enzyme produced by the chief or zymogenic cells is *pepsin*. This is released, as with all extracellular proteolytic enzymes, as an inactive precursor, *pepsinogen*. It is activated by hydrolysis of a single peptide bond, catalysed by hydrogen ions, thereby releasing a 42 amino acid peptide and the active enzyme. Pepsin has a very acidic pH optimum, around 2. It acts preferentially on peptide bonds in the middle of peptide chains (i.e. it is an *endopeptidase*), to the C-terminal side of aromatic amino acids. Thus proteins are broken down into shorter chains.

Little absorption into the bloodstream occurs from the stomach: ethanol and some lipid-soluble drugs are absorbed, but not the normal dietary constituents. The stomach is primarily an organ of mechanical digestion, comparable with a food liquidizer. By the rhythmic contractions of the lower part of the stomach, the food is pounded into a creamy mixture known as *chyme*. Entry to the duodenum is regulated by a circular muscle, the pyloric sphincter. It opens at regular intervals (about twice each minute) and about 3 ml of chyme is squirted into the duodenum. The *pyloric sphincter* only opens partially, so large particles are retained for further pummelling. Thus a creamy acidic mixture of lightly digested starch, partially digested protein and coarsely emulsified fat enters the duodenum.

2.2.3   The small intestine
2.2.3.1   General description

It is often said that the small intestine is about 6 m (20 feet) long and about 2.5 cm (1 inch) in diameter. This is a generalization and its length actually differs in life and after death; in life it is somewhat contracted by virtue of the 'tone' of its muscular walls. Measurements made by passing tubes through the small intestine in adult, living humans show the length to vary between about 3 m and 4.5 m. Of this, the first 25 cm (or so) is the duodenum, curving downwards after leaving the stomach and running roughly horizontally across the middle of the abdomen. (It gets its name from the Latin *duodecim* for 12, because it is about 12 inches or 12 finger-breadths long.) The jejunum begins after a sharp downward bend; it accounts for around another 2 m, and is the site of much of the absorption of the macronutrients. Finally, the ileum, about 2.5–3 m in length, leads to the large intestine at the ileo-caecal valve.

Two important organs discharge into the small intestine. The *gall bladder*, the storage reservoir for bile salts produced in the liver, discharges its contents via the *common bile duct*, and the exocrine part of the pancreas releases its secretions through the *pancreatic duct*; the common bile duct joins this, and they both discharge into the duodenum. The regulation and the content of their secretions will be covered in detail later.

The small intestine, like all parts of the intestine, has layers of smooth muscle running lengthways and around its circumference. The inner surface, or mucosal layer, is folded into finger-like projections (*villi*), each villus being about 1 mm long. There are 20–40 villi per mm². This increases enormously the surface area where absorption takes place, to a total of about 300 m². The surface area is increased still further by the presence of the *brush border*. Each cell making up the surface of a villus has its own microscopic finger-like projections, the *microvilli*, which give a brush-like appearance under the electron microscope. There are around 2000–4000 microvilli per cell. The presence of the microvilli further increases the surface area about thirty-fold.

Each villus has a characteristic structure (Figure 2.3). Within its core there is a dense network of capillaries surrounding a channel (the *lacteal*) which is a branch of the lymphatic system. (The name, from the Latin *lactis*, means related to milk; we shall see why as we discuss the absorption of fat.) The venous blood vessels leave the intestinal mucosa, merge and eventually form the hepatic portal vein. The lymphatic vessels also merge and form a single vessel, the thoracic duct (see Section 1.3.3), so called because it leads upwards through the thorax (chest), and finally discharges its contents into the great veins in the neck, near where they return to the heart (Figure 2.4).

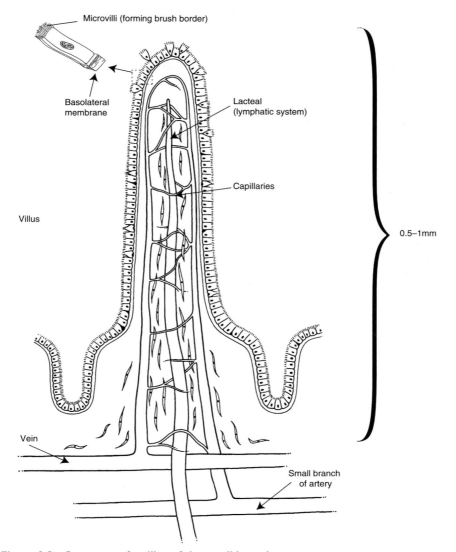

Figure 2.3   Structure of a villus of the small intestine
One of the absorptive cells (enterocytes) on the surface is enlarged to illustrate the microvilli of the brush-border membrane.

There are four important sources of digestive agents in the small intestine: the gall bladder, which provides the bile salts necessary for emulsification of fat; the exocrine pancreas, which provides bicarbonate, to neutralize the acidic chyme entering through the pylorus, and a mixture of digestive enzymes; secretory cells, in glands located throughout the small intestinal wall, which produce an isotonic, neutral, mucus-containing juice; and the brush-border membrane, in which are incorporated several digestive enzymes. These, and the other digestive juices, are summarized in Table 2.2.

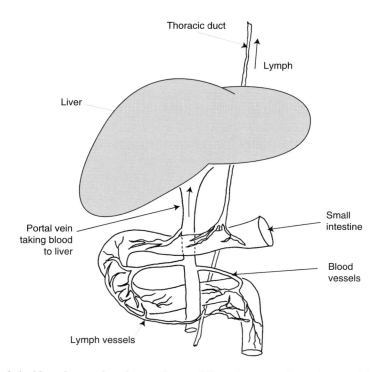

Figure 2.4   Vessels carrying the products of digestion away from the small intestine
Substances entering the bloodstream reach the hepatic portal vein and are thus carried to the
liver. The products of fat digestion are carried in the vessels of the lymphatic system.

2.2.3.2   Regulation of digestive processes in the small intestine

The first aspect of regulation of small intestinal digestion affects not the small
intestine as such, but the stomach. The presence of chyme in the duodenum
activates receptors in its walls via both stretch and chemical effects. These
receptors trigger the *enterogastric reflex*, in which the brain reduces parasympathetic activity (one of the main stimulants of gastric secretion and
contraction) and increases sympathetic nervous stimulation of the pyloric
sphincter, which causes it to contract; these effects combine to retain food in
the stomach and reduce the loading of the small intestine until it is ready for
more. Acidity in the duodenum also causes the secretion of *secretin*, a 27
amino acid peptide, into the bloodstream from cells in the duodenal and
jejunal mucosa. Secretin was the first hormone to be discovered, by Bayless
and Starling in 1902. Its name comes from its effects on pancreatic secretion
(see below), but it has an additional effect in inhibiting gastric contractions and
secretion; these effects are reinforced by other hormones, *cholecystokinin* and
gastric inhibitory peptide, both also secreted in response to distension of the
duodenum and the presence of acidic chyme. This is another example of
negative feedback: the entry of chyme into the duodenum is inhibited as it
accumulates there.

Table 2.2 Digestive enzymes and juices

Source	Enzyme/juice	Function
Mouth		
Salivary glands	α-Amylase	Initial digestion of starch
Glands on tongue	Lingual lipase	Possibly some lipid hydrolysis in stomach
Stomach		
Gastric glands	HCl	Denaturation/swelling of proteins
		Acidification for pepsin action
		Antibacterial
		Activation of pepsinogen
	Pepsin (secreted as pepsinogen)	Initial digestion of proteins
Small intestine and associated organs		
Small intestinal wall	*Succus entericus* (intestinal juice)	Dilution, lubrication
Gall bladder	Bile	Neutralization of acidic chyme
	Bile salts	Emulsification of fats
Exocrine pancreas	Pancreatic juice	Neutralization of acidic chyme
	Proteases	Digestion of protein to oligopeptides and free amino acids
	Trypsin (secreted as trypsinogen)	
	Chymotrypsin (secreted as chymotrypsinogen)	
	Carboxypeptidases A,B (secreted as procarboxypeptidase)	
	Pancreatic lipase	Triacylglycerol hydrolysis
Brush-border membrane	Disaccharidases	Disaccharide hydrolysis
	Peptidases	Hydrolysis of peptides to di- and tripeptides

Two of these hormones, secretin and cholecystokinin, have other, probably more important, effects. Secretin stimulates the exocrine pancreas to produce a fluid that is high in bicarbonate (and is thus alkaline, to neutralize the acidic chyme) but relatively low in enzyme content. Cholecystokinin stimulates the exocrine pancreas to produce a digestive juice that is lower in bicarbonate but higher in enzyme content. The name cholecystokinin, however, relates to its effect on the gall bladder: it causes the gall bladder to contract, releasing its contents via the common bile duct into the duodenum. (At one time there were thought to be two separate hormones: *pancreozymin*, responsible for stimulation of pancreatic juice secretion, and cholecystokinin, acting on the gall bladder. Now they are known to be one and the same.) Thus the arrival of chyme in the duodenum causes the secretion of digestive juices via the release of these two hormones: this is a further example of the role of hormones in integrating events within the body. The role of hormones in integration of digestion is illustrated in Figure 2.5.

Figure 2.5   Hormonal regulation of the secretion of digestive juices
Gastrin stimulates HCl secretion by the oxyntic cells in the gastric glands. Secretin and cholecystokinin promote the secretion of pancreatic juices. In addition, cholecystokinin causes the gall bladder to contract, releasing bile into the duodenum. Abbreviation: CCK, cholecystokinin.

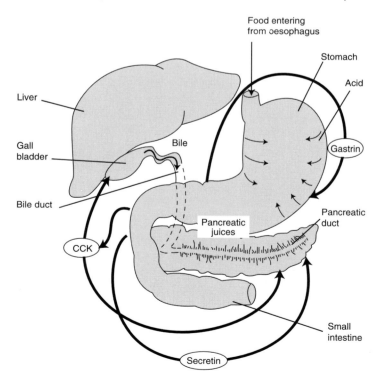

2.2.3.3   Digestive processes in the small intestine

The pancreatic juice contains amylases (for hydrolysis of starch), proteases and a lipase; thus it plays a major role in luminal digestion of each of the macro-nutrients.

1.   Starch digestion. The pancreatic juice contains two α-amylases, enzymes which hydrolyse the α-1,4 glycosidic bonds in starch. Their pH optimum is around 7.0, which is the pH of the contents of the small intestine after the bicarbonate-containing pancreatic juice has neutralized its acidity. These enzymes will not hydrolyse the α-1,6 branch-point in the amylopectin molecule, nor α-1,4 links within two glucosyl units after a branch. Therefore, α-*limit dextrins* — small oligosaccharides which contain the α-1,6 link — are produced, along with tri- and disaccharides such as maltotriose and maltose (three and two α-1,4-linked glucosyl units, respectively). These products, along with other disaccharides ingested in the food, such as sucrose and lactose, are then hydrolysed by the enzymes associated with the microvillus membrane of the absorptive cells. There are at least four different enzymes, which hydrolyse the various remaining bonds (including the α-1,2 linkage in sucrose), to liberate free monosaccharides.

2.   Protein digestion. The pancreatic juice contains a number of enzymes with proteolytic activity. The most important of these are secreted as proenzymes or *zymogens* which are activated by proteolysis in the intestinal lumen, presumably to protect the pancreas from digesting itself. These proteases are *trypsin* (secreted as trypsinogen), *chymotrypsin* (secreted as chymotrypsinogen) and *carboxypeptidases* (the precursor procarboxypeptidase is activated to produce carboxypeptidases A and B). The enzyme trypsin is derived from trypsinogen by the action of an enteropeptidase associated with the brush-border membrane; trypsin then catalyses the activation of the other zymogens. Each of these enzymes has its own characteristic specificity for peptide bonds, but the net result of their combined action is the liberation of some free amino acids and a mixture of oligopeptides. These may be further hydrolysed by membrane-bound enzymes to tri- and dipeptides and amino acids for absorption.

3.   Lipid digestion. This is the most complex process because, as mentioned earlier, it involves both physico-chemical and enzymic processes. Lipid digestion and absorption depend upon emulsification of triacylglycerol, and, finally, formation of particles even smaller than those typical of emulsions, known as micelles. The main emulsifying agents are the *bile salts*, amphipathic molecules secreted in the bile (Box 2.1). Lipid digestion proceeds, further amphipathic molecules are formed that may help in emulsification: these include monoacylglycerols and phospholipids, particularly lysolecithin. Emulsification is brought about by the non-polar tails

Box 2.1 The bile acids and salts

These are derivatives of cholesterol (see Figure 1.7), synthesized in the liver. A typical structure is shown. The acid is *cholic acid*; *chenodeoxycholic acid* lacks the hydroxyl group at C-12. They are secreted in the bile in the form of covalent conjugates, formed with a base: either glycine ($^+H_3NCH_2COO^-$) as shown here, or taurine ($^+H_3NCH_2CH_2SO_3^-$). The conjugate shown is sometimes known as *glycocholate*. They are amphipathic molecules, with a predominantly non-polar ring structure but a highly polar acidic group (especially in the conjugated form).

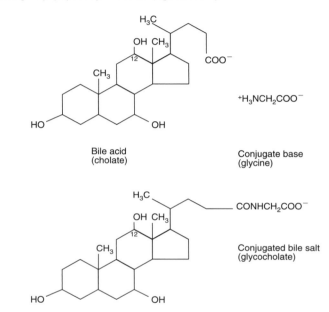

Bile acid
(cholate)

Conjugate base
(glycine)

$^+H_3NCH_2COO^-$

CONHCH_2COO^-

Conjugated bile salt
(glycocholate)

The bile salts are not absorbed with the contents of the mixed micelles. Instead, they are absorbed from the terminal part of the ileum by an energy-requiring process. They then enter the portal vein and are re-utilized in the liver. This salvaging of the bile acids is known as the *enterohepatic circulation*. Bile salts returning to the liver repress the conversion of further cholesterol to bile acids.

If the re-absorption of bile salts is interrupted, they are excreted, after some bacterial modification, in the faeces. As a consequence, more cholesterol is converted to bile acids in the liver, thereby depleting the body's cholesterol pool. The usefulness of this as a treatment for lowering of the serum cholesterol concentration will be discussed further in Chapter 8 (Box 8.3).

of the amphipathic molecules that stabilize small groups of non-polar molecules, predominantly triacylglycerol and a smaller amount of cholesterol; their polar aspects face outwards to the aqueous intestinal contents. A net repulsive action of the outward-facing polar groups also tends to split further the lipid droplets, resulting in a finer and finer emulsion. These emulsified particles are typically 1 μm in diameter. It is in this form that most of the hydrolysis of triacylglycerols proceeds.

Pancreatic lipase (EC 3.1.1.3) is a member of a family of lipases that includes *lipoprotein lipase* (EC 3.1.1.34), an important enzyme in fat metabolism to be discussed in later chapters. These enzymes act on the ester links in the terminal (1 and 3) positions in an acylglycerol, but not the central fatty acid (2-position). Thus fatty acids are liberated and 2-monoacylglycerols

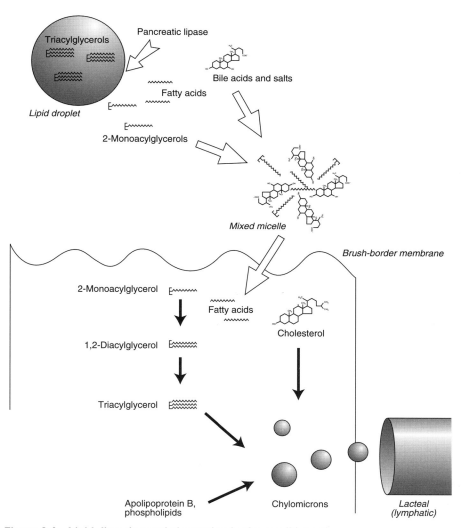

Figure 2.6   Lipid digestion and absorption in the small intestine
Within the mucosal cells, 2-monoacylglycerol and fatty acids are re-esterified largely by the monoacylglycerol pathway (see Figure 2.8) and packaged into chylomicrons. Cholesterol absorption is not shown for simplicity; it is described in the text.

remain. Both fatty acids and monoacylglycerols have amphipathic properties. The monoacylglycerol is an effective emulsifying agent and aids the action of the bile salts, as noted above. Gradually, much smaller groups of molecules are formed: the *mixed micelles* — mixed because they contain both bile salts (which can themselves form micelles) and other molecules, particularly fatty acids and monoacylglycerols. These micelles have a diameter of 4–6 nm; they are so small that they do not scatter light and therefore produce an almost clear solution. They are able to move readily through the aqueous intestinal contents, and thus bring the products of triacylglycerol hydrolysis, i.e. fatty acids and monoacylglycerols, to the surface of the absorptive cells. Lipid digestion in the small intestine is summarized in Figure 2.6.

Other forms of lipid in the diet — phospholipids and cholesteryl esters — are also hydrolysed by pancreatic and other lipases, and the products (fatty acids, monoacylglycerols and free cholesterol) also incorporated into the mixed micelles.

2.3   Absorption from the small intestine

2.3.1   Monosaccharides

The hydrolysis of the digestible carbohydrates proceeds to the stage of monosaccharides, some of which are liberated by the enzymes of the brush-border membrane. These must then enter the *enterocytes*, the absorptive cells of the intestinal mucosa. As monosaccharides are freely water soluble, relatively polar molecules, they cannot cross the cell membrane by free diffusion.

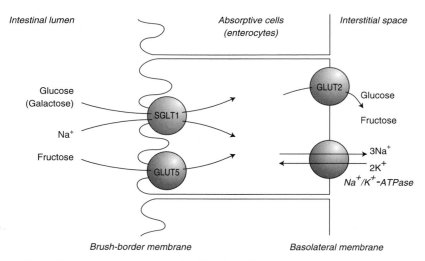

Figure 2.7   Absorption of monosaccharides from the intestine
Monosaccharides enter the enterocytes across the brush-border or apical membrane and leave the cell by the basolateral membrane using specific transport proteins. Based on Thorens (1993) and Wright (1993).

Instead, there are specific transport proteins for their entry, summarized in Figure 2.7. Glucose and galactose enter by active transport mediated by the sodium–glucose co-transporter SGLT1; i.e. these sugar molecules may be absorbed against a concentration gradient (see Box 1.2). During the active phase of digestion, it is likely that the local concentration of free glucose or galactose on the luminal surface of the brush-border membrane is so high that this is unnecessary, but, during the early and late phases of digestion, active transport ensures complete capture of almost all the intestinal sugar molecules. Energy is provided by a concentration gradient of sodium ions across the membrane, maintained in turn by the enzyme Na^+/K^+-exchanging ATPase. This enzyme pumps Na^+ ions out of the cell against a strong concentration gradient, in exchange for K^+ ions brought in against a strong concentration gradient; energy is provided by hydrolysis of ATP. Generation of the ATP will be discussed later. Fructose, in contrast, appears to be taken up into the mucosal cells by a different carrier, by the process of facilitated diffusion; it moves down a concentration gradient with the aid of a (non-energy requiring) transport protein, GLUT5.

From within the mucosal cells, the sugars enter the capillaries, which form a dense network within each villus. They must first cross the cell membrane at the 'back end' of the cell — the *basolateral membrane* (see Figures 2.3 and 2.7) — to enter first the interstitial space and then the blood in the vessels draining the small intestine towards the portal vein. This basolateral transport is by facilitated diffusion rather than active transport, and the transport protein involved is GLUT2, a carrier for both glucose and fructose (Figure 2.7). Active transport of sugar into the cell must raise its intracellular concentration to the extent that it moves out, into the interstitial space, down a concentration gradient. Thus carbohydrate from the diet appears ultimately in the form of monosaccharides in the blood in the hepatic portal vein.

However, not all of the sugars absorbed are liberated into the bloodstream in this way. Some are metabolized by the cells of the intestinal mucosa, which require a constant supply of ATP for maintenance of the sodium gradient. At least a proportion of the glucose used by these cells for ATP generation is metabolized to lactate, which is released into the portal vein. The amount of absorbed carbohydrate that is converted to lactate in this way is presently unknown (and very difficult to estimate). The relevance of this pathway of lactate production will be considered again in Section 3.2.2.1.

2.3.2 Amino acids and peptides

The products of protein digestion are absorbed into the intestinal epithelial cells in two ways: absorption of free amino acids by certain specific transport proteins, and absorption of di- and tripeptides.

Amino acids are actively transported by sodium-linked carriers. Again, therefore, energy is required to pump the sodium ions out and maintain their concentration gradient. There are a number of amino acid transporters, common to the intestinal cells and to many other tissues. Each has a fairly broad specificity and transports a number of amino acids. The transport mechanisms may be grouped as follows:

1. *Neutral amino acid transport*: for monoamino, monocarboxylic acids; this is very rapid (i.e. has a high maximal activity).

2. *Dibasic amino acid transport*: for lysine, arginine, ornithine (and cystine); rapid but only about 10% of the maximal activity of the neutral transporter.

3. *Dicarboxylic amino acid transport*: for glutamic and aspartic acids.

There are further subdivisions and at least seven distinct carriers have been described. However, these are not of direct relevance here and will not be discussed further.

Amino acids thus enter the epithelial cells and eventually the capillaries of the intestinal mucosa. Like glucose, however, they do not escape some metabolism during their passage through the intestinal absorptive cells. Some amino acids are oxidized very effectively to provide energy for the intestinal cells, in particular glutamine, glutamate and aspartate. Glutamine is actually extracted from the blood flowing through the intestinal wall and oxidized. Therefore, as in the case of glucose, the energy required for active absorption of the amino acids is provided to some extent by oxidation of the molecules absorbed.

2.3.3   Lipid absorption

Although the uptake of monoacylglycerols and fatty acids by the intestinal epithelial cells appears to occur by simple diffusion, specific carriers for fatty acids have been identified in recent years in a number of other tissues, and may yet be found in the intestine. Certainly, inside the cell the fatty acids are bound by one or more specific *fatty acid-binding protein(s)* which may aid or direct movement through the cytosol.

Within the enterocytes, fatty acids and monoacylglycerols are re-esterified to form new triacylglycerol molecules. This occurs mainly by the *monoacylglycerol esterification pathway* which begins with monoacylglycerol (Figure 2.8), unlike most other tissues in which the formation of triacylglycerols occurs by the *phosphatidic acid* pathway which begins with glycerol 3-phosphate (Figure 2.8).

The triacylglycerols are packaged with phospholipids and proteins, particularly the protein called *apolipoprotein B*. (For a more detailed discussion, see Chapter 8, Box 8.1.) They form particles approx. 100 nm to 1 μm in diameter, the *chylomicrons*. The chylomicrons are the largest of the lipoprotein particles present in blood. They leave the absorptive cells and pass into the lacteals (Figure 2.6). From there they flow slowly into more major branches of the

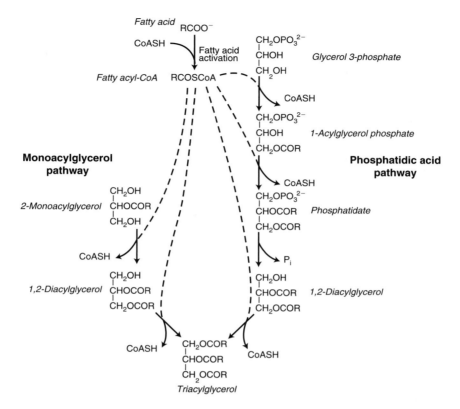

Figure 2.8   Esterification pathways for the formation of triacylglycerol
The monoacylglycerol pathway is prevalent in enterocytes, the phosphatidic acid pathway in
other tissues. Chemical structures are detailed in Figure 1.4. Abbreviations used: CoASH,
coenzyme-A; P_i, inorganic phosphate; R represents the fatty acid hydrocarbon chain.

lymphatic system, up the thoracic duct and thence into the circulation. Because
the diameter of chylomicrons is of the same order as the wavelength of visible
light, they scatter light, resulting in a turbid or milky appearance. Hence the
name lacteal, as mentioned earlier. As chylomicrons enter the plasma they give
it a milky appearance; it is easy to see from visual inspection of the plasma
whether someone has recently eaten a fatty meal.

   Not all fatty acids are re-esterified to form triacylglycerol. Those with a
shorter chain length, below C_{12} to C_{14}, are not good substrates for esterification, because the specific medium-chain acyl-CoA synthetase (EC 6.2.1.2)
required for their activation is not present. They enter the capillary plasma
directly in the form of non-esterified fatty acids. However, except when the
diet contains a large amount of dairy produce rich in short- and medium-chain
fatty acids, most of the dietary fatty acids are long chain (C_{16} or more) and
enter the bloodstream as chylomicron-triacylglycerol.

   One other form of lipid must be considered. We eat a certain amount of
cholesterol (Table 2.1). This becomes incorporated into the mixed micelles

(Figure 2.6). About half enters the absorptive cells by a process that is not clearly understood, although it probably moves freely by passive diffusion. The remainder is lost in the faeces. Within the absorptive cells, some of the cholesterol is esterified with long-chain fatty acids by the action of the enzyme *acyl-CoA:cholesterol O-acyltransferase* (EC 2.3.1.26), to form the hydrophobic cholesteryl esters. Both cholesterol and cholesteryl esters are incorporated into the chylomicron particles and thus enter the bloodstream via the lymphatics.

2.3.4   Other processes in the small intestine

Most of the absorption of sugars, amino acids and peptides, and fatty acids and monoacylglycerols, is completed during passage through the duodenum and jejunum. In the ileum some further specific compounds are absorbed, particularly vitamin B_{12} and the bile salts (left behind when other components of the mixed micelles are taken up higher in the small intestine; see Box 2.1). The re-absorption of bile salts has important implications for the whole-body store of cholesterol, and will be considered again in Chapter 8 (Box 8.3).

2.4   The large intestine

The large intestine is about 1.5 m in length, and extends from the end of the ileum, the ileo-caecal valve, to the anus. An important function of the large intestine is the absorption of water, but it is also the site of considerable bacterial activity on the carbohydrate which has escaped digestion in the small intestine.

There is still some debate about the extent to which carbohydrates which have escaped digestion in the small intestine can be broken down and absorbed in the large intestine. The topic is outside the scope of this book, except to mention that some breakdown undoubtedly occurs, and is brought about by enzymes secreted by the resident bacteria. Among the products of this breakdown are short-chain fatty acids, such as acetate, butyrate and propionate. These are absorbed by the epithelial cells of the large intestine. Acetate enters the bloodstream and can be converted to acetyl-CoA in the liver and other tissues, thus serving as a precursor for lipogenesis (fat synthesis) or as a substrate for oxidation. Butyrate is mostly used as a fuel by the large intestinal cells (often called *colonocytes*) themselves, and little enters the bloodstream; in fact, the short-chain fatty acids are essential for the well-being of the large intestine. There is also considerable evidence that the short-chain fatty acids — butyrate in particular — protect the colon against cancer development. However, the quantitative importance of volatile fatty acids from large intestinal fermentation, in relation to the energy needs of the body as a whole, is probably not great.

Suggestions for further reading

General
Caspary, W.F. (1992) Physiology and pathophysiology of intestinal absorption. *Am. J. Clin. Nutr.* **55 (Suppl.),** 299S–308S
Hunt, S.M. & Groff, J.L. (1990) *Advanced Nutrition and Human Metabolism,* Chapters 2, 4–6 and 10, West Publishing Co, St Paul

Dietary carbohydrate, digestion and absorption
Englyst, H.N. & Kingman, S.M. (1993) Carbohydrates. In *Human Nutrition and Dietetics.* (Garrow, J.S. & James, W.P.T., eds.), pp. 38–55, Churchill Livingstone, Edinburgh. (A useful review of the different forms of dietary carbohydrate and their handling in the intestine.)
Levin, R.J. (1994) Digestion and absorption of carbohydrates: from molecules and membranes to humans. *Am. J. Clin. Nutr.* **59 (Suppl.),** 690S–698S

Lipid digestion and absorption
Carey, M.C., Small, D.M. & Bliss, C.M. (1983) Lipid digestion and absorption. *Annu. Rev. Physiol.* **45,** 651–677
Derewenda, Z.S. & Sharp, A.M. (1993) News from the interface: the molecular structures of triacylglycerol-lipases. *Trends Biochem. Sci.* **18,** 20–25
Sethi, S., Gibney, M.J. & Williams, C.M. (1993) Postprandial lipid metabolism. *Nutr. Res. Rev.* **6,** 161–183. (This review contains some information on digestion and absorption of lipids, although it is mainly on the metabolism of chylomicrons and other lipoproteins.)

3

Metabolic characteristics of the organs and tissues

3.1   Metabolism of tissues and organs

In this chapter we shall look at the specific features of metabolism in different tissues. This will enable us to integrate them more easily in later chapters.

The distinction between an organ and a tissue is not absolute; either may be composed of more than one cell type. For instance, the kidney is composed of two distinctive tissue types, the cortex and medulla, and each of these is composed of various types of cell. The most important tissues in metabolism, such as skeletal muscle and adipose tissue, are arranged in fairly discrete groups, and under many circumstances one type of tissue may behave in a broadly similar manner across the body: thus adipose tissue throughout the body is sometimes referred to as the adipose organ. In this chapter some of the major organs and tissues involved in the utilization and interconversion of substrates for cellular energy generation — energy metabolism — will be described. Some emphasis will be given to the way in which the various organs and tissues are interconnected by blood vessels, since this is essential to a full understanding of the way in which they interact metabolically.

A common theme in this chapter will be the way in which the kinetic properties of metabolic pathways within each tissue reflect the metabolic role of that tissue. One general mechanism is glucose transport into or out of the cell. Further details of individual types of *glucose transporter* and their effects on the kinetics of glucose transport are given in Box 3.1.

Box 3.1 Transport of glucose across cell membranes

It has long been known that glucose enters cells by carrier-mediated diffusion (facilitated diffusion) rather than by free diffusion across the cell membrane (see Box 1.2 for definitions). In recent years the genes for the specific glucose-transport molecules have been cloned and sequenced; the transport proteins have been expressed in cell lines and their characteristics studied. With one exception (the intestinal sodium–glucose co-transporter SGLT1 — see Section 2.3.1) these transporters form a family of related proteins and are all passive transporters, allowing the movement of glucose across cell membranes only down a concentration gradient. In the case of SGLT1, glucose may move up a concentration gradient, i.e. it may be concentrated by the transporter, because sodium ions, co-transported with the glucose, are moving down a concentration gradient. The expression of these transporters is tissue specific, and their properties are an integral part of the regulation of glucose metabolism in the particular tissue.

The effect that the characteristics of the glucose transporter may have on the rate of glucose entry into cells is illustrated in the figure.

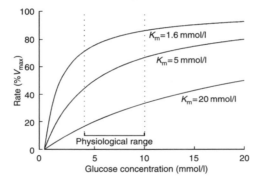

With a glucose transporter whose K_m for glucose entry is 1.6 mmol/l (e.g. GLUT3), the rate of glucose uptake is relatively independent of the extracellular glucose concentration over the normal, physiological range of plasma glucose concentrations. This would be appropriate in, for instance, the brain, where the rate of glucose uptake needs to be constant despite cycles of feeding and fasting. With a K_m for glucose entry of 20 mmol/l (e.g. GLUT2), the rate of glucose entry is almost proportional to the extracellular glucose concentration (the higher the external concentration, the greater the rate of ☞

3.2   The liver

3.2.1   General description

The word liver seems to come from old Norse *lifr*. The adjective hepatic, describing things to do with the liver, comes from the Greek *hepatos*. The adult human liver weighs 1–1.5 kg and lies immediately under the diaphragm. It is supplied with blood from below through two major vessels: the *hepatic*

☞ **Box 3.1 (continued)**

entry). The lines are plotted assuming Michaelis–Menten kinetics. This is oversimplified because it assumes that glucose within the cells is removed as fast as it enters. Therefore, the enzyme responsible for phosphorylation of glucose (hexokinase or glucokinase) must have similar characteristics to, or a greater capacity than, the glucose transporter for these kinetics to be expressed. The removal of glucose 6-phosphate must also occur at approximately the same rate as glucose enters the cell; the pathways of glucose metabolism are regulated hormonally so as to coordinate all these events (e.g. see Figure 3.2).

Name	Tissue distribution	Approximate K_m	No. of amino acids	Important features
GLUT1	Erythrocytes, fetal tissue, placenta, brain	5–7 mmol/l	492	
GLUT2	Liver, kidney, intestine, pancreatic β-cell	High (7–20 mmol/l)	524	High K_m allows glucose to 'equilibrate' across the membrane
GLUT3	Brain	Low (1.6 mmol/l)	496	Low K_m allows relatively constant rate of glucose uptake independent of extracellular concentration over the normal range
GLUT4	Muscle, adipose tissue	5 mmol/l	509	The insulin-sensitive glucose transporter
GLUT5	Jejunum	5 mmol/l for fructose	501	Probably responsible for fructose uptake from intestine
SGLT1	Duodenum, jejunum renal tubules		664	The sodium–glucose co-transporter of the small intestine (not part of the same family as GLUT1–5)

Based on Pilch (1990); Gould & Holman (1993); Thorens (1993); Wright (1993).

artery (which supplies about 20% of the blood) and the *hepatic portal vein*, often called simply the *portal vein*. The portal vein carries blood which has passed through the complex system of blood vessels around the intestinal tract (see Figure 2.4). This unusual feature — that the liver receives its major blood supply via a vein — gives the liver a special role in metabolism.

The portal vein is short, about 7–8 cm in length. It is formed by the joining of veins coming from different parts of the intestinal tract, including the stomach, and also from the spleen. These veins carry the substances absorbed from the intestinal tract into the blood, particularly — from the point of view of energy metabolism — monosaccharides and amino acids. Thus the water-soluble substrates arising from the diet are transported first to the liver, before entering the general circulation.

Another important, although small, group of veins joins the portal vein just before it enters the liver: the *pancreatic veins*. These veins carry blood containing the pancreatic hormones insulin and glucagon from the endocrine part of the pancreas (described in more detail in Chapter 4). These hormones, therefore, exert their effects first on the liver, before being diluted in the general circulation.

Blood leaves the liver through a number of *hepatic veins*, which enter the *inferior vena cava*, the main blood vessel returning blood from the lower part of the body up towards the heart.

Another important system of vessels associated with the liver carries *bile* to the gall bladder. Bile (see Section 2.2.3.3) contains the bile salts, which are essential to the digestion and absorption of fats from the intestine. It is also a route for excretion of organic compounds detoxified in the liver that have a molecular mass greater than 400 Da. The 500–1000 ml of bile produced each day travels through a system of *hepatic ducts* to the gall bladder, a pear-shaped organ (about 8 cm long and 2–3 cm in diameter) located immediately under the liver (see Figure 2.5). Here it is stored between meals, and emptied during digestion through the *common bile duct* to the duodenum.

The major part of the liver (80% by volume) is composed of *hepatocytes*. Other cell types include the phagocytic Kupffer cells and endothelial cells. Hepatocytes are arranged in a very characteristic manner (Figure 3.1) which appears in cross-section as hexagonal units or *lobules*, each around 1 mm across. At each corner of the hexagon is a *triad* of three vessels: tiny branches of the portal vein, the hepatic artery and the bile duct. In the centre of the lobule is a branch of a hepatic vein, which carries blood away. The hepatocytes radiate outwards from the central vein. Blood flows from the triads towards the central vein in small passages between the hepatocytes, the *sinusoids*. Sinusoids are the equivalent of the capillaries found in other tissues and are lined with flat *endothelial cells,* as are all capillaries. The blood in the sinusoids is in intimate contact with the hepatocytes. Bile formed in the hepatocytes passes out to the bile-duct branch in the triad along the lines of hepatocytes in fine tubes called *bile canaliculi* (little canals).

The precise arrangement of hepatocytes within the liver is closely related to the function of the cells; this is known as *metabolic zonation* of hepatic metabolism. The *periportal hepatocytes* on the outside of each lobule are exposed to blood which has recently arrived at the liver in the portal vein and hepatic artery. Thus these cells are well oxygenated and supplied with substrates, and oxidative metabolism predominates. The synthesis of glucose *(gluconeogenesis)* occurs mainly in these cells, whereas the cells nearer the centre of each lobule *(perivenous hepatocytes)* are more involved in glycolysis

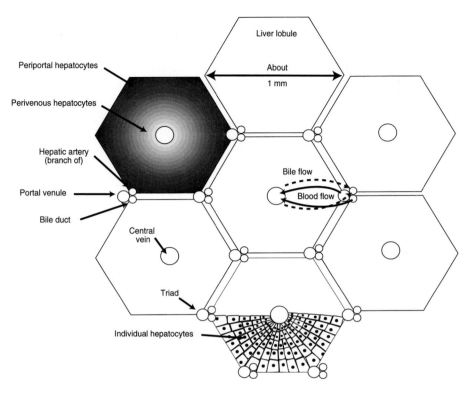

Figure 3.1   Arrangement of hepatocytes
In a cross-section of the liver, the hepatocytes appear to radiate out from the central vein. (Individual hepatocytes are not to scale, they are much magnified.) The anatomical features are described in more detail in the text.

and ketone body production. It appears that this arrangement is quite flexible, and each individual cell can perform either function depending upon its location in the lobule and the prevailing physiological circumstances.

3.2.2   Liver metabolism

By understanding how the liver is placed within the circulatory system, we can understand the rationale behind many of its metabolic functions. It is the first organ to 'get its pick' of the nutrients that enter the body from the intestine after a meal, and we might therefore predict that it would have a major role in energy storage after a meal. This is indeed so, at least for carbohydrate; storage and later release of glucose are major functions of the liver. It also has an important role in amino acid metabolism. Although fats bypass the liver as they enter the circulation (see Section 2.3.3), the liver does have important roles in fat metabolism.

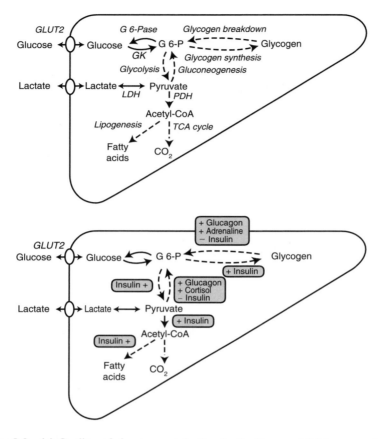

Figure 3.2   (a) Outline of glucose metabolism in the liver and (b) hormonal regulation of glucose metabolism
Abbreviations used: GK, glucokinase; GLUT2, hepatic glucose transporter (see Box 3.1); G 6-P, glucose 6-phosphate; G 6-Pase, glucose-6-phosphatase; LDH, lactate dehydrogenase; PDH, pyruvate dehydrogenase; TCA cycle, tricarboxylic acid (Krebs) cycle. (b) A plus sign (+) indicates stimulation; a minus sign (−) indicates inhibition. Shaded boxes show hormonal regulation.

3.2.2.1   Carbohydrate metabolism in the liver

The major pathways of glucose metabolism in the liver and their hormonal regulation are summarized in Figure 3.2. Glucose is absorbed from the intestine into the portal vein, where its concentration may reach almost 10 mmol/l after a meal. (Arterial blood glucose concentration is normally around 5 mmol/l.) The hepatocytes, especially the periportal cells, are therefore exposed to high concentrations of glucose during the absorptive phase. Liver cells have predominantly the GLUT2 type of glucose transporter (Box 3.1), which is not responsive to insulin and has a relatively high K_m for glucose so that it normally operates well below saturation. In addition, because there are many transport molecules, there is a high maximal activity (V_{max}) for glucose transport. This means that the rate and direction of movement of glucose across the hepatocyte membrane are determined by the relative glucose concentrations inside and outside the cell.

Within the hepatocyte, glucose is phosphorylated to form glucose 6-phosphate — the initial step in its metabolism by any pathway — by the enzyme *glucokinase* (EC 2.7.1.1-2). This enzyme belongs to the family of hexokinases (hexokinase Type IV), but differs from the hexokinases found in muscle and other tissues in that it has a high K_m for glucose (12 mmol/l) and is not inhibited by its product, glucose 6-phosphate, at physiological concentrations[1]. Like the GLUT2 transporter it has a high capacity (high V_{max}) and is unaffected, in the short term, by insulin.

The overall result is that when the glucose concentration outside the hepatocyte rises, glucose will be rapidly taken into cells and phosphorylated; the liver is often described as acting as a 'sink' for glucose. Another way of expressing this is to say that it acts as a buffer, taking up glucose when the concentration outside is high (e.g. after ingestion of a carbohydrate-containing meal) and releasing it, by specific mechanisms discussed below, when it is required elsewhere in the body.

The presence of the high-K_m glucose transport protein and the high-K_m glucokinase would not, alone, enable the hepatocyte to take up unlimited quantities of glucose, as glucose 6-phosphate would simply accumulate within the cell until glucose phosphorylation ceased. Instead, there are specific mechanisms for stimulating the storage of glucose as glycogen. The most important of these mechanisms is direct regulation of the enzymes of glycogen metabolism by insulin and by glucose itself. Insulin has reciprocal actions, activating the rate-controlling enzyme of glycogen synthesis (*glycogen synthase*; EC 2.4.1.11) and inhibiting that of glycogen breakdown (*glycogen phosphorylase*; EC 2.4.1.1). These are brought about in both cases by changes in the phosphorylation of the enzyme (Box 3.2). They are reinforced by the effect of glucose on glycogen phosphorylase (Box 3.2, Figure a). The result is a rapid stimulation of glycogen synthesis and suppression of glycogen breakdown, so that net storage of glycogen occurs. It will be apparent that because insulin is secreted from the pancreas, and reaches the liver directly, it may give precise coordination to this system.

Glucose 6-phosphate can also be metabolized to pyruvate via glycolysis in hepatocytes. Some of the resulting pyruvate may be oxidized directly in the tricarboxylic acid cycle, some released as lactate. Most of the energy required

---

[1]*It is more correct to say that glucokinase has a low affinity for glucose (and other hexoses): the term K_m implies strict Michaelis–Menten kinetics, which is not true. Although glucokinase is not inhibited by glucose 6-phosphate at concentrations found in the cell, it is regulated by fructose 6-phosphate, acting via a regulatory protein. [See Cornish-Bowden & Cárdenas (1991) and further reading at the end of this chapter.]*

Box 3.2 Hormonal regulation of glycogen breakdown (glycogen-olysis) and synthesis (glycogenesis) in the liver

The pathways and their regulation are similar in muscle: see Figure 7.7.

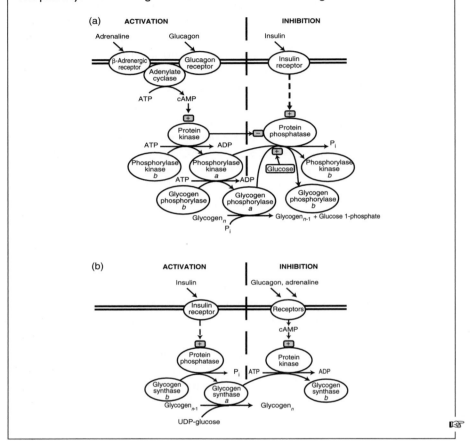

by the liver for its multiple metabolic purposes is, however, derived from the oxidation of amino acids and fatty acids rather than glucose.

Glycogen breakdown, controlled by reciprocal activation of glycogen phosphorylase and inhibition of glycogen synthase, is brought about by a change in the balance of hormones. The activation (by phosphorylation) of glycogen phosphorylase is regulated by a number of hormones, including glucagon, and by the catecholamines, adrenaline and noradrenaline (Box 3.2, Figure a). (The role of the catecholamines in metabolic regulation during normal daily life is probably small, although it becomes important in stress situations; this will be considered in Chapters 6 and 7.) Activation of glycogen phosphorylase is opposed by insulin and glucose, as we have seen. As the absorption of a meal is completed, tissues such as brain and muscle will still be using glucose, and the blood glucose concentration will begin to fall, albeit

☞ **Box 3.2 (continued)**

Glycogen breakdown (Figure a): Adrenaline, acting via β-adrenergic receptors, and glucagon activate adenylate cyclase (EC 4.6.1.1) via G-proteins (not shown). Cyclic AMP activates cyclic AMP-dependent protein kinase (also known as protein kinase A; EC 2.7.1.37) which phosphorylates phosphorylase kinase (EC 2.7.1.38), converting it from its dephosphorylated, inactive form (b) to its phosphorylated, active form (a). Phosphorylase kinase then phosphorylates and activates glycogen phosphorylase (EC 2.4.1.1), converting it from its dephosphorylated, inactive form (b) to its phosphorylated, active form (a). Glycogen phosphorylase acts on glycogen, releasing by phosphorolysis one molecule at a time of glucose 1-phosphate; this may be converted to glucose and released into the circulation. Glycogenolysis is inhibited by insulin, which activates protein phosphatase-1 (EC 3.1.3.16) by phosphorylation at a particular site; this dephosphorylates (and thus inactivates) phosphorylase kinase and phosphorylase itself.

A further form of regulation is brought about by glucose itself. Glucose binds to a specific site on phosphorylase *a*, causing a conformational change which makes the enzyme a better substrate for dephosphorylation by protein phosphatase-1. Thus in the liver an increase in the intracellular glucose concentration will itself lead to inactivation of phosphorylase.

Glycogen synthesis (Figure b). Many of the enzymes are common to glycogen synthesis and glycogenolysis. Insulin, via activation of protein phosphatase-1, brings about the dephosphorylation (and thus activation) of glycogen synthase (EC 2.4.1.11), by conversion from its inactive, phosphorylated form (b) to its active, dephosphorylated form (a). This is opposed by the hormones which stimulate glycogenolysis (e.g. adrenaline and glucagon), which activate the cyclic AMP-dependent protein kinase and lead to phosphorylation (and inactivation) of glycogen synthase. Thus there is coordinated control of glycogen synthesis and breakdown: when one process is stimulated, the other is inhibited.

very slightly; the balance of the hormones — insulin and glucagon — secreted by the pancreas will then change in favour of glucagon. Again, the anatomical relationship of the liver to the endocrine pancreas means that hepatic metabolism is very directly regulated by this balance.

Glycogen will be broken down when the concentration of glucose in the blood falls. The purpose of this is to liberate carbohydrate, stored in the liver after meals, into the bloodstream. The breakdown of glycogen leads to the production of glucose 1-phosphate, which is in equilibrium with glucose 6-phosphate (catalysed by *phosphoglucomutase*; EC 5.4.2.2). Glucose 6-phosphate cannot be converted to glucose by glucokinase, which catalyses an essentially irreversible reaction, and the formation of glucose from glucose 6-phosphate is instead brought about by *glucose-6-phosphatase* (EC 3.1.3.9) (Figure 3.2). Like that of glucokinase, the K_m of glucose-6-phosphatase is high relative to normal concentrations of its substrate, glucose 6-phosphate. Neither glucokinase nor glucose-6-phosphatase is directly regulated in the short term by hormonal signals (they are regulated over a matter of some hours, by changes in the amount of enzyme protein present), and the net flux between glucose and glucose 6-phosphate is therefore determined by their relative concentrations. During glycogen breakdown, brought about because the plasma glucose concentration is falling, the net flux will be towards the formation and export from the cell of glucose.

The properties of the hepatic glucose transporter and enzymes of glucose metabolism, as well as the anatomical relationship of the liver to the endocrine pancreas and the small intestine, give the liver a very important role as a buffer to take up glucose after a meal, when it is in plentiful supply, and to release it later when required elsewhere in the body.

The other important function of the liver in glucose metabolism is gluconeogenesis, the synthesis of glucose from other precursors. In terms of function, the pathway of gluconeogenesis is like glycolysis in reverse, but there are some essential differences in the enzymic steps and these are the points at which regulation occurs (Box 3.3). The substrates for gluconeogenesis are smaller molecules: usually, in increasing order of importance, lactate, alanine and glycerol. Other amino acids can also serve as gluconeogenic precursors, although alanine is by far the most important, for reasons that will be discussed in Section 5.4.2.

The pathway of gluconeogenesis is regulated by two major factors: (i) the rate of supply of substrate and (ii) hormonal regulation of the enzymes concerned (discussed in detail in Box 3.3). Overall, gluconeogenesis is stimulated by glucagon and inhibited by insulin, while glycolysis is favoured under the opposite conditions. The stimulation of gluconeogenesis by glucagon also occurs in part because of direct stimulation of the transporters for uptake of substrates (particularly alanine) from the blood into the liver cell. The net result is, again, that in conditions where glucagon predominates over insulin the liver will become a producer of glucose 6-phosphate and thus, by the mechanisms discussed earlier, an exporter of glucose into the circulation. It will be apparent that glycogenolysis and gluconeogenesis tend to be active at the same time in normal daily life. This is not so in more prolonged starvation, a condition in which gluconeogenesis becomes particularly important but there is little glycogen in the liver to mobilize; this will be discussed fully in Chapter 7.

Hepatic gluconeogenesis can also be stimulated by an increase in the supply of substrate from other tissues. One example is the period after physical exercise when there is an elevated concentration of lactate in the blood, some of which will be reconverted to glucose in the liver. During starvation, an increased concentration of blood glycerol arising from adipose tissue lipolysis (see Section 3.6.2.2) will have the same effect. However, there is one common situation in which hormonal factors tend to suppress gluconeogenesis, whereas substrate supply increases it. This is the situation after a meal and is at the heart of a phenomenon known as the *glucose paradox*. It was noted some years ago that an isolated liver, perfused with an artificial 'blood' medium, will synthesize glycogen under appropriate conditions. However, the highest rates of glycogen synthesis are observed not when glucose alone is supplied at high concentration in the perfusate, but when it is supplied together with a precursor of gluconeogenesis, such as lactate. Under these conditions lactate rather than glucose appears to be the true substrate for glycogen synthesis. (Lactate must first be converted to glucose 6-phosphate by the pathway of gluconeogenesis, see Box 3.3.) Findings in an isolated tissue such as the perfused liver must be interpreted with caution for the reason discussed earlier, i.e. in the body there are special relationships between different organs and tissues that are not reproduced in this laboratory situation. However, the result has since been confirmed in humans, i.e. hepatic glycogen synthesis after a meal comes about by a combination of the 'direct pathway' (glucose uptake; glucose 6-phosphate formation; and glycogen synthesis) and the 'indirect pathway' (uptake of 3-carbon gluconeogenic substrates, particularly lactate; formation of glucose 6-phosphate; and glycogen synthesis). The origin of the lactate in this situation is not yet completely clear. One suggestion is that the small intestine itself, during the process of glucose absorption, metabolizes a portion of the glucose to lactate, which passes to the liver through the portal vein. Again, the anatomical relationship of liver to intestine is important. Other tissues may produce some lactate from glucose in the plasma: red blood cells, adipose tissue and muscle play some part in this, although it is not yet clear how important any particular tissue is in the post-prandial period (the period after a meal). The essential point, however, is still that glycogen is synthesized by the liver after a meal, although the pathways involved are not quite as straightforward as would have been thought 10 years ago.

3.2.2.2 Fatty acid metabolism in the liver

The main pathways of fatty acid metabolism in the liver, and their hormonal regulation, are shown in Figure 3.3. The liver may, like other tissues, take up non-esterified fatty acids from the plasma. These fatty acids have two major fates within the liver: oxidation or triacylglycerol formation.

The liver may oxidize fatty acids by the mitochondrial β-oxidation pathway to produce energy for its many metabolic activities. (An alternative β-oxidation pathway in peroxisomes seems to operate mainly to shorten long-chain fatty acids. It uses different enzymes, but the same metabolic steps. It has been estimated to contribute 5–30% of the total rate of hepatic fatty acid oxidation, and will not be considered here.) In particular, gluconeogenesis, a pathway which requires energy, appears to be fuelled by oxidation of fatty acids. If fatty acid oxidation is prevented experimentally by using a specific inhibitor, gluconeogenesis is suppressed. During the oxidation of fatty acids in

Box 3.3 The pathways of glycolysis and gluconeogenesis and their hormonal regulation

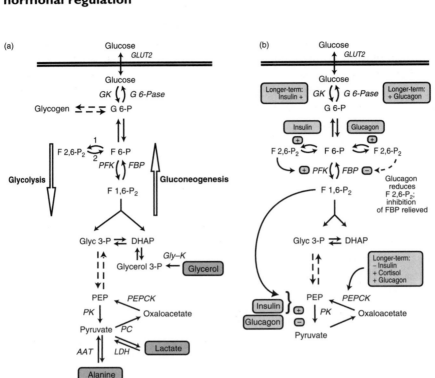

The pathways (Figure a). The pathways are shown as they occur in the liver. Dashed arrows indicate multiple steps. Note that there are three places in which the pathways of glycolysis and gluconeogenesis diverge. Co-substrates including ATP, ADP, P_i, GTP and CO_2 are not shown for simplicity. The three major substrates for gluconeogenesis are shown (dark boxes) together with the places at which they enter the pathway. They arise from tissues outside the liver. Substrates: G 6-P, glucose 6-phosphate; F 6-P, fructose 6-phosphate; F 1,6-P_2, fructose 1,6-bisphosphate; F 2,6-P_2, fructose 2,6-bisphosphate; Glyc 3-P, glyceraldehyde 3-phosphate; DHAP, dihydroxyacetone phosphate; PEP, phosphoenolpyruvate. Enzymes: GK, glucokinase; G 6-Pase, glucose-6-phosphatase; PFK, phosphofructokinase; FBP, fructose-1,6-bisphosphatase; PK, pyruvate kinase; PC, pyruvate carboxylase; PEPCK, phosphoenolpyruvate carboxykinase; Gly-K, glycerol kinase; LDH, lactate dehydrogenase; AAT, alanine aminotransferase. The enzymes marked 1 and 2 are part of a single, bifunctional enzyme known as 6-phospho-fructo-2-kinase/fructose-2,6-bisphosphatase, responsible for formation and breakdown of F 2,6-P_2, a compound with a crucial role in regulation of these pathways.   ☞

☞ **Box 3.3 (continued)**

Regulation (Figure b). The pathways of glycolysis and gluconeogenesis catalyse opposite functions, and it is not surprising that conditions which favour one tend to suppress the other. In general, glycolysis is favoured under 'fed' conditions, gluconeogenesis under 'starved' conditions. There are three major modes of regulation: allosteric, covalent (phosphorylation) and gene expression. The last of these is relatively long term (hours rather than minutes) and affects GK, G-6-Pase and PEPCK activities as shown. Allosteric and covalent regulation by hormones works mainly through adenylate cyclase/cyclic AMP (see Box 3.2 for more details). The principal features are as follows:

- The bifunctional 6-phosphofructo-2-kinase/fructose-2,6-bisphosphatase is regulated by phosphorylation by cyclic AMP-dependent protein kinase (glucagon high) and dephosphorylation by protein phosphatase-2A (insulin high). In the phosphorylated form it catalyses breakdown of F 2,6-P_2; in the dephosphorylated form it catalyses formation of F 2,6-P_2.

- F 2,6-P_2 is a potent activator of PFK and inhibitor of FBP; thus when insulin is elevated glycolysis is favoured; when glucagon is high relative to insulin, the F 2,6-P_2 concentration falls and gluconeogenesis is favoured.

- PK (glycolysis pathway) is inhibited by phosphorylation by cyclic AMP-dependent protein kinase (glucagon high); insulin inhibits this phosphorylation (i.e. maintains the enzyme active).

- In addition, PK is activated allosterically by F 1,6-P_2 (thus its activity is maintained when glycolytic flux is high).

- Other compounds within the cell also play a role in allosteric regulation. Of these, the most important are probably: (i) the adenine nucleotides (ATP, ADP, AMP), which regulate several steps such that when the cellular energy state is low (low ATP/ADP ratio) glycolysis is favoured; (ii) citrate, which inhibits PFK. The importance of these additional controls may lie in the fact that when cellular energy is plentiful, e.g. because the cell is oxidizing fatty acids (and thus citrate concentrations are also high), gluconeogenesis will be favoured. There is much experimental evidence that an increased rate of fatty acid oxidation in the liver increases the rate of gluconeogenesis.

Glucagon is an example of a hormone counteracting insulin (a *counter-regulatory* hormone). In certain 'stress' conditions (see Section 6.3.1) adrenaline and noradrenaline may play the equivalent role, raising cyclic AMP concentrations through β-adrenergic receptors.

Based in part on Hue & Rider (1987) and Pilkis & Granner (1992); see also Krauss-Friedmann (1984) for details of short-term control.

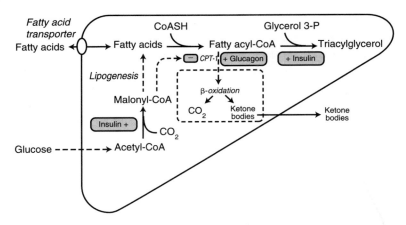

Figure 3.3   Fatty acid metabolism in the liver
Fatty acids cross the hepatocyte membrane by a carrier-mediated process. Inside the liver cell
they are transported through the cytosol by binding to specific fatty acid-binding proteins, and
activated by esterification to coenzyme-A (CoASH). To enter the mitochondrion (dotted box)
for oxidation, fatty acyl-CoA esters are converted to acyl-carnitine derivatives by the action of
carnitine O-palmitoyltransferase-1 (CPT-1). This enzyme is inhibited by malonyl-CoA, an intermediate in the pathway of *de novo* lipogenesis. Insulin inhibits fatty acid oxidation by increasing
the concentration of malonyl-CoA and stimulating fatty acid esterification to form triacylglycerol. Glucagon increases fatty acid oxidation, possibly by a direct effect on CPT-1.

the liver, the ketone bodies *acetoacetate* and *3-hydroxybutyrate* are produced
and exported into the circulation. The regulation of *ketogenesis* is complex,
although it is clear that to a major extent ketone body production in the liver is
determined by the rate of fatty acid oxidation. There may be some modulation
by oxaloacetate availability, regulating the rate at which acetyl-CoA is
oxidized in the tricarboxylic acid cycle rather than forming ketone bodies. The
rate of fatty acid oxidation is regulated, in turn, by two factors: the availability
of fatty acids, and the balance between their two fates in the liver.

The alternative fate for fatty acids taken up by the liver is esterification to
form triacylglycerol, which is stored within hepatocytes. This triacylglycerol
pool is not a major energy store for the rest of the body (that function is
performed by the triacylglycerol stored in adipose tissue) but appears to be a
local store for hepatic needs.[2] The stored triacylglycerol acts as the substrate
for hepatic secretion of fat into the bloodstream, in the form of the lipoprotein
particles known as *very-low-density lipoprotein* (VLDL). The bulk of the lipid
in VLDL is in the form of triacylglycerol, derived from the hepatic store. (The

---

[2]*In certain conditions, the hepatic fat content can become much greater and result in the
pathological condition known as fatty liver (characterized, as its name suggests, by the
large fat deposits seen under the microscope). This happens in alcoholism. Fat can build
up to the extent that it disrupts the normal functioning of the liver.*

details and the regulation of lipoprotein metabolism will be discussed in detail in Chapter 8.)

The balance between fatty acid oxidation and esterification in the liver is controlled mainly by insulin and glucagon. (The special relationship of pancreatic hormones to hepatic metabolism will again be apparent.) A major site for regulation is that of entry of fatty acids into the mitochondrion for oxidation. This is brought about by the action of the enzyme *carnitine O-palmitoyltransferase-1* (CPT-1; EC 2.3.1.21) as shown in Figure 3.3. The activity of this enzyme is controlled by the cellular level of the compound *malonyl-CoA*, which is a potent inhibitor of CPT-1. Thus in 'fed' conditions, when insulin is elevated, malonyl-CoA levels will be high and fatty acid oxidation (and hence ketogenesis) will be inhibited. Fatty acids will tend to be esterified, a process that also appears to be stimulated by insulin (although the exact locus of control is not clear). Hence in the fed state the liver tends to store fatty acids as triacylglycerol rather than to oxidize them. Hepatic energy requirements under these circumstances will be met mainly by amino acid oxidation. The physiological importance of *de novo* lipogenesis as a means of producing new fatty acids will be considered further in a later chapter (see Section 5.4.1.1). In normal circumstances it is probably not great, but the pathway is nevertheless very important in metabolic regulation because it is the source of malonyl-CoA, and hence is a major means by which insulin inhibits fatty acid oxidation.

The liver has other specialized roles in fat metabolism. These include its production of bile salts (Box 2.1) and its role in cholesterol metabolism (see Chapter 8).

3.2.2.3 Amino acid metabolism in the liver

Under normal circumstances in adult life, the body does not continuously accumulate or lose protein in a net sense. The rate of amino acid oxidation must, therefore, balance the rate of entry of dietary protein (typically 70–100 g of protein per day on a Western diet). General features of amino acid metabolism will be covered later (see Section 5.3). The liver plays a special role in amino acid oxidation, not least because it is the organ which first receives the dietary amino acids, which enter the circulation via the portal vein. It is also the only organ capable of eliminating the amino acid nitrogen by synthesis of urea. Therefore, with a few exceptions, amino acid catabolism occurs predominantly in the liver. (An important exception is catabolism of the group of branched-chain amino acids which is largely initiated in muscle; see Section 5.3.2.2.) Amino acid oxidation provides about half the liver's energy requirements. Figure 3.4 gives a general overview of hepatic amino acid metabolism.

Amino acids are not merely substrates for energy production in the liver. They also provide a substrate for synthesis of glucose (particularly alanine; see Box 3.3), of fatty acids and of ketone bodies. Of course, amino acids also serve

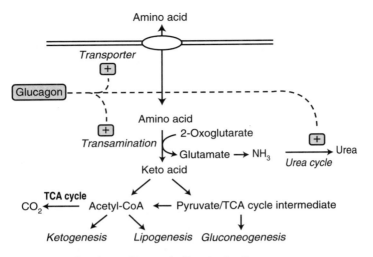

Figure 3.4 Outline of amino acid metabolism in the liver
The intracellular effects of glucagon are relatively long term, particularly increased expression of the enzymes for transamination and of the urea cycle. Abbreviation: TCA cycle, tricarboxylic acid (Krebs) cycle.

as precursors for hepatic protein synthesis, both proteins required within the liver and proteins exported into the circulation such as albumin.

An important general reaction in amino acid catabolism is the loss of the amino group by the process of *transamination* (see Figure 3.4; this will be described in detail in Box 5.3). The *keto acid* that results may enter a catabolic pathway directly: for instance, the keto acid of alanine is pyruvate, the end-product of glycolysis; that of glutamic acid is 2-oxoglutarate; and that of aspartic acid is oxaloacetate. The last two are intermediates in the tricarboxylic acid cycle. Alternatively, the keto acid may undergo further metabolic transformations leading to a compound (acetyl-CoA for many amino acids) which can enter one of the catabolic pathways.

Catabolism of amino acids by the liver is mainly regulated on a short-term basis by substrate supply. Substrate supply depends in the fed state on the arrival of dietary amino acids, and in the starved state on the net rate of body protein breakdown. The latter is itself under hormonal control, discussed in Section 5.3.3. On a longer-term basis, it is regulated by the hormones glucagon and cortisol. These hormones stimulate the synthesis of the enzymes of amino acid catabolism and urea synthesis. Glucagon has a short-term effect by activating amino acid transport proteins, particularly that for alanine, to increase amino acid uptake. In addition, there is long-term control by the amount of dietary protein; when the dietary protein content is low, the hepatic enzymes of amino acid catabolism are repressed; when dietary protein is more than adequate, their expression is stimulated. Thus the liver regulates the body's overall store of amino acids.

3.3   The brain

The brain is a very heterogeneous structure and different regions may have very different patterns of metabolism. Some generalizations may be made, however, which are relevant for understanding energy metabolism in the body as a whole. Some more-specialized functions of the brain — coordination of the autonomic nervous system and production of hormones, for instance — will be dealt with in Chapters 4 and 6.

The adult human brain weighs about 1.5 kg. It consists of a large number of cell types (Section 6.2.1), although the bulk consists of nerve cells: an outer layer of *grey matter*, largely nerve cell bodies, surrounding the *white matter*, largely myelinated fibres bundled into large tracts (like electrical cables). These terms, and the structure of the brain, will be amplified in Chapter 6. The head is supplied with blood through the two *common carotid arteries* (one on either side of the neck). Each divides in the neck into an internal and an external carotid artery: the internal supplies blood to the brain; the external supplies more to the face, neck and exterior of the head. Blood returns from the brain in the *internal jugular veins*, eventually reaching the heart via the superior vena cava. The rate of blood supply to the brain is high, about 750 ml/min (50 ml of blood/min per 100 g of tissue). This can be compared with about 5 ml of blood/min per 100 g of tissue for resting skeletal muscle and for adipose tissue, or around 50 ml of blood/min per 100 g of tissue for skeletal muscle during vigorous exercise. This high rate of blood flow to the brain reflects its high metabolic rate.

The brain oxidizes about 120 g of glucose/day, equivalent to about 2 MJ of energy, or 20% of the whole body energy expenditure in a typical day. This is known from studies in which samples of blood have been taken from jugular veins and compared with arterial blood. It is not possible to detect any increase in this overall rate of metabolism during mental activities (such as mental arithmetic), presumably because the actual increase in metabolic rate in a small area adds very little to the overall rate of metabolism, although with specialized techniques for scanning metabolic activity (based on glucose utilization) it is possible to show local increases in metabolic activity when a subject performs certain tasks.

Many substances, such as metabolites and drugs, which gain ready access to other tissues from the blood, seem to be excluded from the brain. This gave rise to the concept of a *blood–brain barrier* which some substances cannot cross. In general, the blood–brain barrier seems to prevent the access of lipid-soluble (hydrophobic) molecules to the brain, including the plasma non-esterified fatty acids. The brain as a whole does not appear to use fatty acids as a metabolic fuel. Instead, it uses almost entirely glucose under normal circumstances, although in prolonged starvation (see Section 7.3) it can use the ketone bodies. The glucose is for the most part completely oxidized (a small proportion is released as lactate), so the brain has a correspondingly high rate of oxygen consumption and carbon dioxide production. In general, the rate of utilization of glucose by the brain is not affected by insulin, although there are particular insulin-sensitive areas where insulin receptors exist. Glucose is transported into nerve cells by the glucose transporter GLUT3, which has characteristics that make it particularly suitable for this role. It has a low K_m for glucose transport into the cell so that at normal plasma glucose concentrations it is saturated with substrate (Box 3.1): thus quite wide variations in glucose concentration cause little change in the rate at which it is taken up by the brain. This is, of course, eminently sensible; if the rate of glucose uptake by the brain were to rise in response to increased plasma glucose concentrations after a meal, we might experience some strange effects! More importantly, the brain is protected against a fall in the plasma glucose concentration: not until the plasma glucose concentration falls below about 2 mmol/l does the rate of glucose uptake decrease so much that mental function is impaired. Again, therefore, the metabolic characteristics of the tissue seem ideally matched to its function.

The glucose transport protein GLUT1 (Box 3.1) is also expressed in the brain. It appears to mediate glucose transport at the blood–brain barrier. Since its K_m for glucose is considerably higher than that of GLUT3, it might appear that it would pose a limitation to glucose entry to the interstitial fluid at low plasma glucose concentrations. However, it may be that its capacity is sufficiently high that this does not limit the rate of glucose utilization by brain cells.

3.4   Skeletal muscle

3.4.1   General description and structure of skeletal muscle

Skeletal or *striated muscle* is also known as voluntary muscle since we have conscious control over its use. Other muscles, such as those lining the wall of the intestine, are involuntary *smooth muscle*, which lacks striations. The molecular basis of muscle contraction will not be covered here. What does concern us is that a supply of chemical energy in the form of ATP is required at the point of action at the appropriate time. There is a 'buffer store' in the form of phosphocreatine, which is in equilibrium with ATP through the action of creatine kinase (EC 2.7.3.2) (Figure 3.5). Since this is an equilibrium reaction, any fall in the ATP concentration will lead to the formation of further ATP from ADP, using the energy of phosphocreatine. This section covers the major fuels used by skeletal muscle to form the ATP required for contraction, and for the many other functions involved in cellular metabolism.

The cells of skeletal muscle are also known as *muscle fibres* since they are long and fibril-like — they may be a few centimetres long. Individual cells are grouped together into bundles known as *fasciculi* (sing. *fasciculus*), each surrounded by a sheath of connective tissue. A number of fasciculi are grouped

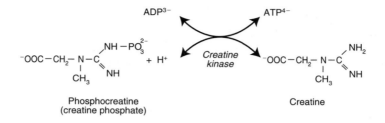

Figure 3.5 The creatine kinase reaction in muscle
The reaction is referred to as the Lohmann reaction after the German biochemist who elucidated it. Creatine kinase operates near to equilibrium; therefore, as ATP is utilized rapidly at the beginning of contraction, the phosphocreatine pool is used to maintain the ATP concentration. In resting muscle, typical concentrations of ATP and phosphocreatine are 5 mmol/kg of muscle and 17 mmol/kg of muscle, respectively; therefore, the presence of phosphocreatine approximately quadruples the ability to produce rapid contraction, before more ATP can be generated by other routes.

together and surrounded by a covering of connecting tissue, the *epimysium* or *deep fascia*; this whole structure is what we call a muscle (Figure 3.6).

3.4.2 Metabolism of skeletal muscle: general features

Muscle cells differ according to their relative capacity for oxidative metabolism, as opposed to anaerobic, glycolytic metabolism. If a cross-section of muscle is stained for one of the enzymes associated with aerobic metabolism (for instance, succinate dehydrogenase; EC 1.3.99.1) then it can be seen that individual fibres differ in the extent of their staining (Figure 3.7).

Broadly, there are two major types of muscle fibre (Table 3.1). Oxidative or *red* fibres are so-called because of their high content of *myoglobin*, a pigment related to haemoglobin which assists the diffusion of oxygen into the muscle. They have a high density of capillaries perfusing them, and many mitochondria. Red fibres use substrates largely from the blood, and oxidize

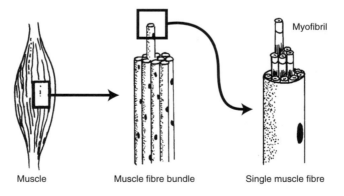

Figure 3.6 Structural organization of skeletal muscle
One cell is a muscle fibre. The whole muscle is made up of bundles of fibres, each filled with myofibrils. Reproduced from Jones & Round (1990) with permission.

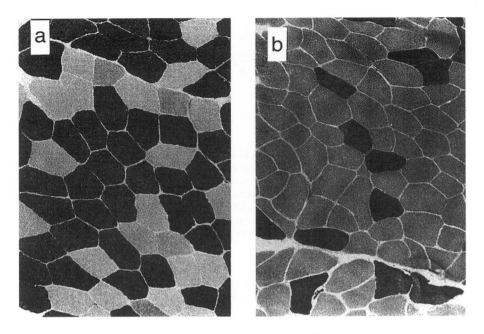

Figure 3.7   Fibre-type composition of leg muscles in athletes
Different types of muscle fibre (muscle cell) are shown in a cross-section of muscle, by staining for the enzyme myosin ATPase (EC 3.6.1.23), which reflects fast-twitch muscles: dark-stained fibres are Type II, lighter fibres are Type I. The Figure shows quadriceps muscle from (a) a high-jumper and (b) a marathon runner. Reproduced from Jones & Round (1990) with permission.

them to yield energy. Because the supply of substrate from the blood can be maintained for a long time — for instance, most of us have plenty of fat which can be supplied in this way — these muscle fibres are particularly important for sustained but relatively low-intensity exercise, such as walking or long-distance running. The oxidation of substrates from the blood requires time for diffusion of the substrate to the cell, diffusion of oxygen to the cell, and diffusion of CO_2 out of the cell. Therefore, contraction of this type of fibre, when it is stimulated, is relatively slow. These fibres are called *slow-twitch* or *Type I* fibres.

At the other extreme are the *white* fibres, which lack myoglobin. These fibres have fewer mitochondria, and are more equipped for anaerobic glycolysis than for oxidative metabolism. Their main substrate for glycolysis is glucose 6-phosphate produced by the breakdown of glycogen stored within the same cells. The sequence of glycogen breakdown and generation of energy by glycolysis can be extremely rapid, since everything is 'on site'. Hence these are the *fast-twitch* or *Type IIb* fibres (Table 3.1). Their role is to produce energy quickly, but, because they largely depend upon stored substrate, they cannot maintain this for long. They are therefore particularly important in the rapid generation of energy over short periods, such as that required for

Table 3.1	Characteristics of fibre types in skeletal muscle	
Property	**Type I** **(slow-twitch) fibre**	**Type II** **(fast-twitch) fibre**
Speed of contraction	Slow	Fast
Myoglobin content	High	Low
Capillary density	High	Low
Myofibrillar ATPase activity	Low	High
Mitochondrial enzyme activity	High	Low
Glycogenolytic enzyme activity	Low	High
Glycogen content		May be somewhat higher
Triacylglycerol content	High	Low
Lipoprotein lipase activity	High	Low

Based partly on Åstrand & Rodahl (1977). The terms high and low are relative. Type II fibres are adapted to fast work using their endogenous stores (ATP, phosphocreatine and glycogen, using anaerobic glycolysis), but have limited endurance. Type I fibres are adapted to slower work using energy generated by the complete oxidation of fuels (their own glycogen and triacylglycerol, and also glucose and non-esterified fatty acids taken up from the plasma).

sprinting. A third type of muscle fibre is described as fast-twitch oxidative glycolytic or Type IIa, as distinct from the very fast, anaerobic glycolytic Type IIb fibres.

In some animals, individual muscles are fairly uniform in their fibre type. In the rat, for example, there are some muscles that are composed almost entirely of red or white muscle types. For instance, the soleus muscle in the calf is used during movement such as running, and it is uniformly composed of slow-twitch fibres. The adductor longus muscle in the thigh plays an intermittent role in maintaining posture and is mainly composed of fast-twitch muscle. In humans, most muscles are composed of a variety of fibre types. The composition of any particular muscle is not the same in everybody; some people have a preponderance of oxidative fibre types, some an abundance of white, fast-twitch fibre types. This pattern is inherited to some extent. This is one reason why some people are naturally better than others at certain types of athletic event; for instance, someone with a lot of oxidative fibres will be better at endurance exercise than someone with more white, glycolytic fibres (Figure 3.7).

3.4.3   Routes of ATP generation in skeletal muscle

The major pathways for generation of ATP in muscle are illustrated in Figure 3.8. Skeletal muscle uses both stored fuel (glycogen and triacylglycerol) and substrates (glucose and fatty acids) taken up from the blood. The fatty acids may be either plasma non-esterified fatty acids, or esterified fatty acids carried in the form of triacylglycerol in lipoproteins.

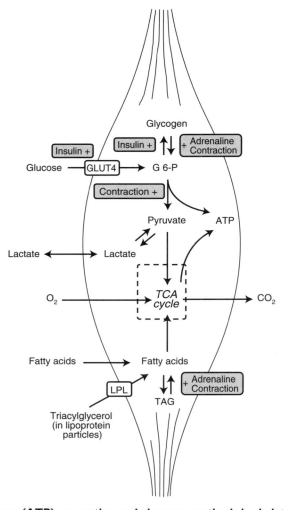

Figure 3.8   Energy (ATP) generation and glycogen synthesis in skeletal muscle
Only major pathways are shown: each arrow may represent one or more steps in a pathway.
The major sites of regulation are shown: a plus sign (+) indicates stimulation. Abbreviations
used: G 6-P, glucose 6-phosphate; LPL, lipoprotein lipase (situated in capillaries); TAG, triacylglycerol; TCA cycle, tricarboxylic acid (Krebs) cycle. The way in which muscle contraction is
coordinated with metabolism is discussed in Section 7.4.3.

3.4.3.1   Glucose metabolism in skeletal muscle

Glucose uptake is mainly mediated by the insulin-sensitive glucose transporter, GLUT4 (see Box 3.1). GLUT1 is also expressed in skeletal muscle and
may play a role in uptake of glucose at a 'basal' rate. Glucose uptake by
GLUT4 has certain characteristics which are relevant to its role in skeletal
muscle. The K_m is within the physiological range of plasma glucose concentrations. In the presence of low concentrations of insulin the V_{max} of glucose

uptake is low. Raising the insulin concentration brings more transporters into action at the cell membrane, and hence increases the V_{max}. Insulin thus increases the rate at which muscle takes up glucose from the blood. This glucose may be used for glycogen synthesis or metabolism via the pathway of glycolysis. As in the liver, insulin stimulates glycogen synthase in muscle, and inhibits glycogen phosphorylase. Therefore, when the plasma insulin concentration is high after a meal, glucose will be stored as glycogen in skeletal muscle. Glycogen synthesis is also stimulated after exercise when the glycogen store has been depleted.

3.4.3.2 Fatty acid metabolism in skeletal muscle

Fatty acids are taken up by muscle, particularly in the oxidative fibres. These are either the plasma non-esterified fatty acids, which have arisen from stored triacylglycerol in adipose tissue, or fatty acids carried as triacylglycerol in lipoprotein particles.

It is probable that non-esterified fatty acids are taken up across the cell membrane by a specific transport mechanism, although this is currently under investigation. The activity of the transporter does not appear to be regulated, however, since the rate of uptake is usually closely related to the concentration of non-esterified fatty acids in the plasma. Similarly, within the cell, fatty acids are oxidized in accordance with their rate of uptake. During exercise, however, there is clearly a need to increase the rate of uptake of substrates for oxidation. In the case of fatty acids, this is brought about mainly by increasing the rate of blood flow through muscle. The rate at which blood flows through any particular muscle increases several-fold when that muscle is exercising, resulting in the 'delivery' of more fatty acids to the muscle. Experiments with perfused muscle preparations in which the delivery of fatty acids is altered, either by altering their concentration or by altering the blood flow, show that the rate of fatty acid uptake is determined by the delivery rate (i.e. blood flow × concentration).

Apart from during exercise, increased uptake of fatty acids by muscle will occur when the plasma non-esterified fatty acid concentration is raised — for instance, during fasting. Under these conditions the muscle will not need to use so much glucose. Mechanisms by which the use of one fuel is regulated in response to the availability of another will be considered later (see Section 5.4).

Plasma triacylglycerol cannot be taken up directly. The fatty acids must first be released by the action of an enzyme, lipoprotein lipase, which is attached to the endothelial cells lining the capillaries. This process is therefore similar to the absorption of triacylglycerol from the intestine, and indeed lipoprotein lipase and pancreatic lipase (EC 3.1.1.3) belong to the same family of lipolytic enzymes. Lipoprotein lipase is also present in other tissues, especially adipose tissue. Since more is known about its action in adipose tissue, it will be described in more detail later (see Section 3.6.2.1; Figure 3.10). The fatty acids it releases from triacylglycerol in the capillaries enter the muscle cells, probably by the same means as do plasma non-esterified fatty acids. Thereafter their fate may be either oxidation or re-esterification to replenish the muscle triacylglycerol store.

3.5   The heart

Here we will be concerned with the metabolism of the muscular walls of the chambers of the heart — the *myocardium*. These walls are responsible for pumping blood through the lungs, and around the rest of the body. It is clearly important that they maintain their activity under all conditions. Blood is supplied to the heart muscle via arteries which branch from the aorta as it emerges from the left ventricle. These arteries encircle the heart rather like a crown, hence their name the *coronary arteries*. If these arteries should become blocked by a blood clot (a *coronary thrombosis*), some of the myocardium will be starved of blood and, therefore, of its supply of fuel and oxygen, and the heart will have difficulty in pumping blood around the body. This situation is a heart attack or *myocardial infarction* (infarction means blockage).

From the description of skeletal muscle metabolism, it will be clear that the myocardium is an extreme example of a muscle which must be able to keep contracting over long periods, i.e. a red or oxidative muscle. It has striations under the microscope that are not dissimilar from those of skeletal muscle, and the contractile mechanism is the same.

The fuels used by the heart have been studied by threading a fine tube (catheterization) into the great coronary vein which carries venous blood away from the myocardium. The blood in this vein can then be compared with blood in the arteries to see what has happened to it during passage through the myocardium. The heart is able to use a number of fuels, which it takes up from the blood. These include non-esterified fatty acids, glucose and ketone bodies. It can also take up lactate and oxidize it, via lactate dehydrogenase (EC 1.1.1.27) and the tricarboxylic acid cycle. Use of the different fuels by the heart depends to a large extent upon their concentrations in blood, although its uptake of glucose, by the insulin-sensitive GLUT4, is stimulated by insulin. In 'fed' conditions (high insulin concentrations) the myocardium tends to use carbohydrate rather than fat. The activity of lipoprotein lipase is also relatively high in the heart compared with skeletal muscle, implying that it may utilize fatty acids transported as plasma triacylglycerol in lipoprotein particles.

3.6   Adipose tissue

Adipose tissue has a number of functions which include mechanical cushioning (e.g. in the buttocks and around some internal organs) and thermal insulation; however, its main role from a metabolic point of view is storage of chemical energy in the form of triacylglycerol, and release in the form of non-esterified fatty acids when it is needed by other tissues.

3.6.1 White and brown adipose tissue

Two types of adipose tissue can be distinguished by their gross characteristics, by their appearance under the microscope and by their metabolic pattern. These are *brown adipose tissue* and *white adipose tissue*. Brown adipose tissue gets its colour from the presence of large numbers of mitochondria in the cytoplasm. Under the microscope, the major difference is in the way that triacylglycerol is stored. In brown fat cells (*brown adipocytes*), the stored lipid is present in multiple droplets. In white fat cells (*white adipocytes*), it is stored as one droplet which typically almost fills the cell; the cytoplasm, mitochondria and nucleus are confined to a thin 'crust' around the outside. In function, the similarity is that both types of cell store triacylglycerol and may release fatty acids. However, brown fat cells have a much higher oxidative capacity, and may oxidize a large proportion of the fatty acids released from storage.

Brown adipose tissue has a unique metabolic feature. Like most other tissues it can oxidize substrates, via the tricarboxylic acid cycle, in the mitochondria; unlike in any other tissue, this process can be uncoupled from the generation of ATP. Normally the electron-transport chain generates a proton gradient across the mitochondrial inner membrane, the energy of which is used to bring about synthesis of ATP from ADP. In the mitochondria of brown adipose tissue this process is uncoupled by the *uncoupling protein* (also known as *thermogenin*), which allows the proton gradient across the mitochondrial inner membrane to be dissipated or 'short-circuited'. This results in the liberation of heat from oxidation of substrates without trapping the free energy in high-energy compounds, and indeed the role of brown adipose tissue is specifically to generate heat. It does not do this all the time; it can be activated via the sympathetic nervous system, to bring about an increase in the liberation of fatty acids from the stored triacylglycerol and a large increase in the flow of blood through the tissue. It is very highly vascularized, i.e. it has many capillaries per unit cross-sectional area. The increased blood flow brings an increased supply of oxygen, and carries the heat produced to the rest of the body.

Brown adipose tissue is important in organisms that have a particular need to generate heat, for instance hibernating mammals. During hibernation the body temperature falls and metabolism slows, to preserve fuel stores. Awakening from hibernation is helped by the generation of heat in brown adipose tissue. Large adult mammals such as humans do not usually have a problem in generating heat, since the ratio of body mass (in which heat is generated) to body surface area (through which heat is lost) is in favour of generating too much heat, and instead adult humans have a variety of means of losing excess heat: sweating and dilatation of blood vessels in the skin, for example. Correspondingly, there is no good evidence that adult humans have significant amounts of brown adipose tissue. In contrast, infants have a different surface area/body mass ratio and have a need for a mechanism to generate heat, thus in infant humans brown adipose tissue has a clear role. It is lost during development. There is considerable controversy over whether it can be 'reawakened' in adults, or whether white adipose tissue can ever be converted into brown.

3.6.2 White adipose tissue metabolism

In the adult human, then, adipose tissue is virtually all 'white'.[3] Its major metabolic role is the regulated storage and release of fat, stored in the form of triacylglycerol and released to the rest of the body in the form of non-esterified fatty acids. Adipose tissue is sometimes described as an inert tissue metabolically. This is true in one restricted sense only: it has a very low consumption of oxygen. But the flow of fatty acids in and out of adipose tissue represents a large proportion of the energy metabolism of the body, and this is regulated on a minute-by-minute basis.

It is worth here re-emphasizing the point that lipid fuels — triacylglycerol and non-esterified fatty acids — are not water-soluble, and their presence in the plasma is dependent on specialized transport mechanisms. Excess concentrations of lipid fuels in the plasma can have adverse consequences, outlined in Box 3.4. Therefore, the regulatory role of white adipose tissue is essential to normal health as well as to the coordination of fat metabolism in everyday life, responding to meals and overnight fasting.

Two distinct aspects of the metabolism of white adipose tissue will be considered: the storage of triacylglycerol when there is an excess of chemical energy present in the circulation (as after a meal), and the liberation of fatty acids — fat mobilization — when other tissues in the body require it, e.g. during exercise or after an overnight fast. Although it is simplest to consider these separately, both are actively regulated all the time; if fat storage is occurring, fat mobilization is suppressed, and vice versa.

The major pathways of metabolism in white adipose tissue are illustrated in Figure 3.9.

3.6.2.1 Triacylglycerol storage

The triacylglycerol droplet within an adipocyte represents a very concentrated form of energy storage, usually accumulated over a period of some years. Metabolic pathways exist for 'laying down' triacylglycerol by two major routes: (i) uptake of triacylglycerol from plasma, and (ii) *de novo* lipogenesis, the synthesis of lipid (triacylglycerol) from other sources, particularly glucose.

---

[3]*In fact it is distinctly yellow because fat-soluble pigments are stored along with the triacylglycerol; these include carotenoids — compounds related to Vitamin A — and some breakdown products of haemoglobin.*

Box 3.4 Adverse consequences of excessive concentrations of lipids in the circulation

Prolonged exposure of the blood vessels to high concentrations of cholesterol and tri-acylglycerol can lead to the build up of fatty deposits, *atheroma*, in arterial walls — the process known as *atherosclerosis* (see Section 8.4.1 for more details).

Excessive release of non-esterified fatty acids can also have adverse effects. This can occur in stressful situations (see Section 6.3.3.2). Excessive fatty acid concentrations have adverse effects on the heart and may predispose it to irregular patterns of con-traction, and, in severe cases, to *ventricular fibrillation* — an uncoordinated fluttering in which the pumping of blood effectively ceases. This is a possible link between an acutely stressful situation and a heart attack. In addition, elevated non-esterified fatty acid con-centrations lead to increased hepatic secretion of triacylglycerol in the very-low-density lipoproteins, thus exacerbating any tendency to atherosclerosis. [See Oliver & Opie (1994) for a review of this topic.]

One dramatic (although unusual) example of excessive lipid concentrations is *fat embolus*. If excess fat in the form of triacylglycerol is liberated into the plasma, droplets of fat will circulate and may block blood vessels. This can occur after injury, when long bones such as the femur are fractured. Loosely connected fat cells are present in bone marrow; if the bone fractures, the cells (and their triacylglycerol contents) may be liberated in an entirely uncontrolled manner into the bloodstream. Globules of this fat may block blood vessels, particularly in the lung, leading to difficulties with breathing.

These features of excessive concentrations of lipid fuels in the circulation highlight the need to regulate their entry to, and removal from, the bloodstream. White adipose tissue plays an essential role in these processes.

Both will be outlined, although there is no doubt that in humans — at least on a typical Western diet in which there is no shortage of fatty acids — the uptake of triacylglycerol from the plasma is by far the more important.

Triacylglycerol in the plasma is present in lipoprotein particles (covered fully in Chapter 8). The larger particles, which carry most of the triacylglyc-erol, are too big to escape from the capillaries into the interstitial fluid; therefore, the adipocytes cannot take them up directly. There is an interesting mechanism to overcome this difficulty. Adipocytes produce lipoprotein lipase, which hydrolyses the triacylglycerol in lipoprotein particles to release fatty acids, which can then diffuse into the interstitial space and so reach the adipocytes. However, since lipoprotein lipase must act in the capillaries, it is exported from the adipocytes to the endothelial cells lining the capillaries of adipose tissue. Here it is attached by chains of the complex glycosaminoglycan *heparan sulphate*, a carbohydrate with highly negatively charged groups to which the enzyme molecules attach through a charge interaction. Lipoprotein lipase can thus come into contact with, and act upon, passing lipoprotein

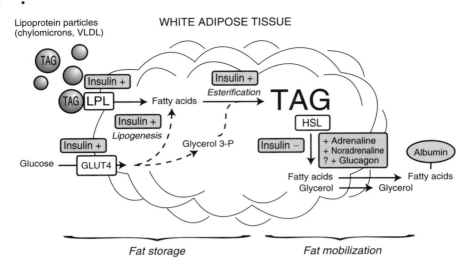

Figure 3.9　**Fatty acid and glucose metabolism in white adipose tissue**
The body's main store of chemical energy is in the form of triacylglycerol in white adipose tissue. Fat storage is the process of deposition of triacylglycerol; fat mobilization (or lipolysis) is the process of hydrolysis of the stored triacylglycerol to release non-esterified fatty acids into the plasma (bound to the carrier protein albumin), so that they can be taken up by other tissues. The major pathways and main sites of hormonal regulation are shown: a plus sign (+) indicates stimulation; a minus sign (−) inhibition. Abbreviations used: glycerol 3-P, glycerol 3-phosphate; HSL, hormone-sensitive lipase; LPL, lipoprotein lipase; TAG, triacylglycerol; VLDL, very-low-density lipoprotein.

particles (Figure 3.10). It acts on them to hydrolyse their triacylglycerol, thus releasing fatty acids. These fatty acids diffuse a short distance through the interstitial space towards the adipocytes, which take them up.[4] The fatty acids are taken up into the cells by a carrier-mediated process, an area of current research. The process of diffusion of the fatty acids from the site of lipoprotein lipase action and their entry into the cells is probably regulated for the most part by concentration gradients. The concentration gradient from capillary to cell will be produced, after a meal, by the activation of lipoprotein lipase and suppression of the release of fatty acids from the triacylglycerol store within the cell.

Once inside the cells, the fatty acids are esterified to form triacylglycerol which joins the lipid droplet for storage. The pathway of esterification is the usual one in which the fatty acids are first activated by formation of CoA-derivatives, then linked to glycerol 3-phosphate (the *phosphatidic acid pathway*; see Figure 2.8). The glycerol 3-phosphate is formed through glycolysis; it is in equilibrium with dihydroxyacetone phosphate, an inter-

---

[4]*Because the fatty acids are not water-soluble, the term 'diffuse' here may include some sort of structured pathway in which the fatty acids bind to albumin or to an extension of the cell membrane.*

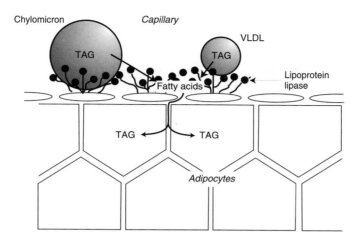

Figure 3.10 The action of lipoprotein lipase in white adipose tissue
Lipoprotein lipase (small black circles) is attached to the branching glycosaminoglycan chains which form the glycocalyx (a fuzzy surface lining the capillary). It acts on lipoprotein particles in the capillaries which contain triacylglycerol, hydrolysing this triacylglycerol to release fatty acids which are taken up into adipocytes and re-esterified for storage as triacylglycerol. Note that more than one molecule of the enzyme acts on a lipoprotein particle at once. Abbreviations used: TAG, triacylglycerol; VLDL, very-low-density lipoprotein.

mediate in glycolysis, the interconversion being catalysed by *glycerol-3-phosphate dehydrogenase* (EC 1.1.1.8).

The activity of lipoprotein lipase in adipose tissue is stimulated by insulin, which is released in response to an elevation in the blood glucose concentration. Since we rarely eat fat alone, this means that after a typical meal containing both fat and carbohydrate the uptake of fat into adipose tissue will be stimulated. The activation of lipoprotein lipase by insulin is rather more complex than a simple dephosphorylation, because of the rather complicated 'life cycle' of this enzyme: it involves increased transcription, altered processing of the enzyme within adipocytes and probably increased export to the endothelial cells. It is therefore not a rapid process and takes a matter of 3–4 h. This time-course will be highly relevant when we consider the co-ordination of metabolism in different tissues by insulin (Chapter 5). Within adipose tissue the esterification of fatty acids is also stimulated by the production of glycerol 3-phosphate through glycolysis, which is increased by insulin (Figure 3.9). Thus insulin stimulates both the uptake and storage in adipose tissue of fat circulating as triacylglycerol in the plasma.

The other potential pathway of fat deposition in adipose tissue is that of *de novo* lipogenesis (outlined in Box 3.5). It is stimulated by insulin at multiple points. Thus, again, insulin acts to promote fat storage in adipose tissue.

Box 3.5 The pathway of *de novo* lipogenesis

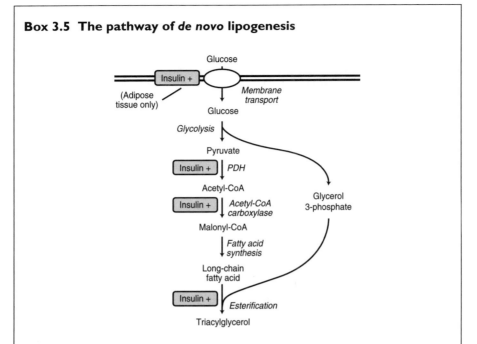

The starting point may be glucose (as shown) or amino acids, which can form pyruvate or acetyl-CoA by their degradation. The pathway occurs in both liver and adipose tissue (although its physiological importance may be small in humans). Most of the arrows involve a number of enzymic steps — for clarity not all of these are shown.

- Acetyl-CoA carboxylase (EC 6.4.1.2) is the first committed step in fatty acid synthesis, and a major site for regulation by insulin.

- Fatty acid synthesis proceeds by sequential addition of 2-carbon units.

- Esterification by the phosphatidic acid pathway (see Figure 2.8) utilizes glycerol 3-phosphate. In the liver this may arise from phosphorylation of glycerol taken up from blood; in adipose tissue it is produced via glycolysis.

- The pathway is over-simplified: acetyl-CoA is produced by pyruvate dehydrogenase (PDH) in the mitochondrion, but subsequent steps take place in the cytosol. There is a 'shuttle' for transfer of acetyl-CoA from the mitochondrion to the cytoplasm.

3.6.2.2 Fat mobilization

The mobilization of fat results in the liberation of fatty acids from the stored triacylglycerol; these fatty acids are released into the plasma as non-esterified fatty acids bound to albumin, and so are made available to other tissues. Since the mobilization of fat involves the hydrolysis of stored lipid, it is also called *lipolysis*. The breakdown of triacylglycerol is catalysed by a lipase (EC 3.1.1.3),

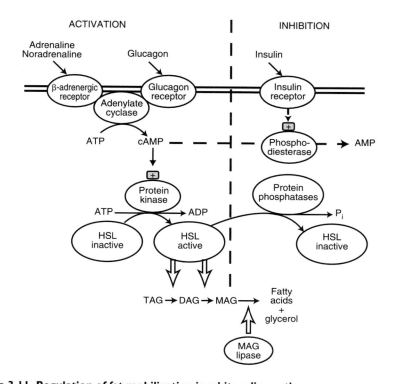

Figure 3.11 Regulation of fat mobilization in white adipose tissue
Triacylglycerol is broken down to its constituent fatty acids and glycerol by a process stimulated by hormones and by noradrenaline released from sympathetic nerve terminals. Notice the similarities with the control of glycogen breakdown (Box 3.2, Figure a). Abbreviations used: DAG, diacylglycerol; HSL, hormone-sensitive lipase; MAG, monoacylglycerol; TAG, triacylglycerol.

although this enzyme is necessarily situated within the adipocytes, in contrast with lipoprotein lipase which is exported to the capillaries. It is known as *hormone-sensitive lipase*, because its responsiveness to hormones was recognized before that of lipoprotein lipase. (It is better, perhaps, to think of this enzyme as the intracellular lipase.) It acts at the surface of the triacylglycerol droplet, and catalyses the hydrolysis of the ester bonds of two fatty acids. Another enzyme, a *monoacylglycerol lipase* (EC 3.1.1.23), present in high activity, is responsible for removal of the third fatty acid. Thus three fatty acids and one glycerol molecule are produced from each molecule of stored triacylglycerol. The fatty acids for the most part leave the cells and enter the plasma non-esterified fatty acid pool. The glycerol also leaves the cell; it cannot be utilized for esterification of fatty acids, since adipose tissue almost lacks glycerol kinase (EC 2.7.1.30) which would be necessary for this.

The activity of hormone-sensitive lipase must clearly be regulated very precisely, such that it is inactive when insulin levels are high. Hormone-

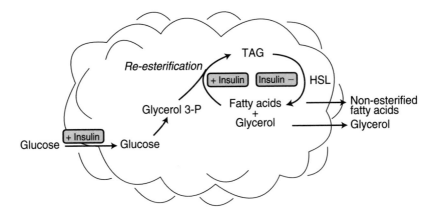

Figure 3.12 Insulin effects on fat mobilization in white adipose tissue
Insulin restrains fat mobilization by two mechanisms: suppression of the activity of hormone-sensitive lipase and stimulation of the re-esterification of fatty acids within the adipocytes. Abbreviations used: glycerol 3-P; glycerol 3-phosphate; HSL, hormone-sensitive lipase; TAG, triacylglycerol.

sensitive lipase is regulated by phosphorylation in a manner similar to glycogen phosphorylase in the liver (Figure 3.11). This phosphorylation is brought about by elevation of the cellular level of cyclic AMP, in response to a number of regulators. It is probable in humans that the most important of these are adrenaline (in the plasma) and noradrenaline (released by sympathetic nerves). Glucagon has a potent effect in isolated fat cells in the laboratory, but appears not to affect fat mobilization in humans *in vivo*. Equally important is the inactivation of hormone-sensitive lipase by dephosphorylation, which is a function of insulin. The mechanism by which insulin brings this about appears to involve increased breakdown of cyclic AMP by a specific phosphodiesterase. This is a very potent effect — it responds to relatively low concentrations of insulin — and very rapid, occurring within a matter of minutes of raising the insulin concentration. Therefore, insulin not only promotes fat storage, but it restrains fat mobilization.

Insulin has a further effect in restraining fat mobilization. The fatty acids released by the action of hormone-sensitive lipase are available for esterification by the phosphatidic acid pathway already described. Insulin, as we have seen, stimulates this pathway by increasing the provision of glycerol 3-phosphate. Hence insulin both inhibits the activity of hormone-sensitive lipase and 'mops up' any fatty acids it may liberate by increasing their re-esterification. These two actions are illustrated in Figure 3.12.

3.7   The kidneys

3.7.1   General description

The two kidneys sit fairly high up towards the back of the abdomen. Strictly speaking they are not in the abdominal cavity; they are behind the *peritoneum*, the membrane which surrounds the other abdominal organs such as the liver and intestines. The kidneys each weigh about 150 g in the adult human.

The adjective *renal* (from the Latin *renes*, the kidneys) is used to describe the properties and functions of the kidneys. The kidneys are supplied with blood through the *renal arteries* which branch off the aorta, and the blood is returned to the inferior vena cava through the *renal veins*. The major purpose of the kidneys is to produce urine. This is a vehicle for excretion of (i) those products of metabolism which the body needs to dispose of and (ii) regulated amounts of water, to maintain the correct osmolarity of the body fluids.

The details of renal physiology are outside the scope of this book, although a brief outline is necessary to understand the energy requirements of the kidneys. Blood flows through a series of complex structures known as the *glomeruli*, where 'tangles' of blood vessels are surrounded by a cup-shaped structure, the *glomerular capsule* or *Bowman's capsule*. The endothelium of these blood capillaries is highly fenestrated (see Section 1.3.1) to allow ready passage of molecules out of the blood into the capsule: this process is known as *glomerular filtration*. It is aided by the fact that blood in the glomerular capillaries is under higher pressure than usual in capillaries. Thus some of the plasma water, together with its complement of the smaller molecules dissolved in plasma, is lost into the capsule. The capsule is the termination of a tube, the *renal tubule*; the complete assembly of glomerular capsule and tubule is called a *nephron*. The fluid thus entering the renal tubule is the beginning of urine. However, before the urine is fully formed, much of the water and many of the solutes filtered at the glomerulus will be re-absorbed into the blood. In contrast with filtration, re-absorption is a very selective process and much of it involves active transport — energy-requiring transport of substances up a concentration gradient back into the plasma. The renal tubule forms a long loop, the *loop of Henle*, with descending and ascending limbs, following it in order from the glomerular capsule towards its end, where it joins a larger duct that collects urine from a number of tubules. The *collecting ducts* merge and eventually form the *ureter*, the tube carrying fully formed urine from the kidney to the bladder.

3.7.2   The scale of kidney function

About 1 litre of blood passes each minute through the glomeruli, or almost 800 litres each day. Of this about 20% is filtered through into the nephrons, producing almost 200 litres of filtrate each day. About 99% of the volume of this filtrate is re-absorbed, so that only 1–2 litres leaves the body as urine.

Water-soluble substances in the plasma are filtered along with the plasma water. Consider glucose as an example. A typical concentration of glucose in the plasma is about 5 mmol/l, or 0.9 g/l. Thus almost 1000 mmol (180 g) of glucose are lost into the glomerular filtrate each day. Since the body does not want to excrete glucose, virtually all of this is re-absorbed from the renal tubule.

Re-absorption of glucose has many similarities to the absorption of glucose from the intestine, as discussed in Chapter 2. The epithelial cells lining the tubules have microvilli, like the intestinal mucosal cells, increasing their absorptive surface area. At least in the first part of the tubule, glucose is carried into the cells mainly by the sodium–glucose co-transporter SGLT1, and leaves — into the interstitial fluid and thus the venous plasma — by the facilitated transporter GLUT2 (see Figure 2.7). Thus the energy for glucose re-absorption again comes from a gradient of concentration for sodium ions, which is maintained by the activity of Na^+/K^+-exchanging ATPase, and ultimately from hydrolysis of ATP.

3.7.3   Energy metabolism in the kidney

Given the very large quantities of solutes other than glucose which also have to be re-absorbed, it should not surprise us to learn that the kidneys have a high demand for energy. In fact they consume about 10% of the total oxygen consumption of the body at rest, although they contribute less than 0.5% of body mass. However, this metabolic activity is not spread evenly throughout the kidney.

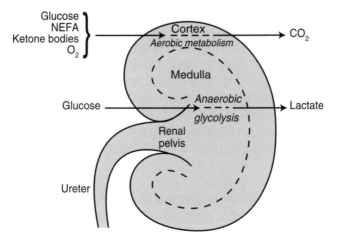

Figure 3.13 Schematic view of energy metabolism in different regions of the kidney
The cortex (outer layer) is well supplied with blood, has a high energy demand and is largely aerobic; the medulla has a poor blood supply and is largely anaerobic. It may derive its glucose by re-absorption from the tubules. Abbreviation: NEFA, non-esterified fatty acid.

In cross-section, the kidney can be seen to be formed of three fairly distinct parts. There is an outer, lighter-coloured layer, the *renal cortex*, surrounding a darker centre, the *renal medulla*. In the concave part of the 'bean' shape is the *renal pelvis*, the area where the collecting ducts gather together and form the ureter. The glomeruli are situated in the cortex, and some nephrons are completely contained in the cortex. Others have their loops 'dipping down' into the medulla; but most of the energy-requiring reabsorption of solutes goes on in the cortex. As we already know, the cortex has a high blood supply and it has a correspondingly aerobic pattern of metabolism; it oxidizes glucose, fatty acids and ketone bodies to provide its metabolic energy. The medulla, on the other hand, is much less well supplied with blood and derives its metabolic energy from the anaerobic metabolism of glucose. This is illustrated in Figure 3.13.

During starvation, the kidney becomes a relatively important site of gluconeogenesis. This process seems to take a few days of starvation to adapt, but may then contribute up to half the body's need for glucose.

Suggestions for further reading

Glucose transporters

Barnard, R.J. & Youngren, J.F. (1992) Regulation of glucose transport in skeletal muscle. *FASEB J.* **6**, 3238–3244

Gould, G.W. & Holman, G.D. (1993) The glucose transporter family: structure, function and tissue-specific expression. *Biochem. J.* **295**, 329–341

Liver metabolism: cellular organization

Gebhardt, R. (1992) Metabolic zonation of the liver: regulation and implications for liver function. *Pharmacol. Ther.* **53**, 275–354

Liver metabolism: control of metabolism

Brady, P.S., Ramsay, R.R. & Brady, L.J. (1993) Regulation of the long-chain carnitine acyltransferases. *FASEB J.* **7**, 1039–1044

Hue, L. & Rider, M.H. (1987) Role of fructose 2,6-bisphosphate in the control of glycolysis in mammalian tissues. *Biochem. J.* **245**, 313–324

Iynedjian, P.B. (1993) Mammalian glucokinase and its gene. *Biochem. J.* **293**, 1–13

Jungas, R.L., Halperin, M.L. & Brosnan, J.T. (1992) Quantitative analysis of amino acid oxidation and related gluconeogenesis in humans. *Physiol. Rev.* **72**, 419–448

McGrane, M.M., Yun, J.S., Patel, Y.M. & Hanson, R.W. (1992) Metabolic control of gene expression: *in vivo* studies with transgenic mice. *Trends Biochem. Sci.* **17**, 40–44. (Studies of the expression of enzymes including those of gluconeogenesis.)

van Schaftingen, E. (1994) Short-term regulation of glucokinase. *Diabetologia* **37 (Suppl. 2)**, S43–S47. (Glucokinase is inhibited by the binding of a specific regulatory protein.)

Regulation of glycogen metabolism (liver and muscle)

Barford, D. & Johnson, L.N. (1989) The allosteric transition of glycogen phosphorylase. *Nature (London)* **340**, 609–616

Dent, P., Lavoinne, A., Nakielny, S., Caudwell, F.B., Watt, P. & Cohen, P. (1990) The molecular mechanism by which insulin stimulates glycogen synthesis in mammalian skeletal muscle. *Nature (London)* **348**, 302–308

Shulman, G.I. & Landau, R. (1992) Pathways of glycogen repletion. *Physiol. Rev.* **72**, 1019–1035. (Discusses the indirect pathway for glycogen repletion.)

Woodgett, J.R. (1991) A common denominator linking glycogen metabolism, nuclear oncogenes and development. *Trends Biochem. Sci.* **16**, 177–181

Brain metabolism

Amiel, S. (1995) Organ fuel selection: brain. *Proc. Nutr. Soc.* **54**, 151–155

Owen, O.E., Morgan, A.P., Kemp, H.G., Sullivan, J.M., Herrera, M.G. & Cahill, G.F. (1967) Brain metabolism during fasting. *J. Clin. Invest.* **46**, 1589–1595. (The 'classic' paper on brain metabolism during fasting.)

Muscle metabolism including heart

Jones, D.A. & Round, J.M. (1990) *Skeletal Muscle in Health and Disease: A Textbook of Muscle Physiology*, Manchester University Press, Manchester. (A small book giving more detail on skeletal muscle structure and function.)

van der Vusse, G.J., Glatz, J.F.C., Stam, H.C.G. & Reneman, R.S. (1992) Fatty acid homeostasis in the normoxic and ischemic heart. *Physiol. Rev.* **72**, 881–940. [A useful review of the pathways for fatty acid uptake (from plasma non-esterified fatty acids and triacylglycerol) and oxidation in heart, but much also applies to skeletal muscle.]

White adipose tissue metabolism

Braun, J.E.A. & Severson, D.L. (1992) Regulation of the synthesis, processing and translocation of lipoprotein lipase. *Biochem. J.* **287**, 337–347. (A review of the regulation of lipoprotein lipase.)

Frayn, K.N., Coppack, S.W. & Humphreys, S.M. (1995) Fuel selection in white adipose tissue. *Proc. Nutr. Soc.* **54**, 177–189

Hollenberg, C.H. (1990) Perspectives in adipose tissue physiology. *Int. J. Obesity* **14 (Suppl. 3)**, 135–152

Brown adipose tissue metabolism

Klingenberg, M. (1990) Mechanism and evolution of the uncoupling protein of brown adipose tissue. *Trends Biochem. Sci.* **15**, 108–112. (A review of molecular aspects of the uncoupling protein or thermogenin.)

Trayhurn, P. (1995) Fuel selection in brown adipose tissue. *Proc. Nutr. Soc.* **54**, 39–47

Kidney metabolism

Baverel, G., Ferrier, B. & Martin, M. (1995) Fuel selection by the kidney: adaptation to starvation. *Proc. Nutr. Soc.* **54**, 197–212

Owen, O.E., Felig, P., Morgan, A.P., Wahren, J. & Cahill, G.F. (1969) Liver and kidney metabolism during prolonged starvation. *J. Clin. Invest.* **48**, 574–583. (A 'classic' paper showing the increased contribution of renal gluconeogenesis during starvation.)

4

Some important endocrine organs and hormones

4.1   Endocrine glands and hormones

A *gland* is an organ that produces a secretion, such as a hormone, which may enter the bloodstream; a juice which enters the digestive tract; or a substance, such as sweat, which enters the external environment. Other terms used in this connection are *endocrine* and *exocrine*: endocrine refers to internal secretions or hormones and exocrine refers to the production of juices to be delivered to the outside world. (The tube of the intestine is regarded as the outside world, since it connects with it at either end.)

The term *hormone* comes from the Greek *hormao*, meaning to urge on or excite. Hormones are released into the bloodstream from one tissue and cause an effect in another. However, the way in which they exert their effect must be distinguished from that of a metabolite — for example, the ketone body 3-hydroxybutyrate is also produced in one organ (the liver) and causes an effect (uptake and oxidation) in another (e.g. skeletal muscle). But the essence of hormone action is that the hormone affects substances other than itself, typically by causing regulation of a metabolic pathway. Hormones consist of a variety of types of chemical: peptides, glycoproteins, steroids and other small molecules, mostly derivatives of amino acids. At their target tissue they act by binding to a specific receptor, itself a protein. For peptide and protein hormones this receptor is usually part of the cell membrane. For steroid hormones and thyroid hormones it is within the cell; the hormone/hormone receptor complex enters the nucleus (or is formed in the nucleus) and affects DNA transcription, and thus synthesis of specific proteins.

The endocrine and exocrine glands are not in themselves major consumers of energy relative to other tissues in the body. Nevertheless, their products clearly have important effects in regulating energy supply and storage in the body. Here the major hormone-producing glands, and some exocrine tissues, relevant to energy metabolism will be considered. The location of the glands to be discussed is shown in Figure 4.1.

4.2   The pancreas

4.2.1   General description of the pancreas and its anatomy

The pancreas is a fish-shaped organ, about 15–20 cm long, lying under the liver (Figure 4.1). It has a distinct 'head' and a narrow 'tail', and the head end is wrapped around the small intestine. The pancreas is a complex organ since it contains both exocrine and endocrine tissues. The exocrine function of the pancreas consists of the liberation of digestive juices into the small intestine; the endocrine function consists of the production and secretion of hormones into the bloodstream, most importantly *insulin* and *glucagon*.

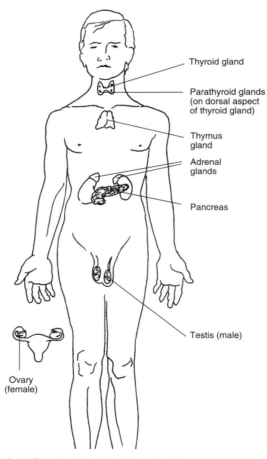

Figure 4.1   The location of endocrine glands involved in energy metabolism

The vast majority of cells in the pancreas are exocrine. These cells produce an alkaline digestive juice which contains a number of enzymes, particularly amylase, pancreatic lipase (EC 3.1.1.3) and the proteases, trypsin (EC 3.4.21.4) and chymotrypsin (EC 3.4.21.1). The juice is collected into small ducts which merge to form one main *pancreatic duct*. This is joined by the common bile duct just before it enters the duodenum; thus bile salts and pancreatic enzymes are liberated together into the small intestine. (The digestive function of the pancreas, and its regulation, are discussed in Chapter 2; see Table 2.2.)

Scattered among the exocrine tissue are little groups of cells, appearing like islands under the microscope. They were first described by a German medical student, Paul Langerhans, in 1869, and are known as the *islets of Langerhans* (Figure 4.2). These are the endocrine cells. There are around one million islets in the adult pancreas, although they constitute only 1–2% of the total mass of the pancreas. Within the islets there are three types of endocrine cell: the α-cells or A cells, which secrete glucagon; the β-cells or B cells, which secrete insulin; and the D cells, which secrete *somatostatin*. The β-cells occupy about 60% of the volume of the islet. Somatostatin in the pancreas probably has a local regulatory role, affecting the secretion of insulin and glucagon, but this is not entirely clear and it will not be considered further. Each islet is supplied with blood by a branch of the *pancreatic artery*, and venous blood leaves the islet in tiny veins (venules) which merge to form the *pancreatic* and *pancreatico-duodenal veins*. As discussed in Section 3.2.1, they discharge their contents into the hepatic portal vein, so the liver is in a unique position as regards its exposure to the pancreatic hormones.

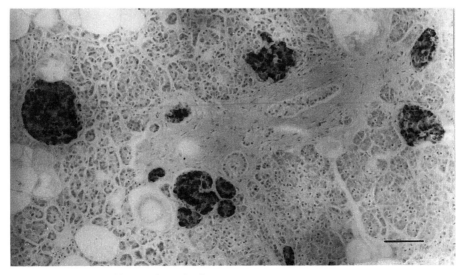

Figure 4.2   Islets of Langerhans in the pancreas
The pancreatic tissue has been immuno-stained to show the presence of insulin (and hence the islets). Scale bar = 100 μm. Courtesy of Dr Anne Clark; reproduced with permission from Frayn (1991).

4.2.2   Insulin

Insulin is a peptide hormone. It consists of two peptide chains, the A and B chains, linked by disulphide bonds: the A chain contains 21 amino acids, and the B chain 30 amino acids. Insulin is synthesized within the β-cells as a single polypeptide chain, and the connecting peptide or C-peptide is removed by proteolytic action before secretion (Figure 4.3).

Clearly, for insulin to have a useful signalling function, its rate of secretion must vary according to the metabolic or nutritional state. The mechanism by which this is achieved in the pancreatic β-cells is reasonably well understood. The most important regulator of the rate of insulin secretion is the concentration of glucose in the plasma. The β-cell responds to an elevation in glucose concentration by an increase in its own rate of glucose metabolism, leading to the production of ATP, which regulates events at the cell membrane. Insulin, which is synthesized within the cell and stored in secretory granules, is released by exocytosis of these granules — the granule membrane fuses with the cell membrane and its contents are discharged into the extracellular space. The synthesis of new insulin is also stimulated, and, if the stimulus (elevated glucose concentration) persists, insulin secretion will be maintained by increased synthesis.

The response of the β-cells to the surrounding glucose concentration may be studied by isolating pancreatic islets and incubating them with medium containing different concentrations of glucose. The characteristic sigmoid dose-response curve for insulin secretion rate against glucose concentration is

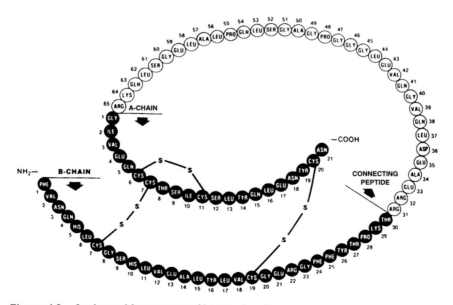

Figure 4.3   Amino acid sequence of human insulin
Reproduced with permission from Johnson (1982).

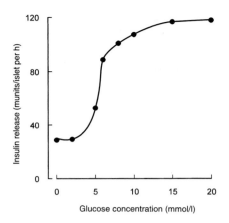

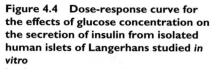

Figure 4.4 Dose-response curve for the effects of glucose concentration on the secretion of insulin from isolated human islets of Langerhans studied *in vitro*

Insulin secretion is stimulated as the glucose concentration rises above about 5 mmol/l (a typical concentration of glucose in the plasma). Based on Harrison *et al.* (1985); reproduced with permission from Springer-Verlag and the authors.

shown in Figure 4.4. Insulin secretion is not much increased until the glucose concentration rises above 5 mmol/l, which (by no coincidence) is the normal concentration of glucose in plasma. In other words, an elevation of the concentration of glucose in the plasma above its normal level will result in increased secretion of insulin.

Glucose is not the only stimulus to insulin secretion. Insulin secretion is also responsive to most amino acids (to somewhat differing extents), so that after a meal containing protein there is a stimulus for net protein synthesis. Insulin secretion may also respond weakly to ketone bodies. There is conflicting evidence on whether insulin secretion responds to non-esterified fatty acids; different fatty acids affect it differently, and overall this is probably not an effect of great physiological importance. Insulin secretion is also modulated by the nervous system, in ways which will be discussed in more detail in Chapter 6.

Insulin circulates free in the bloodstream; it is not bound to a carrier protein. It affects tissues by binding to specific *insulin receptors*, proteins consisting of four subunits (two α- and two β-chains), embedded in cell membranes. How insulin receptors affect intracellular metabolism is complex and will not be discussed in detail here. Ultimately most processes regulated by insulin are regulated via dephosphorylation of specific enzymes — e.g. glycogen synthase (EC 2.4.1.21) and glycogen phosphorylase (EC 2.4.1.1) — but in some cases phosphorylation is involved; the chain of events between insulin binding to a receptor and a change in some intracellular pathway is initiated by phosphorylation, since the insulin receptor β-subunit is itself a tyrosine kinase.

Insulin is removed from the circulation after binding to the cell-surface insulin receptors. These, with their bound insulin, become *internalized*, i.e. taken up into the cell, and eventually the insulin is proteolytically degraded. The process of internalization may have some role in bringing about insulin's actions, but this is not clear. It is also not clear whether some insulin is removed from the bloodstream by processes that do not result directly in metabolic effects. However, what is clear is that almost 50% of the insulin reaching the liver is removed in its 'first passage'. This means that the liver is exposed to much higher concentrations of insulin than other tissues or organs. It also means that swings in insulin concentration are to some extent 'damped down' by the time the insulin reaches the general circulation. This emphasizes the special relationship between endocrine pancreas and liver.

4.2.3 Glucagon

Glucagon is a single polypeptide chain of 29 amino acids. Unlike insulin, its major action is to elevate the blood glucose concentration. In fact, it was first discovered as a contaminant of preparations of insulin made from animal pancreases, which caused some batches to have the opposite of the desired blood glucose-lowering effect.

Its secretion from the pancreatic α-cells, like that of insulin from the β-cells, responds to both glucose and amino acids. However, unlike insulin, glucagon secretion is suppressed by a rise in glucose concentration (although it is stimulated by amino acids). Thus a rise in the plasma glucose concentration will lead to an increased ratio of insulin to glucagon secretion, and a fall in the plasma glucose concentration will lead to an increased ratio of glucagon to insulin. Again, some glucagon is removed on its first passage through the liver, although probably rather less than for insulin (animal experiments suggest around 5–10%); nevertheless, glucagon probably has no important metabolic effects in any tissue other than the liver.

Glucagon also produces its effects on intracellular metabolic pathways by binding to receptors in the cell membrane. These receptors are coupled, via G-proteins, to adenylate cyclase (EC 4.6.1.1), and intracellular effects of glucagon are mediated via cyclic AMP.

4.3   The pituitary gland

The pituitary gland is about the size of a pea and is situated on the under-surface of the brain. It is attached through a little stalk to the area of the brain known as the *hypothalamus*. The pituitary gland is also known as the *hypophysis*, or 'growth underneath'; the operation to remove the pituitary gland is called hypophysectomy. The hypothalamus, which itself lies under the thalamus, is the seat of integration of incoming signals from nerves with specialized 'sensing' functions, and outgoing nervous activity, particularly in the sympathetic nervous system; it will be discussed in more detail in Section 6.2.1.1. The location of the pituitary gland in close proximity to the hypothalamus is no mere chance.

The pituitary gland has two major parts, or lobes: the *anterior pituitary*, also called the *adenohypophysis*, and the *posterior pituitary*, or *neurohypophysis*. The adenohypophysis contains cells that manufacture and secrete hormones. Regulation of the synthesis and secretion of its hormones is controlled, however, by other signals (local hormones) coming down a system of blood vessels in the stalk from the hypothalamus. The neurohypophysis is composed mainly of nerve cells which have their cell bodies in the hypothalamus. It is not a true endocrine organ; rather, the hormones which it releases are synthesized in the hypothalamus, transported along axons and stored temporarily before being secreted in response to nervous stimuli from the hypothalamus. Thus the hypothalamus controls nervous signals and hormonal signals to the rest of the body.

The hormones produced by the pituitary gland and their target organs are shown in Figure 4.5.

4.3.1 Hormones of the anterior pituitary

The anterior pituitary secretes at least six distinct peptide and glycoprotein hormones. Several act on other hormone-producing organs to influence the secretion of further hormones: they are known as *tropic* (or *trophic*) hormones. Of these, *follicle-stimulating hormone* (FSH) and *luteinizing*

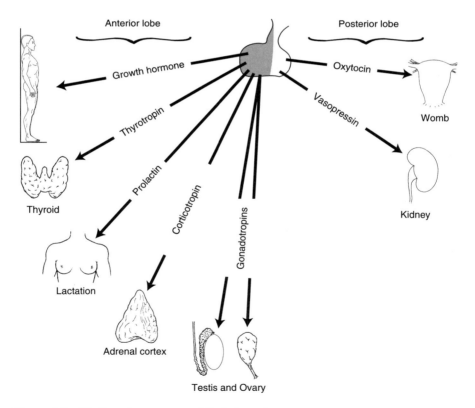

Figure 4.5 Pituitary hormones and their target organs
Based on Mason (1960) with permission.

hormone (LH), known together as *gonadotropins*, have functions in the reproductive system which will not be considered further.

Corticotropin (adrenocorticotropic hormone; ACTH) is a peptide hormone (of 39 amino acids) which acts on the adrenal cortex to stimulate release of glucocorticoids, particularly cortisol. Corticotropin is released in response to stress. It also has an important circadian rhythm (24 h cycle); it is at its highest, as is cortisol secretion, in the morning at about the time of waking. There is feedback control of corticotropin secretion: high levels of cortisol suppress corticotropin secretion.

Thyroid-stimulating hormone (TSH) — sometimes called *thyrotropin* — acts on the thyroid gland to stimulate the production of thyroid hormones and to stimulate growth of the gland (discussed further below). Again there is a feedback system, so that in thyroid deficiency, for example, TSH levels in blood are high; this is usually a clearer diagnostic test than direct measurement of thyroid hormone levels themselves.

Two more hormones secreted by the anterior pituitary act on other non-endocrine tissues: *prolactin* and *growth hormone*. Prolactin stimulates milk production, and will not be considered further.

Growth hormone is a peptide hormone (of 190 amino acids in humans), sometimes called *somatotropin* because of its major role in regulating growth and development (somato- refers to the body). It does not do this directly. Growth hormone stimulates the production in the liver of other peptide hormones, known as the *insulin-like growth factors* IGF-1 and IGF-2, formerly known as the somatomedins since they mediate the effects of somatotropin. As their name implies, the insulin-like growth factors have structural similarities with insulin. They exert stimulatory effects on growth, whereas growth hormone has no direct effect. Even in adults, however, growth hormone is secreted. This occurs mainly overnight, in discrete bursts during sleep. It has some direct metabolic functions, although their significance in adults is not fully understood. The most important effect is probably a stimulation of fat mobilization. This is not a rapid effect (unlike the effects of adrenaline or noradrenaline acting through the cyclic AMP system; see Figure 3.11); after a single injection of growth hormone, there is a stimulation of lipolysis after 2–3 hours. Growth hormone also has an effect on hepatic glucose production, probably involving stimulation of both gluconeogenesis and glycogenolysis. Again, this is probably not an effect of short-term importance. Adults who have had their pituitary gland removed surgically (usually because of a tumour) are usually not given growth hormone replacement, as it is expensive and has not until recently been thought necessary. Recently, a number of trials of growth hormone replacement have shown that such treatment results in a loss of body fat and an increase in lean body mass, including muscle, reflecting a combination of the lipolytic and anabolic (growth-promoting) effects. It may also result in a feeling of well-being, which is thought to reflect in part increased availability of fuels for physical work — i.e. non-esterified fatty acids and glucose in the plasma.

4.3.2 Hormones of the posterior pituitary

The posterior pituitary secretes two structurally similar, nine amino acid, peptide hormones: *oxytocin* (which causes the uterus to contract) and *vasopressin*, also called *antidiuretic hormone* (ADH). The latter name suggests an obvious function in regulating urine production (more specifically in regulating urine concentration), but the name vasopressin shows that this hormone also has a potent effect in constricting certain blood vessels. It may also, under certain conditions (particularly stress states), have a role in metabolic regulation; it has been suggested that vasopressin can stimulate glycogen breakdown in the liver. This is brought about by a change in the cytosolic Ca^{2+} concentration rather than through an increase in cyclic AMP. An interesting relationship between the different effects of vasopressin may be seen. We have already seen (Section 1.2.2.1) that glycogen is stored with about three times its own weight of water: the liver glycogen store of about 100 g is accompanied by 300 g water. Mobilization of glycogen, therefore, liberates water into the circulation. In a severe stress state brought about by loss of blood, for example, vasopressin might have multiple actions: further loss of water through the kidney is prevented by its antidiuretic action; extra water is mobilized along with glycogen; fuel (glucose) is provided for the organism to help deal with the stress, e.g. to provide energy to run away from an aggressor; and the vasoconstrictive action helps maintain blood pressure despite the loss of blood.

4.4 The thyroid gland

The thyroid gland weighs about 25 g and is made up of two lobes, joined by a bridge, situated on either side of the trachea (windpipe) in the throat (Figure 4.6). It has a rich blood supply. It is responsible for secretion of the thyroid hormones and the protein, *thyroglobulin*, which carries them in the circulation. The thyroid hormones are iodinated amino acid derivatives; they are formed from tyrosine residues within thyroglobulin and iodine which is taken up avidly by the gland from the blood (Figure 4.7). There are two thyroid hormones, known as *thyroxine* or T_4 (with four iodine atoms per molecule) and *tri-iodothyronine* or T_3 (with three iodine atoms). Both are secreted by the gland and are present in blood, although it appears that T_3 is the active hormone. Most tissues possess the enzyme necessary to convert T_4 to T_3.

Synthesis and secretion of the thyroid hormones are regulated by the pituitary-derived TSH. TSH also increases thyroid size. In thyroid deficiency owing to, for instance, lack of iodine in the diet, thyroid hormone levels in the blood are low. As discussed earlier (Section 4.3.1), this leads to an increase in

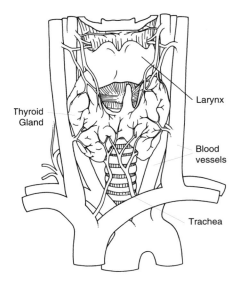

Figure 4.6 The anatomy of the thyroid gland
Based on Mason (1960) with permission.

Thyroid Gland

Larynx

Blood vessels

Trachea

TSH secretion to stimulate more thyroid hormone production. It also leads to enlargement of the thyroid gland, sometimes to a massive growth on the neck known as a *goitre*; hence the apparent paradox of an enlarged gland and a deficient hormone.

Most of the hormones which regulate metabolism do so in a very rapid manner; their secretion is regulated on a minute-to-minute basis and their effects on metabolic pathways are similarly fast, or sometimes somewhat slower if effects on protein synthesis are involved. The thyroid hormones, however, seem to set the general level of metabolism in a long-term way. In parallel with this, the thyroid gland is unusual in that it stores a large amount of hormone — enough for around 3 months' secretion.

Some specific effects of thyroid hormones on metabolism will be covered in later chapters, especially their effect on muscle protein metabolism (see Section 5.3.3). For the most part, however, the thyroid hormones play a 'modulating' role, affecting the level of response to other hormones. In particular, they appear to regulate the sensitivity of metabolic processes to *catecholamines* (adrenaline and noradrenaline): thus an excess of thyroid hormones has many similarities to an excess of adrenaline or noradrenaline. An excess of thyroid hormones is characterized by an increase in the overall metabolic rate; a deficiency is characterized by a depression of metabolic rate.

4.5   The adrenal glands

The two adrenal glands sit like cocked hats over each kidney (Figure 4.8), hence their name — which means additions to the renal organ, or kidney. Each gland has an inner core and an outer layer of cells, the *adrenal medulla* and

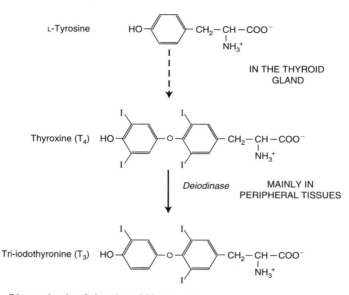

Figure 4.7 Biosynthesis of the thyroid hormones
Thyroxine (T_4) and tri-iodothyronine (T_3) are synthesized in the thyroid gland from tyrosine residues in the protein thyroglobulin. The conversion of T_4 to T_3, the active hormone, occurs mainly in peripheral tissues.

adrenal cortex respectively. The cortex (outer layer) makes up about nine-tenths of the bulk of the gland; under the microscope its cells are seen to be rich in lipid. The medulla stains darkly for microscopy with chromic salts, showing the presence of so-called *chromaffin* cells, characterized by the presence of catecholamines.

4.5.1 The adrenal cortex: cortisol secretion

The adrenal cortex secretes a number of steroid hormones which are synthesized from cholesterol. Some of these affect mainly mineral metabolism (salt and water balance) and are known collectively as the *mineralocorticoids*; some affect intermediary metabolism (glucose, fatty acid and amino acid metabolism) and are known as the *glucocorticoids*. The most important of these in humans is *cortisol*.[1]

As we have seen, the synthesis and secretion of cortisol are regulated in turn by corticotropin from the anterior pituitary. Cortisol has both short- and longer-term metabolic effects on a number of tissues. Even the short-term effects are, for the most part, mediated by changes in protein synthesis and therefore take a matter of hours rather than minutes. These short-term effects include: a stimulation of fat mobilization, by increased activity of the enzyme

---

[1] *Cortisol is also known as hydrocortisone. The latter name is more commonly used when referring to a medicinal product, but chemically they are identical.*

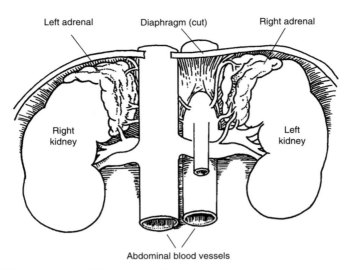

Left adrenal   Diaphragm (cut)   Right adrenal

Right
kidney   Left
                                     kidney

Abdominal blood vessels

Figure 4.8 The anatomy of the adrenal glands
Based on Mason (1960) with permission.

hormone-sensitive lipase (this probably involves synthesis of additional enzyme protein); a stimulation of gluconeogenesis (again via synthesis of key enzymes, see Box 3.3); inhibition of the uptake of glucose by muscle (mechanism not clear); and an increase in the breakdown of muscle protein.

These effects of cortisol are often difficult to demonstrate in isolated tissues, and it is thought that many of cortisol's effects are more *permissive* than direct. A permissive effect means that a process cannot occur (or activation by another hormone cannot occur) in the absence of the 'permitting agent' — in this case cortisol — but the actual level of the permitting agent is not important. Thus, in people or animals whose adrenal cortex has been removed, some effects of adrenaline, for instance, do not occur (particularly stimulation of glycogen breakdown). Responsiveness to adrenaline can be reinstated by giving a glucocorticoid hormone such as cortisol; however, the level achieved is not important, just its presence. This is certainly an over-simplification for most of cortisol's effects, but it is probably true that cortisol 'sets the tone' of response to other hormones.

4.5.2 The adrenal medulla, adrenaline secretion and adrenaline action

The adrenal medulla develops as part of the nervous system. It is supplied with nerves which are part of the sympathetic nervous system. (They are pre-ganglionic fibres whose neurotransmitter is acetylcholine; this will be discussed in detail in Section 6.2.2.1.) Its secretory activity is controlled directly by the brain through these nerves, and not by substances in the blood. It secretes adrenaline (named, of course, after the adrenal gland; in American literature this hormone is called *epinephrine*). Some more will be said about adrenaline and the related compound noradrenaline (*norepinephrine* in

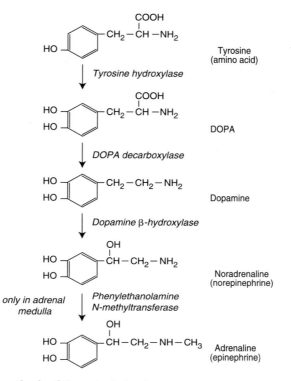

Figure 4.9 Biosynthesis of the catecholamines
Noradrenaline is released from sympathetic nerve terminals, whereas adrenaline is a true hormone, released into the bloodstream from the adrenal medulla.

American) in a later chapter (Section 6.2.3.1); but for now it is satisfactory to think of them as having similar effects, although noradrenaline is almost entirely liberated as a neurotransmitter from sympathetic nerve terminals, and is thus not a true hormone, whereas adrenaline is a hormone in every sense. They are both referred to as catecholamines because they are amine derivatives of the catechol nucleus. Their structures and the route of synthesis are shown in Figure 4.9.

Adrenaline and noradrenaline act on *adrenergic receptors* (or *adrenoceptors*), found in the plasma membranes of most tissues. There are different types of adrenergic receptor, first recognized because of the different potencies of adrenaline-like substances in bringing about various effects in specific tissues. Broadly, they may be divided into the α- and β-receptors, which are themselves subdivided into α_1, α_2 and β_{1-3} subtypes; in humans the β_3-subtype is mainly found in brown adipose tissue. The subtypes of adrenergic receptors are summarized in Table 4.1. The adrenergic receptors are all single polypeptide chains, related structurally, and belong to the superfamily of G-protein-coupled receptors.

Table 4.1 Adrenergic receptors and their effects

	Receptor type		
	β	α_1	α_2
Second messenger system	Adenylate cyclase/ cyclic AMP	Phospholipase C/ intracellular Ca^{2+}	Inhibition of adenylate cyclase
Metabolic effects	Glycogenolysis Lipolysis	Glycogenolysis	Inhibition of lipolysis
Circulatory effects	Increased heart rate and force Dilation of blood vessels	Constriction of blood vessels	Constriction of blood vessels

Note that the β-adrenergic receptors have not been subdivided here: see text Section 4.5.2.

Binding of adrenaline and noradrenaline to adrenergic receptors brings about a variety of effects. From the point of view of energy metabolism, we will divide these into two groups: circulatory effects and direct metabolic effects. The two are not independent, as will become clear in later sections.

β-Adrenergic receptors are linked, via the stimulatory G_s-proteins, to the membrane-bound enzyme adenylate cyclase (EC 4.6.1.1), which produces cyclic AMP from ATP (see Box 3.2). Binding of adrenaline or noradrenaline to a β-adrenergic receptor thus causes an increase in cytosolic cyclic AMP concentration, and activation of the *cyclic AMP-dependent protein kinase* (also known as *protein kinase A; EC 2.7.1.37*). This may lead (directly or through other protein kinases) to phosphorylation of a key regulatory enzyme: glycogen phosphorylase and hormone-sensitive lipase are two examples (see Box 3.2 and Figure 3.11). Thus catecholamines acting through β-adrenergic receptors tend to lead to breakdown of stored fuels, triacylglycerol and glycogen. The circulatory effects of β-adrenergic receptors are mainly stimulatory, especially stimulation of the heart to beat both more rapidly (the *chronotropic* effect) and more strongly (the *inotropic* effect). Broadly, β_1-receptors mediate the effects on the heart and on lipolysis, β_2 those on blood vessels and on glycogenolysis. In rodents, lipolysis is stimulated mainly by a third type, known as the *atypical β-receptor* or simply the β_3-receptor. In humans the significance of the β_3-receptor is still unclear. Its one certain role is in stimulation of thermogenesis in brown adipose tissue.

α-Adrenergic receptors may produce similar or opposite effects, depending upon the tissue. α_1-Receptors are linked to the secondary messenger system which involves hydrolysis of phosphatidylinositol 4,5-bis-phosphate. One of the products of this is inositol 1,4,5-trisphosphate (IP_3), which causes the release of Ca^{2+} from intracellular stores into the cytoplasm. This is involved, for instance, in an alternative route for the activation of glycogen breakdown by adrenaline: an increased cytosolic Ca^{2+} concentration will directly activate phosphorylase kinase (EC 2.7.1.38) (see Figure 7.7). α_2-Receptors are linked to adenylate cyclase through the inhibitory G_i-proteins, and thus adrenaline binding to such receptors will reduce the production of cyclic AMP and oppose effects caused by its binding to β-receptors. α_2-Receptors are important in adipocytes and seem to exert a 'moderating influence' on the activation of fat mobilization brought about by adrenaline acting on β-receptors. α-Receptors (especially α_1) also mediate the constriction of blood vessels and this has some repercussions on metabolism in stress states.

This sounds a complex system and indeed it is: the net effect will depend upon the relative abundance of the different types of adrenergic receptor in a tissue, as well as on the concentrations of other hormones. To put it into perspective, if adrenaline or noradrenaline is injected or infused (given as a slow injection, over perhaps 1 h) into human volunteers to raise the level in the blood to the upper limit of levels seen in normal everyday life, the major changes noted are an increase in heart rate and a rise in the concentrations of glucose and non-esterified fatty acids in the blood; thus the net metabolic effect of catecholamines appears to be mobilization of the stores of glycogen and triacylglycerol. There is also an increase in oxygen consumption, reflecting a general increase in metabolism. If very high levels are infused, then somewhat different changes may be observed, with restriction of blood flow in certain tissues and some inhibition of metabolic processes. These probably reflect the effects (which may be at least as important) of the catecholamines on blood flow in different tissues.

Suggestions for further reading

General reading

Ashcroft, F.M. & Ashcroft, S.J.H. (1992) *Insulin: Molecular Biology to Pathology*, Oxford University Press, Oxford

Bliss, M. (1983) *The Discovery of Insulin*, Paul Harris, Edinburgh. (A wonderful read, giving a feel for the excitement, and competition, of scientific research.)

White, D.A. & Baxter, M. (1994) *Hormones and Metabolic Control* (2nd edn), Edward Arnold, London

Insulin secretion and islet structure

Holz, G.G. & Habener, J.F. (1992) Signal transduction crosstalk in the endocrine system: pancreatic β-cells and the glucose competence concept. *Trends Biochem. Sci.* **17**, 388–393. (Glucose competence in this article refers to the ability to match insulin secretion to the prevailing glucose concentration.)

MacDonald, M.J. (1990) Elusive proximal signals of β-cells for insulin secretion. *Diabetes* **39**, 1461–1466

Weir, G.C. & Bonner-Weir, S. (1990) Islets of Langerhans: the puzzle of intraislet interactions and their relevance to diabetes. *J. Clin. Invest.* **85**, 983–987

Insulin receptor signalling

Exton, J.H. (1991) Some thoughts on the mechanism of action of insulin. *Diabetes* **40**, 521–526

O'Brien, R.M. & Granner, D.K. (1991) Regulation of gene expression by insulin. *Biochem. J.* **278**, 609–619

Growth hormone and the insulin-like growth factors

Langford, K.S. & Miell, J.P. (1993) The insulin-like growth factor-I/binding protein axis: physiology, pathophysiology and therapeutic manipulation. *Eur. J. Clin. Invest.* **23**, 503–516

Rudd, B.T. (1991) Growth, growth hormone and the somatomedins: a historical perspective and current concepts. *Ann. Clin. Biochem.* **28**, 542–555

Catecholamines and metabolism

Lafontan, M. & Berlan, M. (1993) Fat cell adrenergic receptors and the control of white and brown fat cell function. *J. Lipid Res.* **34**, 1057–1091

Macdonald, I.A., Bennett, T. & Fellows, I.W. (1985) Catecholamines and the control of metabolism in man. *Clin. Sci.* **68**, 613–619

5

Integration of carbohydrate, fat and protein metabolism in the whole body

In previous chapters we have looked at carbohydrate, fat and amino acid metabolism in some individual tissues. The aim of this chapter is to show how metabolism in the different tissues is integrated in the whole body. The hormonal system plays an important part in this integration.

Numerical examples will be used to illustrate the turnover of substrates in the blood. These all involve approximations, and should be taken as illustrations only. For most purposes, a fairly typical person of 65 kg body weight will be assumed.

5.1 Carbohydrate metabolism

Glucose is always present in the blood. It is not static; glucose molecules are continually being removed from the blood and replaced, so that the concentration remains relatively constant, at close to 5 mmol/l in humans (Figure 5.1). In fact, of all the energy substrates circulating in the blood, the concentration of glucose is by far the most constant. One reason for this is that it is necessary to provide a constant source of energy for those tissues in which the rate of glucose utilization is regulated primarily by the extracellular glucose concentration. For instance, we have seen that in the brain the rate of glucose utilization is fairly constant over a range of glucose concentrations, but will decrease considerably, with adverse consequences, if the glucose concentration falls below about 3 mmol/l. Furthermore, consistently elevated concentrations of glucose in blood — above about 11 mmol/l — have harmful effects, although these may take a matter of years to develop; this topic will be considered later with reference to diabetes mellitus (Chapter 9).

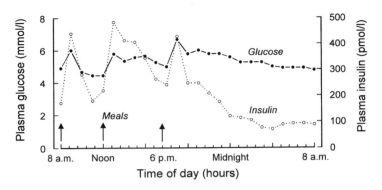

Figure 5.1   Relative constancy of blood glucose concentrations during a typical day, compared with the relative variability of plasma insulin concentrations
For a mechanical analogy, see Figure 5.2. Based on Reaven *et al.* (1988); reproduced with permission from the American Diabetes Association.

Glucose enters the blood in three major ways: by absorption from the intestine, from the breakdown of glycogen in the liver and from gluconeogenesis in the liver. (Remember that muscle glycogen breakdown does not liberate glucose into the blood, since muscle lacks glucose-6-phosphatase.) The relative importance of these routes differs according to the nutritional state. Glucose leaves the blood by uptake into tissues. In normal life very little escapes into the urine; although glucose is filtered at the glomerulus, it is almost completely re-absorbed from the proximal tubules.

During a typical day the average person on a Western diet eats about 300 g of carbohydrate. We can look at this in relation to the amount of free glucose in the body at any one time. The volume of blood is about 5 litres and the glucose concentration about 5 mmol/l, so the amount of glucose in the blood is about 25 mmol or (multiplying by 180, the relative molecular mass) 4.5 g. More correctly, we should look at the amount of glucose in all the extracellular fluid (about 20% of body weight or approx. 13 litres), i.e. about 12 g. Thus in 24 h we eat enough to replace our 'glucose in solution' about 25 times. This illustrates the need for coordinated control; even a single meal (say 100 g of carbohydrate) could elevate the glucose concentration about eight-fold if there were no mechanisms to inhibit the body's own glucose production and to increase the uptake of glucose into tissues.

The constancy of blood glucose concentration is brought about by coordinated control of various aspects of glucose metabolism. It will already be clear that insulin plays a major role in this coordination. The relationship between blood glucose and insulin concentrations is illustrated in Figure 5.1, which shows the relative constancy of glucose compared with the variability of insulin. This is typical of many systems in which one component varies to keep another constant. A useful analogy is with a thermostatically controlled water tank. At its simplest, a thermostat dips into the water. When the water temperature falls below a certain limit, e.g. 2 ° below the desired temperature, an electrical switch is triggered and the heating element is switched on. When the temperature reaches an upper limit, perhaps 2 ° above the desired level, the switch cuts out. The water temperature (the *controlled variable*) stays constant within quite narrow limits (±4 ° in this case), whereas the electrical current through the switch and heater (the *controlling variable*) varies between wide extremes (Figure 5.2). We will reconsider and improve upon this analogy at the end of this chapter.

5.1.1 The post-absorptive state

The phrase *post-absorptive state* implies that all of the last meal has been absorbed from the intestinal tract, but not much further time has elapsed — or the beginnings of starvation would be apparent. In humans, it is typically represented by the state after an overnight fast before breakfast is consumed.

In the post-absorptive state the blood glucose concentration is usually a little under 5 mmol/l. The concentration of insulin in plasma varies widely between individuals, but is typically around 60 pmol/l. The concentration of glucagon will be about 20–25 pmol/l. (There are difficulties in giving typical glucagon concentrations. First, the methods used to measure it in different laboratories tend to give varying results. Secondly, glucagon exerts its metabolic effects mainly, if not entirely, in the liver, and the relevant concentration is that in the hepatic portal vein: this is not easy to measure in normal volunteers.)

The rate of turnover of glucose in the post-absorptive state is close to 2 mg of glucose/kg of body weight per min, or 130 mg of glucose/min entering and leaving the circulation. Where does it come from, and where does it go? The pattern of glucose metabolism after an overnight fast is illustrated in Figure 5.3.

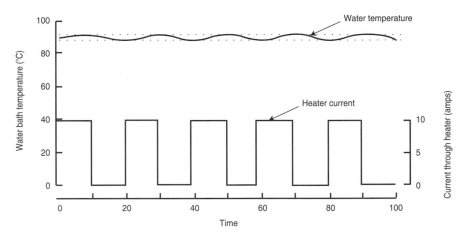

Figure 5.2 An analogy for metabolic regulation
The temperature in a thermostatically controlled water bath (the controlled variable) is relatively constant, whereas the electrical current flowing through the heater (the controlling variable) varies between much wider extremes.

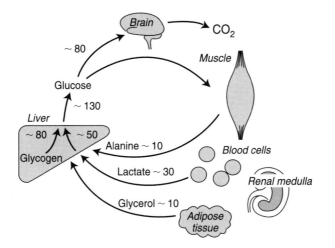

Figure 5.3   The pattern of glucose metabolism after an overnight fast
The numbers are approximations only, in mg/min, for a typical person of 65 kg body weight.
Much of the glucose delivered to peripheral tissues (muscle, adipose tissue, blood cells, etc.) is
'recycled' as lactate, which returns to the liver as a substrate for gluconeogenesis. However, a
large portion is oxidized, especially in the brain, and this constitutes an irreversible loss from the
body's store of carbohydrate. Note that this picture shows only glucose metabolism: muscle and
other tissues (e.g. renal cortex) also oxidize non-esterified fatty acids from the plasma.

In the post-absorptive state, glucose enters the blood almost exclusively
from the liver. Some of this glucose arises from glycogen breakdown and some
from gluconeogenesis. These proportions vary a lot according to how much
glycogen there was the evening before, which in turn depends on previous diet
and other factors, such as the amount of exercise taken. A reasonable approximation is that about two-thirds is from glycogen breakdown, say 80 mg of
glucose/min. The stimulus for glycogen breakdown (in contrast to the
situation after the last meal the previous evening, when glycogen was being
stored) is a decreased insulin/glucagon ratio — a little less insulin, a little more
glucagon. The remainder of glucose entry (say 50 mg/min) must result from
gluconeogenesis. What are the substrates for this? Lactate will constitute a
little over a half, and alanine (largely from muscle) and glycerol (from adipose
tissue lipolysis) most of the remainder. The lactate arises from a variety of
tissues. First, it comes from those tissues which use glucose almost entirely by
anaerobic glycolysis, such as the red blood cells and renal medulla. Note that
this constitutes a recycling of glucose; e.g. red blood cells use about 25 mg of
glucose/min, and return that amount of lactate to the liver for synthesis of new
glucose. Secondly, there will be some breakdown of muscle glycogen releasing
lactate from anaerobic glycolysis. The stimulus for gluconeogenesis (again
comparing with the previous evening when it was suppressed) is mainly the
decreased insulin/glucagon ratio.

On the disappearance side, the brain uses about 120 g of glucose/day (see Section 3.3) or about 80 mg/min, more than half of the total glucose utilization. The remainder is used by a number of tissues, including red blood cells (about 25 mg of glucose/min), skeletal muscle, renal medulla and adipose tissue.

5.1.2 Breakfast

The post-absorptive state usually only lasts a matter of a few hours before it is interrupted by the arrival of a meal. The first meal of the day gives the most dramatic switch from 'production' to 'storage' mode, and we will consider here how this comes about. For simplicity, we will consider a breakfast containing mostly carbohydrate, e.g. cereals and skimmed milk.

The carbohydrate is digested and absorbed from the intestine as described in Chapter 2. An increase in the concentration of glucose in the blood can be detected within about 15 min, and this increase continues to a peak at around 30–60 min after a

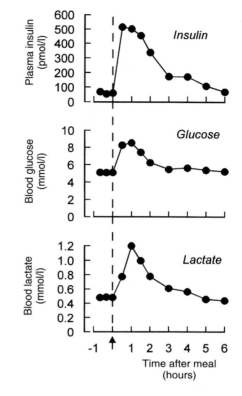

Figure 5.4 Concentrations of insulin, glucose and lactate in blood after an overnight fast and following a single meal The meal, shown by the arrow, contained 86 g of carbohydrate and 33 g of fat. Mean values for eight normal subjects are shown; based on data in Frayn et al. (1993).

moderate breakfast (Figure 5.4). (The exact timing depends upon factors such as the size of the meal and the amount of complex carbohydrate, fibre and simple sugars in the meal.) As the concentration of blood glucose rises, the endocrine pancreas responds: insulin secretion is stimulated and the concentration of insulin in plasma rises (Figure 5.4). The glucagon concentration in 'peripheral' blood (e.g. taken from an arm vein) may not fall after a typical meal, although we do not know directly what happens to glucagon secretion or to the glucagon concentration in the portal vein. Nevertheless, the insulin/glucagon ratio in plasma rises. How does this affect metabolism in individual tissues?

5.1.2.1 Carbohydrate metabolism in the liver after breakfast

The liver receives the blood draining the small intestine in the hepatic portal vein, and so it sees the largest change in blood glucose concentration. This leads to an inflow of glucose into hepatocytes via the transport protein GLUT2. The elevation of intracellular glucose concentration in hepatocytes, together with the change in insulin/glucagon ratio, leads to inactivation of glycogen phosphorylase and activation of glycogen synthase, and thus a switch from glycogen breakdown to glycogen storage (see Box 3.2).

We might expect that the pathway of gluconeogenesis would be inhibited by this hormonal switch, but this does not occur in practice. There is always an elevation of the blood lactate concentration after ingestion of carbohydrate (Figure 5.4). This probably represents the effect of a switch to partially anaerobic glucose metabolism in a number of tissues, including muscle and adipose tissue. The increase in blood lactate concentration is probably sufficient in itself to maintain the activity of the pathway of gluconeogenesis. The overall effect is that some of the glucose arriving in the blood is used by tissues, released into the blood as lactate, taken up by the liver and converted to glucose 6-phosphate and then glycogen — the 'indirect pathway' of glycogen deposition (discussed in Section 3.2.2.1). Note, however, that unlike gluconeogenesis after an overnight fast this gluconeogenic flux does not lead to release of glucose into the blood: glucose 6-phosphate is instead directed into glycogen synthesis. The direction of lactate into glycogen in the liver can be seen as part of an intense drive to store as much as possible of the incoming glucose, even if it supplies some energy to other tissues first.

The rate of glucose release from hepatocytes (i.e. release of glucose from glycogen and from gluconeogenesis) falls dramatically, almost to zero, within 1–2 h after a glucose load or carbohydrate meal. This is, of course, yet another mechanism to reduce the increase in blood glucose concentration that might otherwise occur. At the same time, hepatocytes will take up glucose arriving in the portal vein. Total glucose release into the circulation through the hepatic veins, however, increases because of exogenous (dietary) glucose coming from the small intestine (Figure 5.5).

5.1.2.2   Carbohydrate metabolism in other tissues after breakfast

Other tissues respond to the increase in insulin concentration. In skeletal muscle and adipose tissue, glucose uptake will be stimulated by the rise in insulin through increased activity of the transport protein GLUT4 at the cell membrane, and by increased disposal of glucose within the cell. At the same time, the plasma concentration of non-esterified fatty acids falls because fat mobilization in adipose tissue is suppressed; this will be discussed in more detail later. Therefore, tissues such as skeletal muscle, which can use either fatty acids or glucose as their energy source, switch to utilization of glucose. Not all the glucose taken up by muscle is oxidized under these conditions: insulin also activates muscle glycogen synthase, and glycogen storage will replenish muscle glycogen stores (Figure 5.6). Thus after a carbohydrate-containing meal there is a general switch in metabolism to the use of glucose rather than fatty acids, but there is also a major switch to the storage of glucose

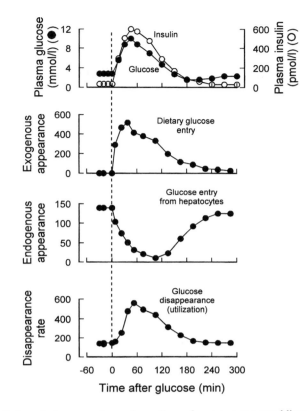

Figure 5.5   Rates of glucose release from liver, from exogenous (dietary) and endogenous (gluconeogenesis + glycogenolysis) sources, in normal subjects before and after drinking 75 g of glucose in water

The rate of glucose disappearance from the circulation (i.e. utilization by all tissues) is also shown. All rates are in mg/min. The measurements were made by radioactive-tracer techniques. Labelled [³H]-glucose was infused into the circulation at a constant rate; the extent to which it was diluted with unlabelled glucose was used to estimate the rate of entry of glucose into the circulation (total glucose appearance). In addition, the glucose drink was labelled with [¹⁴C]-glucose, so that the rate of entry of exogenous glucose into the circulation could be measured. The endogenous glucose production was then calculated by difference. Total glucose entry into the circulation (the sum of exogenous and endogenous appearance) increased after the glucose drink, and hence the blood glucose concentration rose (top panel). Release of endogenous glucose from hepatocytes was markedly suppressed. The rate of disappearance of glucose from the circulation also increased, stimulated by the increased insulin concentration. Based on Féry et al. (1990) with permission from the American Physiological Society.

as glycogen. The pattern of post-prandial glucose metabolism, and some important regulatory points, are illustrated in Figure 5.7.

5.1.2.3   Disposal of glucose after a meal

As we have discussed, the amount of glucose in the meal (typically 80–100 g) would be enough to raise the concentration of glucose in the plasma about eight-fold. In fact, in a normal healthy person, the peak glucose concentration

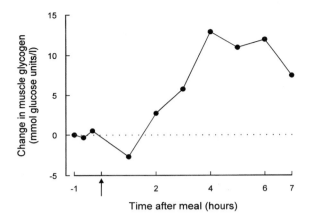

Figure 5.6   Concentrations of muscle glycogen after a single meal in normal subjects, studied using the technique of nuclear magnetic resonance
The meal, shown by the arrow, contained 290 g of carbohydrate and 45 g of fat. Redrawn from Taylor *et al.* (1993) with permission from the American Physiological Society.

after such a breakfast will be about 7–8 mmol/l (Figure 5.4), a rise of only 60% at most from the post-absorptive value of 5 mmol/l. On the other hand, the insulin concentration may have gone from around 60 pmol/l to perhaps

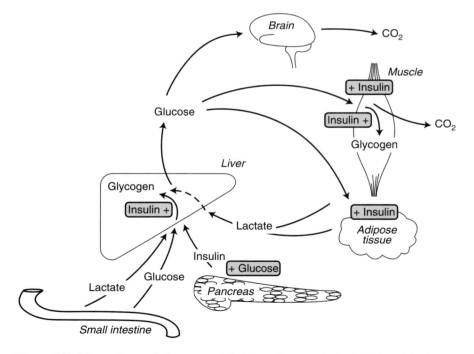

Figure 5.7   The pattern of glucose metabolism after a carbohydrate breakfast
The direct and indirect pathways of glycogen storage are illustrated.

400–500 pmol/l (Figure 5.4), a very much bigger percentage change; this illustrates the relationship between controlling and controlled variables discussed earlier (see Section 5.1). The glucagon concentration in systemic (mixed) blood plasma may not change much, but there will be a change in the insulin/glucagon ratio, possibly greater still in the hepatic portal vein, i.e. in the concentrations of hormones reaching the liver.

By the end of the absorptive period — about 5 h after the meal — approx. 25 g of the 100 g of carbohydrate ingested will have been stored, and 75 g oxidized. Thus although glucose oxidation in tissues was increased after the meal, the drive for glucose storage is such that around one-quarter of the glucose is stored for later use.

What happens towards the end of the absorptive period depends, of course, on what the subject decides to do. It is most likely that another meal will be taken and glucose storage will increase further; however, exercise and other factors (e.g. stress, illness) will influence the disposition of the nutrients. These factors will be considered in later chapters.

5.2   Fat metabolism

Whereas there is one major form of carbohydrate (glucose) circulating in the blood, and its concentration is relatively constant, there are various forms of fat, and their concentrations may vary considerably throughout a normal day. In this section we will consider mainly the regulation of non-esterified fatty acid metabolism in the whole body, along with the fate of fat we eat in the form of triacylglycerol. The transport of triacylglycerol in the blood is closely linked with that of cholesterol, and these aspects will be considered again in more detail in Chapter 8.

Both triacylglycerol and non-esterified fatty acids are always present in the plasma and, like glucose, they are constantly being used and replaced. Non-esterified fatty acids turn over very rapidly; if an injection of a radioactively labelled fatty acid is given, the radioactivity disappears from the blood with a half-life of a few minutes. Triacylglycerol is present in various forms. The form in which it enters the blood after a meal — chylomicron-triacylglycerol — also has a high rate of turnover, with a half-life of 5–10 min. Other forms of triacylglycerol in plasma have half-lives of several hours or days.

5.2.1   Plasma non-esterified fatty acids

Non-esterified fatty acids enter the plasma only from adipose tissue; the process of fat mobilization is catalysed by the enzyme hormone-sensitive lipase (Section 3.6.2.2). Thus regulation of this enzyme and of the opposing process, esterification of fatty acids in adipose tissue, has a major effect on the plasma concentration of non-esterified fatty acids. The rate of utilization of non-esterified fatty acids from the plasma does not appear to be regulated

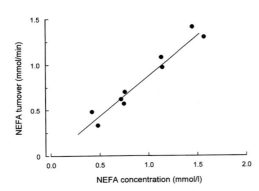

Figure 5.8   Relationship between the concentration and the turnover of non-esterified fatty acids (NEFA) in plasma
Y-axis, rate of turnover of plasma NEFAs measured by infusion of a radioactively labelled fatty acid; X-axis, plasma concentration of NEFAs in normal subjects who had fasted for various periods, from 14 h (left-most points) to 72 h (highest points). Based on Issekutz et al. (1967); reproduced with permission from W.B. Saunders.

directly. It depends almost entirely on the plasma concentration of non-esterified fatty acids: the higher the concentration, the higher the rate of utilization. The relationship is close to proportional over a wide range of concentrations, i.e. utilization of plasma non-esterified fatty acids is a first-order process (Figure 5.8).

Thus the concentration of non-esterified fatty acids in the plasma reflects their rate of release from adipose tissue, and this in turn reflects the regulation of hormone-sensitive lipase and the process of re-esterification (see Section 3.6.2.2).

Non-esterified fatty acids are not water-soluble, and they are carried in plasma bound to the plasma protein albumin (M_r 66 000). The plasma concentration of albumin is ~0.6 mmol/l (~40g of albumin per litre of plasma). Each molecule of albumin has binding sites for about three fatty acid molecules. Multiplying the albumin concentration by the number of binding sites gives the concentration of non-esterified fatty acid that can be comfortably accommodated, approx. 2 mmol/l. (These binding sites are not as specific as, for instance, a hormone receptor binding a hormone. Albumin acts as a carrier for a number of hydrophobic substances, including certain drugs and the amino acid tryptophan. Non-esterified fatty acids, tryptophan and drugs compete for binding, presumably to the same sites.) There is always an equilibrium between fatty acids bound to albumin and a very small concentration (<1 μmol/l) unbound, free in solution. If the plasma concentration of non-esterified fatty acids rises above about 2 mmol/l the concentration of unbound fatty acids rises considerably, and this may have adverse effects, particularly on the heart (see Box 3.4).

The plasma non-esterified fatty acid concentration during a normal day is an inverse reflection of the plasma glucose and insulin concentration: when the body is relatively 'starved', e.g. after overnight fast, the concentrations of glucose and insulin are at their lowest and the concentration of non-esterified fatty acids is at its highest. It can fall dramatically after a carbohydrate meal (Figure 5.9). Situations such as exercise or illness may disturb this relationship; exercise will be considered in Chapter 7.

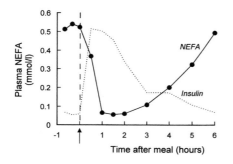

Figure 5.9   Plasma non-esterified fatty acid (NEFA) concentrations after an overnight fast and after a meal
The meal was the same as described in Figure 5.4. The plasma insulin concentration (expressed in nmol/l) is shown as a dotted line. Mean values for eight normal subjects are shown; data taken from Frayn *et al.* (1993).

5.2.2   Plasma triacylglycerol

Triacylglycerol is water-insoluble and is carried in the plasma in specialized particulate structures, the lipoproteins (we have already discussed the largest of these, the chylomicrons, which transport triacylglycerol absorbed from the intestine; see Section 2.3.3). The total concentration of triacylglycerol in plasma varies widely between different people (even apparently quite healthy people), depending greatly upon fitness, body build and genetic influences; but a typical figure after an overnight fast is around 1 mmol/l. It should be borne in mind that, since each triacylglycerol molecule contains three fatty acids, this is equivalent in terms of energy delivery to a concentration of 3 mmol/l of non-esterified fatty acids. For now, we shall just consider the triacylglycerol in chylomicron particles. The concentration of chylomicron-triacylglycerol also varies widely between people, but it is close to zero in the overnight-fasted state, and rises after meals to (typically) 0.4–0.6 mmol/l. This figure will depend on the amount of fat in the meal.

5.2.3   The post-absorptive state

After an overnight fast, the concentration of non-esterified fatty acids in plasma is around 0.5 mmol/l, and the total triacylglycerol concentration around 1 mmol/l. The chylomicron-triacylglycerol concentration will be close to zero — usually less than 0.05 mmol/l.

Note that the lipid fuels (non-esterified fatty acids and triacylglycerol) circulate, for the most part, in lower concentrations than glucose (whose concentration is around 5 mmol/l in this state). But it is interesting to think in terms of energy yield. Some calculations are given in Box 5.1. They show that lipid fuels are potentially a more important source of energy than might appear from their concentrations, and that non-esterified fatty acids constitute an important energy source in the post-absorptive state.

The turnover of non-esterified fatty acids in the post-absorptive state involves their liberation from adipose tissue and their uptake by a number of tissues, predominantly skeletal muscle and liver (Figure 5.10). As we have seen, the rate of liberation from adipose tissue reflects mainly the activity of hormone-sensitive lipase. What is the stimulus for activation of this enzyme, in comparison with the state after the previous evening's supper? Unfortunately

Box 5.1 Glucose and lipids as energy sources

Glucose and lipid fuels in the plasma are compared in terms of their potential yield of energy in the post-absorptive state. First, we will use typical concentrations in the plasma (given in the text) and look at the potential yield of energy per litre of plasma.

Substrate	Typical concentration (mmol/l)	Energy yield on complete oxidation (kJ/g)	Relative molecular mass	Energy concentration in plasma (kJ/l)
Glucose	5	17	180	14
NEFA	0.5	38	280	5
TAG	1	40	850	34

Abbreviations used: NEFA, non-esterified fatty acid; TAG, triacylglycerol.

Lipid fuels carry more energy than might appear from their molar concentrations; this is partly because they consist of bigger molecules than glucose, and partly because, per gram, they yield more energy on oxidation.

Even this is still not a fair comparison, however, because the bulk of triacylglycerol turns over relatively slowly in plasma, whereas plasma non-esterified fatty acids turn over very rapidly. Because triacylglycerol is so heterogeneous in plasma, we shall just compare glucose and non-esterified fatty acids in terms of 'energy turnover', or transport of energy into tissues, in the post-absorptive state.

	Glucose	Non-esterified fatty acids
Rate of turnover (μmol/kg of body weight per min)	10	6
Rate of turnover (mg/kg of body weight per min)	2	1.7
Turnover in mg/min for a 65 kg person	130	112
Energy yield* (kJ/g)	17	38
Energy value of turnover (kJ/min)	2.2	4.3
Energy value of turnover per day (kJ)	3200	6100
Percentage contribution to total energy accounted for	34%	66%

* These figures assume complete oxidation whereas, as discussed in the text, this is not completely true for either glucose or non-esterified fatty acids.

Glucose turnover delivers about one-third, and non-esterified fatty acid turnover about two-thirds, of the energy delivery to tissues calculated in this way. Even this over-emphasizes the contribution of glucose, since a proportion of that glucose (perhaps 20–30%) will not be completely oxidized, but will be returned as lactate. Thus we see that non-esterified fatty acids contribute an important energy source in the post-absorptive state.

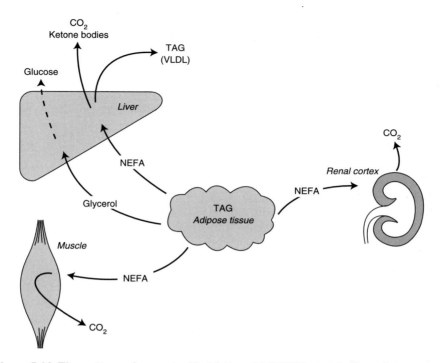

Figure 5.10 The pattern of non-esterified fatty acid (NEFA) metabolism after an overnight fast
Fatty acids are released by the action of hormone-sensitive lipase on the triacylglycerol stores in adipose tissue. Abbreviations used: TAG, triacylglycerol; VLDL, very-low-density lipoprotein.

the answer is not entirely clear, but a major factor is undoubtedly the fall in insulin concentration; since insulin suppresses the activity of hormone-sensitive lipase (see Figure 3.12), a fall in insulin concentration will in itself lead to activation. In addition, it is probable that the enzyme is activated by the influence of adrenaline in the plasma and noradrenaline released from sympathetic nerve terminals within adipose tissue. This is an area of current research activity.

The rate of non-esterified fatty acid release from adipose tissue is also regulated by the process of fatty acid re-esterification within the tissue (see Figure 3.12). However, the process of re-esterification requires glycerol 3-phosphate produced from glycolysis, and this will be occurring at a relatively low rate, so most of the fatty acids will escape from the adipocyte. The best estimates available suggest that around 10% of the fatty acids released by hormone-sensitive lipase action are retained by re-esterification in the overnight-fasted state. This figure falls to near zero if the fast extends another few hours.

No discussion of fat metabolism is complete without some mention of the ketone bodies. These metabolites are produced during the hepatic oxidation of fatty acids (see Figure 3.3) and released into the blood. Their production is favoured in states of relatively low insulin/glucagon. After an overnight fast their concentration in blood is low — usually less than 0.2 mmol/l for 3-hydroxybutyrate and acetoacetate combined; however, their turnover is rapid, typically 0.25–0.30 mmol/min per person. In 'energy' terms, oxidation of these ketone bodies would contribute around 750–800 kJ/day (if this rate of ketone body turnover were continued throughout 24 h) or perhaps 8% of total resting energy expenditure. This contribution increases markedly during more prolonged starvation.

5.2.4   Breakfast

The effects of a meal on non-esterified fatty acid and triacylglycerol metabolism may be quite different. Initially it will be simplest, as before, to consider a mainly carbohydrate breakfast and its effects on non-esterified fatty acid metabolism. Then we shall see how a fatty meal, e.g. fried bacon and eggs, affects the responses.

5.2.4.1   Non-esterified fatty acid metabolism after breakfast

As the meal is absorbed, the rising glucose concentration stimulates insulin secretion and the plasma insulin concentration rises. This has a direct suppressive effect on hormone-sensitive lipase. The dose-response curve for this process is such that relatively low concentrations of insulin almost maximally suppress hormone-sensitive lipase: half-maximal suppression is seen at an insulin concentration around 120 pmol/l, and at the peak concentration of insulin (say 400–500 pmol/l) after a typical carbohydrate breakfast hormone-sensitive lipase will be maximally suppressed. Its activity does not appear to be completely suppressed whatever the insulin concentration, so some hydrolysis of stored triacylglycerol proceeds within adipose tissue. However, the rising glucose and insulin concentrations will also increase adipose tissue glucose uptake and glycolysis, and therefore production of glycerol 3-phosphate and re-esterification of fatty acids within the tissue (see Figure 3.12). Thus release of non-esterified fatty acids from adipose tissue will be almost completely suppressed after a meal and the plasma non-esterified fatty acid concentration will fall markedly, from its post-absorptive level of ~0.5 mmol/l to less than 0.1 mmol/l (Figure 5.9). Notice that the variations in plasma non-esterified fatty acid concentration are much greater than those in plasma glucose; the organism appears to have no need to regulate the plasma non-esterified fatty acid concentration more precisely, other than to avoid the hazards of particularly elevated concentrations.

   The fall in plasma non-esterified fatty acid concentration affects the metabolism of tissues which use fatty acids as an oxidative fuel after the overnight fast. Skeletal muscle is a good example. As discussed earlier, the rate of uptake of non-esterified fatty acids by muscle is a function primarily of fatty acid delivery, i.e. plasma concentration and blood flow. On the other hand, when glucose becomes available in the plasma after a meal, its utilization is stimulated by the rise in insulin concentration. The muscle has no direct way of turning off fatty acid utilization, but the coordinated control of metabolism in the whole body leads instead to its supply being cut off.

Along with the reduction in plasma non-esterified fatty acid concentration there is a switch in liver metabolism, also brought about by the increased insulin/glucagon ratio, leading to a reduction in the rate of ketone body formation and release. The blood ketone body concentration will therefore fall, typically from about 0.1–0.2 mmol/l after overnight fast to almost undetectable low levels — perhaps around 0.02 mmol/l. Their importance as a fuel decreases in proportion, so that ketone bodies are quite unimportant in the fed state.

As the absorptive phase declines, after about 3–5 h, so insulin concentrations begin to decline and the restraint of fat mobilization is relaxed; plasma non-esterified fatty acid concentrations rise again (Figure 5.9).

5.2.4.2 Triacylglycerol

If the meal contains a significant amount of fat it will produce additional responses. However, the processing of dietary fat does not affect the co-ordinated responses of glucose and non-esterified fatty acids already described.

Consider a meal which contains both carbohydrate and fat — say around 30 g of fat and 50 g of carbohydrate — for example, a cheese sandwich. The plasma glucose and insulin concentrations will rise as described before, and the release of non-esterified fatty acids from adipose tissue will be suppressed so that their concentration in plasma falls. Dietary fat is almost entirely in the form of triacylglycerol (usually more than 95% triacylglycerol). This is absorbed in the small intestine and processed in the intestinal cells to produce chylomicron particles, which are liberated into the bloodstream through the lymphatic system. This process is much slower than the absorption of glucose or amino acids, so that the peak in plasma triacylglycerol concentration after a fatty meal does not occur until 3–5 h after the meal.

A typical post-absorptive plasma triacylglycerol concentration of 1.0 mmol/l might rise to 1.5 mmol/l, or perhaps 2.0 mmol/l after a particularly fatty meal (Figure 5.11). The total amount of triacylglycerol (M_r 900) in the plasma (volume ~3 litres) at a concentration of 1 mmol/l, is about $3 \times 900 = 2700$ mg or 2.7 g. Thus, again, the amount eaten (typically 30–40 g in a meal) is sufficient to raise the plasma triacylglycerol concentration many times; however, the rise is minimized by coordinated regulation of the mechanisms for its disposal.

The proportional rise in plasma triacylglycerol concentration after a meal is also lessened by the fact that only a small proportion of the plasma triacylglycerol represents that in chylomicrons. The plasma chylomicron-triacylglycerol concentration will rise from near zero to perhaps 0.3–0.4 mmol/l after a very fatty meal, a big percentage change (Figure 5.11). The rise in total plasma triacylglycerol is usually greater than the rise in chylomicron-triacylglycerol

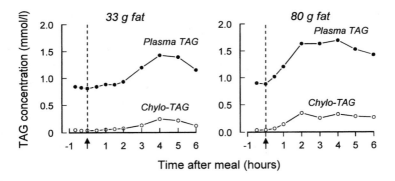

Figure 5.11 Concentrations of triacylglycerol (TAG) in whole plasma and in chylomicrons after overnight fast and after meals in groups of normal subjects
●, whole plasma; ○, chylomicrons. Meals (shown by arrows) contained either 33 g of fat (a typical mixed meal) or 80 g of fat (a high-fat meal). Data from Griffiths *et al.* (1994) and Coppack *et al.* (1990).

concentration, because there is also an increase in the concentration of other lipoproteins containing triacylglycerol, but still the proportional increase is smaller than might be expected.

The route of absorption of dietary fat means that, alone among nutrients, it escapes the liver on its entry into the circulation. In fact, most of the triacylglycerol is removed from chylomicrons in tissues outside the liver, particularly adipose tissue and, to a lesser extent, skeletal muscle and heart. Adipose tissue contains the enzyme lipoprotein lipase in its capillaries, and this is the enzyme responsible for hydrolysis of the chylomicron-triacylglycerol (see Figure 3.10). The activity of lipoprotein lipase is stimulated by insulin (see Figure 3.9), so that it will be increased after the meal. Insulin stimulation of lipoprotein lipase in adipose tissue is a complex process involving both increased gene transcription and increased export of an active form of the enzyme from adipocytes to endothelial cells. Lipoprotein lipase activity in adipose tissue does not reach its peak until after around 3–4 h of insulin stimulation. It is surely no coincidence that this leads to peak lipoprotein lipase activity which corresponds with the entry of chylomicron-triacylglycerol into the plasma; this represents another facet of the remarkable way in which insulin coordinates metabolism of different fuels in different tissues after a meal.

Lipoprotein lipase in adipose tissue hydrolyses the chylomicron-triacylglycerol, leading to the liberation of fatty acids which, for the most part, enter the adipocytes and are esterified to form new triacylglycerol for storage. This process is facilitated by the fact that hormone-sensitive lipase activity is suppressed after the meal, and fatty acid esterification increased by the increased insulin and glucose concentrations (and thus increased glycolytic flux and glycerol 3-phosphate production). The concentration gradient of fatty acids will, therefore, be in favour of their storage rather than diffusion out of the tissue. In this way, the metabolism of triacylglycerol is influenced by the metabolism of glucose and non-esterified fatty acids.

Adipose tissue is not the only tissue that expresses lipoprotein lipase. In skeletal muscle, the enzyme is regulated in different ways. Insulin has a suppressive effect on muscle lipoprotein lipase, although this is fairly weak; it is also, like the stimulation of lipoprotein lipase in adipose tissue, rather slow, taking a matter of hours. Muscle lipoprotein lipase activity is probably influenced mostly by the fitness of the muscle for aerobic exercise. It is present at higher activity in red (oxidative) than white (glycolytic) fibres (see Table 3.1), and its activity is increased by training. These features lead us to believe that the role of muscle lipoprotein lipase is not so much storage of fat, as utilization of fat for energy production. The amount of chylomicron-triacylglycerol removed in skeletal muscle is not known definitely; it is likely to be rather less than the amount removed by adipose tissue in most people, but this might be very different in a fit, muscular person with less adipose tissue than average. The cellular organization is the same as in adipose tissue: the enzyme is present not in the muscle cells themselves, but attached to the endothelial cells lining the capillaries. It hydrolyses circulating lipoprotein-triacylglycerol (mainly chylomicron-triacylglycerol for the present discussion), to liberate fatty acids which reach the muscle cells along some sort of structured diffusion pathway. Muscle is not a tissue in which triacylglycerol is stored for the rest of the body (although muscle cells do contain intracellular triacylglycerol stores)

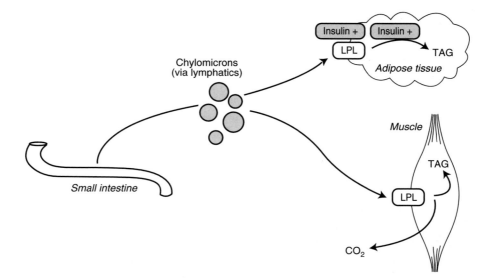

Figure 5.12 The pattern of plasma triacylglycerol metabolism after a breakfast containing both fat and carbohydrate
Triacylglycerol (TAG) enters the circulation in the form of chylomicron particles and is hydrolysed by the enzyme lipoprotein lipase (LPL) in the capillaries of tissues (see Figure 3.12 for more details of this process).

and most fatty acids entering muscle cells are oxidized. However, there is evidence from experiments with chylomicrons containing radioactively labelled fatty acids that chylomicron-triacylglycerol fatty acids which are taken up by muscle are largely esterified. Presumably this is how the muscle cells replete their own local triacylglycerol store for energy production at a later time. It is only fair to say, however, that we understand very little of the regulation of lipoprotein-triacylglycerol utilization by muscle.

The pattern of triacylglycerol metabolism after a meal containing fat is illustrated in Figure 5.12.

5.3   Amino acid and protein metabolism

5.3.1   General features

The topic of amino acid and protein metabolism is vast; twenty different amino acids can be incorporated into proteins and several others exist in the body, and each has its own pathway for synthesis and degradation (except that the so-called essential amino acids are not synthesized in the human body). Furthermore, the synthesis and degradation of individual proteins (e.g. enzymes under hormonal control) is so specific that it may appear very difficult to make generalizations. The emphasis here will be on aspects that relate to energy metabolism, and aspects of the regulation of protein turnover at a whole-body and tissue level where general control by hormones can be distinguished.

Amino acids can be oxidized just as can glucose and fatty acids. In fact, very little amino acid is lost from the body intact — we shed some in skin cells and lose a tiny amount of free amino acid and some protein in the urine. Therefore, most of the amino acids we ingest are ultimately oxidized. At a whole-body level, the total oxidation of amino acids (per day) roughly balances the daily intake of protein, around 70–100 g in the typical Western diet. Amino acid oxidation contributes around 10–20% of the total oxidative metabolism of the body under normal conditions.[1]

The total content of amino acids in the body (stored as constituents of proteins) could, therefore, represent a large store of energy. One important difference between amino acids and carbohydrates and fatty acids, however, is that (in mammals) amino acids are not stored simply for energy production: all proteins have some biological function other than storage. For this reason, body protein is largely preserved during normal conditions; the amount does

[1]*The term 'amino acid oxidation' can cause difficulties. In the liver, for example, much of the carbon from amino acid degradation ends up in glucose. The glucose may be oxidized in the liver or in other tissues. The overall effect is that of amino acid oxidation — but wherever that term is used in connection with a particular tissue, it should strictly be read as 'partial amino acid oxidation'.*

not fluctuate like the glycogen store, for instance. However, unlike fatty acids, amino acids can be converted into glucose. This gives the body protein a special role during starvation when the body must maintain the availability of circulating glucose despite the absence of an external carbohydrate supply. (The utilization of protein in starvation will be considered further in Chapter 7.)

Protein is a constituent of all tissues, but some tissues play more important roles than others in amino acid metabolism. Skeletal muscle, in particular, is important mainly because of its bulk — about 40% of body weight. The liver is important for a number of reasons: it is the first organ through which amino acids pass after absorption from the intestine; some important links between amino acid and carbohydrate metabolism occur there; and it is the organ where urea synthesis takes place.

Both protein and the pools of individual amino acids turn over in a constant cycle of breakdown, or utilization, and replenishment. The rate of protein turnover varies from tissue to tissue. It is normally measured in terms of percentage replacement per day. Estimations are made by studying the incorporation of isotopically labelled amino acids into protein. Usually the turnover of mixed proteins is measured. More specific measurements of the turnover of individual proteins can be made (e.g. by isolating them with immunological techniques after incorporation of an isotopically labelled amino acid), and of course the turnover of some individual proteins is controlled on a very specific basis. We can generalize, however, about rates of protein turnover in different tissues (Table 5.1). The percentage replacement rates are very high in liver and the intestine, but muscle makes the greatest contribution to whole-body protein turnover because of its large protein mass.

Table 5.1 Protein turnover in the whole body and in various tissues

Organ	Replacement per day (%)	Total protein synthesis (g/day)	Contribution to whole body protein synthesis (%)
Whole body	18%	4.7	(100)
Skeletal muscle	12%	1.9	41%
Liver	59%*	1.2	25%
	41%†		
Small intestine	82%	1.1	23%
Large intestine	41%	0.13	3%
Kidneys	32%	0.04	2%
Heart	12%	0.02	0.4%

*Includes proteins synthesized for export (e.g. albumin); †protein retained in liver.
Data are for adult (8-week-old) rats. Based on Goldspink & Kelly (1984); Lewis, Kelly & Goldspink (1984); and Goldspink, Lewis & Kelly (1984). Data for skeletal muscle are calculated assuming that muscle represents 40% body weight, and 'red' (soleus-type) and 'white' (anterior tibialis-type) fibres represent 50% each of this.

Box 5.2 Free amino acids in skeletal muscle

Amino acids are found free (i.e. not as constituents of proteins) both in plasma and in the intracellular water of tissues. They may be present at considerably higher concentrations inside cells than out, reflecting the presence of active transport mechanisms for their entry into cells. The best data are available for skeletal muscle, since small samples (biopsies) can be taken from human subjects with a special needle with a cutting edge. The biopsy is then frozen rapidly in liquid nitrogen to prevent further metabolism, and the amino acids analysed. A correction is made for the amount of amino acid present in extracellular fluid (using the measurement of Cl^- ions, which are present mainly in the extracellular fluid). Some typical results are given in the table:

Amino acid	Plasma concentration (mmol/l)	Intracellular concentration (mmol/l)	Ratio intracellular/ extracellular concentrations
Glutamine	0.57	19.5	34:1
Glutamic acid	0.06	4.4	73:1
Alanine	0.33	2.3	7:1
Serine	0.12	0.98	7:1
Asparagine	0.05	0.47	10:1

A mass of 1 kg of skeletal muscle contains about 650 g of intracellular water. Skeletal muscle represents about 40% of the body weight. In the whole body, the intracellular pool of free amino acids in muscle will be about 80 g, of which glutamine, glutamic acid and alanine contribute almost 80%. Based on Bergström *et al.* (1974).

Free amino acids, i.e. those not bound in proteins, are found both in tissues and in the blood. They are taken up into tissues by specific carrier mechanisms, and their concentration inside tissues may be many times greater than that in blood, so that the concentration in blood is a poor indicator of the amount of free amino acid in the body (Box 5.2). The body pool of free amino acids, like that of protein, is constantly being utilized and replaced. The amount of free amino acid within the body reflects the balance between a number of processes: input into the pool from the intestine (i.e. amino acids from food), from the breakdown of proteins and by synthesis from other amino acids; and loss by incorporation into protein, oxidation and conversion to other amino acids or other metabolites. There appears to be some general control of the rates of protein synthesis and breakdown in particular tissues, and some regulation of the rates of interconversions of amino acids and conversion to non-amino acid metabolites, but little active regulation of amino acid oxidation. This is because the enzymes for degradation and oxidation of amino acids almost exclusively have high K_m values, and thus, when amino acids are in excess, they will be degraded and oxidized in proportion to their concentration.

Box 5.3 Transamination

The reaction of transamination involves the transfer of an amino group from one amino acid (the donor) to a 2-oxo-acid (the recipient), thus forming a new 2-oxo-acid (from the donor) and a new amino acid (from the recipient). The reactions are usually at near-equilibrium (and thus the direction is governed by the relative concentrations of the reactants). One partner is usually either 2-oxoglutarate/glutamic acid, or oxalo-acetate/aspartic acid.

The reaction is illustrated here for pyruvate and glutamic acid.

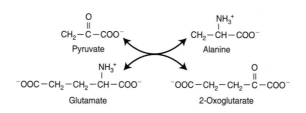

Some amino acids and their 2-oxo-acid derivatives are listed below

Amino acid	2-Oxo-acid	Relevance to energy metabolism
Alanine	Pyruvate	End-product of glycolysis
Glutamate	2-Oxoglutarate	Intermediate in tricarboxylic acid cycle
Aspartate	Oxaloacetate	Intermediate in tricarboxylic acid cycle
Leucine	2-Oxo-3-methylvalerate	May be oxidized in muscle
Isoleucine	2-Oxo-4-methylvalerate	May be oxidized in muscle
Valine	2-Oxo-3-methylbutyrate	May be oxidized in muscle

One reaction that is particularly important in amino acid metabolism is transamination. Pairs of amino acids can be interconverted in what is usually an equilibrium reaction, by transfer of the amino group. An amino acid from which an amino group has been removed is a 2-oxo-acid (often called a keto acid). Each amino acid has a 2-oxo-acid partner. Some examples are alanine and pyruvate, aspartate and oxaloacetate, glutamate and 2-oxoglutarate (Box 5.3). The 2-oxo-acids corresponding to the branched-chain amino acids are less well known, but important nonetheless: they are listed in Box 5.3. Since the 2-oxo-acid partners listed above have obvious roles in other metabolic systems (e.g. pyruvate in glucose metabolism, oxaloacetate and 2-oxoglutarate as inter-mediates of the tricarboxylic acid cycle), it is clear that transamination serves as both a link between amino acid and other aspects of metabolism, and a route for oxidation of amino acids.

5.3.2   Some particular aspects of amino acid metabolism
5.3.2.1   Essential and non-essential amino acids, and other metabolically distinct groups of amino acids

The classification of amino acids into *essential* and *non-essential* was originally based upon the need for them to be supplied in the diet: the non-essential were regarded as those which could be synthesized within the body. A group of *conditionally essential* amino acids was also distinguished. In recent years tracer methodology has led to an improved understanding of the essential nature of amino acids (see Table 5.2).

The 20 amino acids that form proteins occur in reasonably constant proportions in a range of proteins. In some metabolic studies, obvious differences from these proportions are seen and these observations have led to some of our knowledge of amino acid metabolism in individual tissues.

For instance, after eating a meal containing protein, amino acids appear in the portal vein. These broadly reflect the composition of the meal but with some alterations reflecting the metabolic activity of the small intestine. In particular, the proportion of glutamine is reduced, and that of alanine is increased. The amino acids leaving the liver in the hepatic vein after a meal show quite different proportions. They are enriched in the three branched-

---

Table 5.2 Essential and non-essential amino acids

Essential	Non-essential
Arginine (C)	Alanine
Isoleucine	Aspartic acid
Leucine	Asparagine
Valine	Cysteine (C)
Histidine (C)	Glutamic acid
Lysine	Glutamine
Methionine	Glycine (C)
Threonine	Proline (C)
Phenylalanine	Serine (C)
Tryptophan	Tyrosine (C)

Essential amino acids are those which must be supplied in the diet (since they cannot be synthesized within the human body). Non-essential amino acids can be synthesized directly, usually by transamination of a carbon skeleton which is a readily-available metabolic intermediate (e.g. pyruvate, forming alanine). The conditionally essential amino acids (C) may in principle be synthesized from the other essential amino acids; but in nutritional terms, they may be needed in the diet under some circumstances to satisfy requirements. For instance, histidine cannot be synthesized sufficiently rapidly if none is provided in the diet, and arginine is needed by young children. Tyrosine and cysteine can both be synthesized, but from other essential amino acids (phenylalanine and methionine respectively). Thus they become essential if other amino acids are lacking. For a discussion of the classification of amino acids, see Jackson (1989).

chain amino acids: valine, leucine and isoleucine. These three essential amino acids constitute about 20% of dietary protein, but represent about 70% of the amino acids leaving the liver after a meal. The implication is that other amino acids have been preferentially retained in the liver. The branched-chain amino acids are instead preferentially removed by muscle after a meal. Since muscle removes these amino acids preferentially, it cannot require them simply for protein synthesis, or they would not be matched in proportion by other amino acids. In fact, skeletal muscle has the ability to oxidize the branched-chain amino acids.

The pattern of amino acids leaving muscle after an overnight fast also differs from the proportions in protein. There is always a large preponderance of alanine and glutamine (Figure 5.13), much more than would be expected from their occurrence in muscle protein. It is possible to measure the uptake of amino acids across the liver and intestine, and glutamine and alanine are found to contribute the majority of amino acids taken up (Figure 5.13). These observations show us that individual amino acids have specific pathways of metabolism in different tissues, some of which we shall discuss.

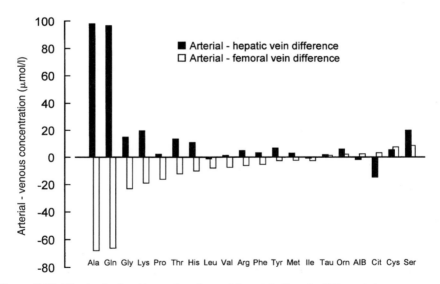

Figure 5.13 The typical pattern of amino acid metabolism in different tissues
The diagram shows the difference in concentration between arterial blood and (1) the blood in a hepatic vein carrying the venous blood from the liver, or (2) a femoral vein, which carries the venous blood mainly from the skeletal muscles of the leg. Solid bars represent the extent to which different amino acids are taken up across the small intestine and liver (the splanchnic bed); open bars show the release of amino acids from muscle into the bloodstream. These observations led to the idea that alanine (Ala) and glutamine (Gln) predominate in transferring both amino groups and carbon atoms from muscle proteolysis, to be taken up by the liver for urea synthesis and gluconeogenesis. The studies were carried out in normal subjects after an overnight fast. Abbreviation: AIB: α-amino-isobutyric acid (a minor amino acid, not incorporated into protein). Based on Felig (1975); reproduced with permission from Annual Reviews Inc.

5.3.2.2 Branched-chain amino acids and muscle amino acid metabolism

The branched-chain amino acids are preferentially taken up by skeletal muscle after a meal. Their uptake is stimulated by insulin. The size of the pool of branched-chain amino acids within muscle reflects the balance between a number of processes: inward transport from plasma and outward release into plasma; utilization for protein synthesis; production from protein breakdown; and loss by transamination and degradation. There is no synthesis from other, essential amino acids.

Muscle possesses a specific branched-chain 2-oxo-acid dehydrogenase, which is a large complex similar in many ways to pyruvate dehydrogenase (EC 1.2.2.2; also a 2-oxo-acid dehydrogenase). Thus branched-chain amino acids in muscle may be transaminated and oxidized, providing a source of energy for the muscle. The amino group is transferred to a 2-oxo-acid. It may then be 'passed around' between recipients, but usually the ultimate acceptor 2-oxo-acid is either pyruvate (forming alanine) or 2-oxoglutarate (forming glutamate). In addition, amino groups may form ammonia (strictly, ammonium ions, NH_4^+) through the action of glutamate dehydrogenase (EC 1.4.1.2) which removes the amino group from glutamate as NH_4^+, producing 2-oxoglutarate again, which may once more participate in transamination reactions. Glutamate and ammonia may also combine to form glutamine through the action of glutamine synthase (EC 6.3.1.2). Thus catabolism of branched-chain and other amino acids leads predominantly to the release of glutamine and alanine (see Figure 5.13). Alanine and glutamine are considered further in the next section. These inter-relationships are shown in Figure 5.14.

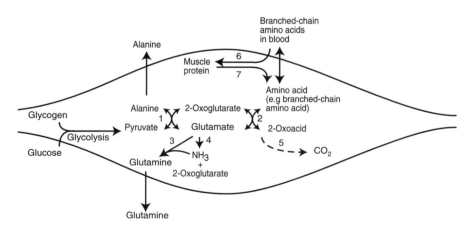

Figure 5.14 Major amino acid interconversions in muscle
Adipose tissue and brain may be similar. 1, alanine aminotransferase (also called glutamate–pyruvate transaminase); 2, leucine, valine or other aminotransferase; 3, glutamine synthase; 4, glutamate dehydrogenase; 5, branched-chain 2-oxo-acid dehydrogenase and further catabolism; 6, muscle protein synthesis; 7, muscle protein breakdown (proteolysis). For simplicity, ionization states are not shown (e.g. NH_3 would be in the form of NH_4^+ at physiological pH).

5.3.2.3 Alanine and glutamine

These amino acids have a special place in a discussion of energy metabolism, as they provide links between amino acid and carbohydrate metabolism.

As discussed above, alanine and glutamine predominate among the amino acids leaving muscle. This is also true of other 'peripheral tissues', including adipose tissue and brain. Since glutamine carries two nitrogen atoms (in its amino group and its amide group), it is usually a larger transporter of nitrogen than is alanine. The preponderance of alanine and glutamine is much greater than would be expected if the amino acids leaving muscle simply reflected the composition of proteins being degraded (Figure 5.13). Therefore, they must be synthesized in the tissues. We will consider their formation a little more deeply. The amino groups for alanine and glutamine, and the amide group of glutamine, may arise from the amino groups of other amino acids as discussed above. What, then, is the origin of their 'carbon skeletons' (i.e. the corresponding 2-oxo-acids)?

For alanine, the corresponding 2-oxo-acid is pyruvate, the end-product of glycolysis. Treatments which increase glycolysis (for instance, in isolated muscle preparations, addition of extra insulin or glucose) usually also increase alanine release. It is possible in principle that the carbon skeletons of some amino acids may form pyruvate, but the evidence that these routes contribute to the carbon skeleton of alanine leaving muscle is not strong, and it is probable that most of the carbon skeleton of the excess alanine leaving peripheral tissues (i.e. in excess of that produced by protein breakdown) arises from glycolysis.

For glutamine, the 2-oxo-acid providing the carbon skeleton is 2-oxo-glutarate, an intermediate in the tricarboxylic acid cycle. It is rather more likely that the carbon skeletons of other amino acids are used for glutamine synthesis, since any amino acid whose breakdown leads to acetyl-CoA may contribute one carbon to 2-oxoglutarate formation (the other being lost as CO_2 in the isocitrate dehydrogenase reaction). However, an intermediate of the tricarboxylic acid cycle like 2-oxoglutarate cannot be tapped off indefinitely without some replenishment of cycle intermediates — or the cycle will stop. It may be that pairs of amino acids contribute to 2-oxoglutarate formation for glutamine synthesis: e.g. catabolism of leucine leads to acetyl-CoA, and catabolism of valine leads to succinyl-CoA, a four-carbon intermediate in the tricarboxylic acid cycle. Thus these two amino acids together may replace the 2-oxoglutarate used in glutamine formation.

Alanine is taken up avidly by the liver, particularly under conditions of active gluconeogenesis when its uptake is stimulated by glucagon. Within the liver, which has very active transaminases, alanine readily passes its amino group to 2-oxoglutarate, leaving its carbon skeleton as pyruvate, a substrate for gluconeogenesis.

Glutamine is not as good a substrate for hepatic uptake, but is removed particularly by the kidney and by the intestinal mucosal cells. In the kidney, the action of glutaminase removes the amide group (forming ammonia) and leaves glutamate; glutamate can be converted to 2-oxoglutarate by the action of glutamine dehydrogenase, again forming ammonia. It is generally believed that this ammonia is a route for urinary excretion of protons (H^+ ions), especially in conditions of excessive acidity in the body; this point is controversial, however, and will not be discussed here. In the intestinal cells, glutamine is an important metabolic fuel. The pathway of metabolism leads to production of alanine, which reaches the liver via the portal vein, for conversion to pyruvate and hence glucose.

Glutamine is also an important fuel for cells capable of undergoing rapid proliferation, such as the cells of the immune system. One reason for this is that it acts as a nitrogen donor in the synthesis of purines and pyrimidines needed for DNA replication and thus cell division.

The major pathways of amino acid flow between tissues discussed in the last two sections are outlined in Figure 5.15.

5.3.3 The overall control of protein synthesis and breakdown

There are some generalizations which can be made about the regulation of protein synthesis and breakdown (summarized in Figure 5.16). Two hormones have a general anabolic role (stimulating net protein synthesis) in the body: insulin and growth hormone. In people with a deficiency of insulin (insulin-

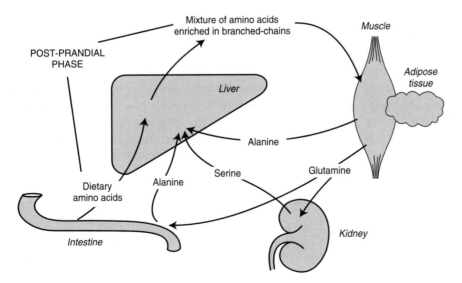

Figure 5.15 Major pathways for amino acid flow between tissues
The pathways are discussed in the text, with the exception of serine release by the kidney. The precursor for this is probably glycine (released from peripheral tissues). In the liver, serine may be converted to D-2-phosphoglycerate (or pyruvate in some species) and thus enter the hepatic pool of gluconeogenic precursors. Based loosely on Felig (1975) and Christensen (1982). For discussion of serine metabolism, see Snell (1986); Snell & Fell (1990).

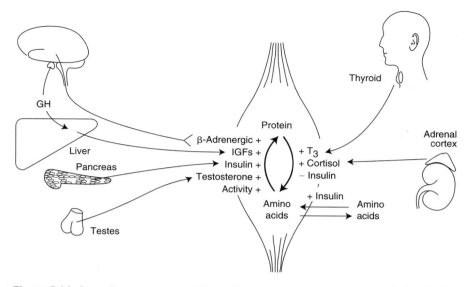

Figure 5.16 Overall control of protein synthesis and breakdown in muscle (and other tissues)
Some of the stimuli here are tissue specific (especially physical activity, testosterone and β-adrenergic stimulation); more details are given in the text. IGFs are the insulin-like growth factors IGF-1 and -2, generated in the liver in response to growth hormone (GH). β-adrenergic represents activation of β-adrenergic receptors, either by noradrenaline released at sympathetic nerve terminals or by adrenaline in the plasma.

dependent diabetes mellitus; see Chapter 9) there is marked loss of protein from the body — the 'melting of flesh into urine'. Treatment with insulin restores body protein. Growth hormone acts through the insulin-like growth factors IGF-1 and IGF-2, and has an important role during development. In the adult this is not of major importance; adults whose pituitaries have been removed do not need growth hormone to be replaced to lead fairly normal lives. However, growth hormone is beneficial in stimulating protein anabolism in patients who have lost protein through severe illness.

The male sex hormone *testosterone* (a steroid hormone produced in the testes) also has a role in promoting protein synthesis, particularly in muscle. This was first realized because of the difference in average muscle strength between men and women. It became clear that this was a function of testosterone. Since that time, synthetic steroids have been developed which have increased *anabolic* tendencies and lesser *androgenic* (masculinizing) tendencies — these are the *anabolic steroids*.

In individual tissues, there are other specific controlling factors. In skeletal muscle the level of activity is an obvious one. The various factors generally work in concert; the combined effects of exercise and anabolic steroids, for instance, are greater than the effect of either alone. Skeletal muscle protein mass is also regulated by adrenergic influences. It has long been known that if a muscle is denervated — has its nerve supply cut — then it wastes away (*atrophies*). It has been assumed that this is because it no longer contracts, and, therefore, there is no 'training stimulus' to growth: so-called *disuse atrophy*. Now it appears that loss of an adrenergic stimulus may also be important. Administration of adrenergic β-stimulating drugs can increase muscle bulk. It is still not clear whether these act through one of the 'classic' β-adrenergic receptors or whether some new type of receptor is involved. One such agent is *clenbuterol*, which has been used in agriculture to increase muscle bulk in cows, and misused in the sports world.

Some endocrine glands are stimulated to growth by their own *tropic* (hormone-releasing) factors. A good example is the stimulation of the thyroid gland by thyroid-stimulating hormone (TSH) from the anterior pituitary. TSH increases thyroid size as well as stimulating thyroid hormone secretion (see Section 4.4). However, this is not of significance for the overall protein metabolism of the body.

The overall rate of protein breakdown to amino acids is also under hormonal control. Insulin may act more by restraining protein breakdown than by stimulating protein synthesis. Since there is continual turnover of protein, the net effect is the same. In addition, two hormones are regarded as having particularly catabolic effects: cortisol and the thyroid hormone tri-iodothyronine (T_3).

The protein catabolic effect of cortisol does not affect all tissues equally. This is clearly seen in *Cushing's syndrome*, the disease caused by overproduction of cortisol from the adrenal cortex.[2] In this condition there is loss of protein from both muscle and bone, and one of the consequences is a liability to bone fractures. The wasting of muscle is, however, somewhat selective and affects the so-called proximal muscles — those nearer the trunk rather than on the lower limbs. It also affects primarily the Type II, fast-twitch muscle fibres.

Loss of body mass including muscle bulk is one of the features of thyroid excess, and it is clear that the thyroid hormones have a net degradative effect on muscle protein. In experimental models, T_3 may also increase the rate of protein synthesis, but less than it increases protein degradation, so the net result is accelerated protein turnover and net loss of protein.

---

[2]*This disease was first described by Harvey Cushing, an American neurosurgeon, in 1932. He linked it to tumours of the pituitary gland. We now understand that these tumours may secrete excessive amounts of corticotropin (ACTH), leading to increased cortisol production. This is true Cushing's disease. Over-activity of the adrenal cortex for any reason produces similar changes, and the term Cushing's syndrome is used to cover the clinical effects without implying a cause.*

5.4   Links between carbohydrate, fat and amino acid metabolism

So far, the topics of carbohydrate, fat and amino acid metabolism have largely been kept separate for clarity. In reality there are many connections between them, as we shall now see.

5.4.1   Carbohydrate and fat metabolism
5.4.1.1 Lipogenesis
Lipogenesis means the synthesis of lipid. More strictly, the term *de novo* lipogenesis means the synthesis of fatty acids and triacylglycerol from substrates other than lipids — particularly glucose, although amino acids which can be converted to acetyl-CoA can in principle also be substrates. The pathway of *de novo* lipogenesis may occur in both liver and adipose tissue. We do not know the relative importance of these tissues in humans; both are thought to play some role, although liver is likely to be more important. The pathway was outlined in Box 3.5 (Section 3.6.2.1). It provides a means by which excess carbohydrate can be laid down for storage as triacylglycerol, since, as we have seen, this is the most energy-dense storage compound.

The regulation of lipogenesis in the liver illustrates some useful points about metabolic regulation and its coordination in the whole body. Fatty acids are synthesized from acetyl-CoA, and the pathway is stimulated by insulin mainly by activation of the rate-controlling enzyme acetyl-CoA carboxylase (EC 6.4.1.2) (see Box 3.5). Acetyl-CoA may be produced from the breakdown of glucose, amino acids or fatty acids. What, then, prevents fat oxidation which produces acetyl-CoA, and lipogenesis which reconverts acetyl-CoA to fatty acids, from occurring simultaneously? The answer is mainly the supply of substrate, regulated by insulin in other tissues. Under conditions when insulin might stimulate lipogenesis, it will also suppress fat mobilization from adipose tissue; thus the supply of fatty acids for oxidation in the liver will be diminished. In addition, an increased concentration of malonyl-CoA will divert those fatty acids reaching the liver into esterification rather than oxidation (via inhibition of carnitine *O*-palmitoyltransferase-1; see Figure 3.3). Thus several different regulatory points act together to direct metabolism in appropriate ways.

The pathway of lipogenesis, although of interest from the point of view of metabolic regulation, is probably not of major importance as a route of fat deposition in humans on a Western type of diet. The evidence for this is reviewed in Box 5.4.

5.4.1.2 Metabolic interactions between fatty acids and glucose: the glucose–fatty acid cycle
The *glucose–fatty acid cycle* refers to important interactions between glucose and fat metabolism (Box 5.5). These interactions occur in adipose tissue and in

---

Box 5.4 The physiological importance of *de novo* lipogenesis in humans on a Western diet

The occurrence of *net* lipogenesis in the body, i.e. a rate of lipogenesis which exceeds the rate of fat oxidation in the body as a whole, can be detected by measuring the consumption of O_2 and production of CO_2 by the body (indirect calorimetry). Net lipogenesis results in a ratio (mol for mol) of CO_2 production to O_2 consumption that is greater than 1.00; this is mainly because pyruvate (C_3) has to be converted to acetyl-CoA (C_2), and for each mole of pyruvate one mole of CO_2 is thus liberated. In contrast, the ratio of CO_2 production to O_2 consumption — called the respiratory quotient — for oxidation of glucose is 1.00, and that for fat is around 0.71.

If normal volunteers are fed a large carbohydrate breakfast (600 g of carbohydrate, 9.6 MJ) and studied over the next 10 h, they continue to oxidize rather than synthesize fat in a net sense (Acheson *et al.*, 1982). If they are fed a very-high-carbohydrate diet for several days beforehand, net lipogenesis will occur for a few hours after a high-carbohydrate meal; it is as though continuing high insulin concentrations have 'primed' the pathway (Acheson *et al.*, 1984).

Another situation in which net lipogenesis is observed is in patients being fed intravenously to help them recover body mass lost during a severe illness. Sometimes these patients are given their energy almost entirely in the form of carbohydrate (glucose in solution), and then over a period of days they begin to show net lipogenesis; the carbohydrate taken in is being laid down as fat for storage (King *et al.*, 1984).

Because these are extreme situations, it seems certain that in normal conditions lipogenesis is not a way in which we lay down fat in a net sense, although the metabolic pathways clearly exist and can be activated under some circumstances. The situation may well be different in people eating more traditional carbohydrate-based diets in developing countries.

---

muscle; the endocrine pancreas is involved via insulin secretion. They were first observed in rat heart muscle, but there is now considerable evidence that they occur in skeletal muscle in humans.

In adipose tissue, we have already seen these mechanisms at work. When the glucose concentration in plasma is high, the plasma insulin concentration responds. Insulin suppresses the release of fatty acids from adipose tissue. Thus a high plasma glucose concentration leads to a low plasma non-esterified fatty acid concentration. In muscle, the rate at which fatty acids are utilized from plasma is dependent almost entirely on the plasma non-esterified fatty acid concentration (and the blood flow) (see Section 3.4.3.2). Thus when additional glucose becomes available in the plasma, e.g. after a meal, the muscle will tend to switch to the use of glucose rather than fatty acids because, first, glucose uptake will be stimulated by insulin, and, secondly, the plasma non-esterified fatty acid concentration will fall and remove that substrate.

On the other hand, between meals (in the post-absorptive phase), the plasma glucose concentration falls a little, insulin secretion decreases and the plasma non-esterified fatty acid concentration rises. In this situation the body's strategy is to 'spare' the use of carbohydrate for tissues such as the brain which cannot use fatty acids. This is achieved by the fact that oxidation of fatty acids in muscle suppresses the uptake and oxidation of glucose. The mechanism for this effect is described in Box 5.5, together with further consequences of the glucose–fatty acid cycle in situations of disturbed metabolism.

The glucose–fatty acid cycle is not a metabolic cycle in the normal sense — it does not involve the interconversion of glucose and fatty acids — but a series of metabolic regulatory events which coordinate glucose and fat metabolism under normal and some abnormal conditions.

5.4.2 Interactions between carbohydrate and amino acid metabolism: the glucose–alanine cycle and gluconeogenesis from amino acids

It has already been mentioned how alanine released from muscle may be 'pyruvate in disguise' — pyruvate onto which has been transferred an amino group from the breakdown of another amino acid. Pyruvate is a potential precursor for gluconeogenesis. Glucose thus formed may be released into the circulation and taken up by muscle, and through glycolysis pyruvate may be formed. This pyruvate may be transaminated, and so on. This has been termed the glucose–alanine cycle. It is very closely related to the glucose–lactate cycle, or Cori cycle, described in the 1920s by Carl and Gertrude Cori (husband and wife, who shared the Nobel Prize for Medicine in 1948). These two cycles are illustrated in Figure 5.17. The glucose–alanine cycle provides a clear link between glucose and amino acid metabolism and attracted a lot of attention when it was first proposed by Philip Felig and colleagues (Felig *et al.*, 1970). But it needs close examination. What does it achieve for the body?

There needs to be a link between amino acid and glucose metabolism. The body's store of carbohydrate is relatively limited and, as has been stressed several times, certain tissues require a supply of glucose. Much of the metabolic regulation we have been considering seems directed at preserving and storing glucose when it is available. But many amino acids can, in principle, be converted to glucose, so that the body's protein reserves — particularly the bulk of skeletal muscle — could maintain glucose production for a considerable time. Thus there needs to be a mechanism for transporting the necessary substrates to the liver (the main site of gluconeogenesis). But the glucose–alanine cycle as just outlined does not do this; it merely recycles pyruvate, derived from glucose. It is a means by which muscle glycogen, which cannot lead directly to glucose release from muscle, may lead to release of glucose into the circulation, i.e. from the liver. It also provides a way for the muscle to export amino-nitrogen, liberated from those amino acids whose 2-oxo-acids it has oxidized, e.g. the branched-chain amino acids. The nitrogen will eventually be excreted as urea, which is synthesized in the liver.

Box 5.5 The glucose–fatty acid cycle

The glucose–fatty acid cycle integrates the utilization of fatty acids and glucose. These interactions between glucose and fatty acid metabolism were first described in 1963 by Philip Randle and colleagues (Randle *et al.*, 1963). Central to this is a mechanism whereby the oxidation of fatty acids in muscle reduces the uptake and oxidation of glucose. The metabolic interactions involved are as follows. A high rate of fatty acid oxidation, and hence acetyl-CoA formation, leads to a high rate of citrate formation (via citrate synthase). In addition, the $NADH/NAD^+$ and ATP/ADP ratios will be increased. The high acetyl-CoA/CoA and $NADH/NAD^+$ ratios inhibit pyruvate dehydrogenase (via phosphorylation by pyruvate dehydrogenase kinase). Thus the oxidation of pyruvate (derived from glycolysis) is suppressed. This is linked with co-ordinated inhibition of glucose uptake and glycolysis. Citrate is an inhibitor of the regulatory glycolytic enzyme phosphofructokinase (it potentiates the inhibition by ATP). Fructose 6-phosphate and correspondingly glucose 6-phosphate build up; glucose 6-phosphate is an allosteric inhibitor of hexokinase. Hence, the pathway of glucose breakdown and oxidation is inhibited. Accumulation of free glucose is assumed to occur within the cell, thus inhibiting the uptake of further glucose. (There is some difficulty here, since free glucose concentrations in muscle are low and difficult to measure, and never seem to approach those in plasma as would be necessary for this story to hold completely. But the evidence for operation of the glucose–fatty acid cycle is so strong that it seems likely that our understanding of free glucose concentrations is at fault rather than the theory.) These interactions are illustrated in the figure.

The glucose–fatty acid cycle may lead to adverse consequences in unusual situations when both non-esterified fatty acids and glucose are elevated. Some such situations will be discussed in later chapters: they include 'stress' and diabetes. This situation can also occur after a particularly large meal of both fat and carbohydrate. The muscle cannot ☞

For the glucose–alanine cycle to function as a means of transporting amino acid carbon to the liver for gluconeogenesis, the carbon skeleton of the alanine also needs to be formed from an amino acid, not from glucose. In fact there is not a lot of evidence that this occurs, although much effort has been devoted to attempting to demonstrate it. Glutamine may be a more likely carrier of such carbon (as discussed earlier, Section 5.3.2.3). Nevertheless, the cycle certainly operates, even if only as an alternative arm of the Cori cycle.

5.5 An integrated view of metabolism: a metabolic diary

The post-absorptive state provides a useful starting point from which to re-examine the patterns of carbohydrate, fat and amino acid metabolism. Some of this will be a recapitulation of the previous sections, but the aim is to show how all facets of energy metabolism interact during two typical days which contrast substrate flow in two extreme lifestyles.

☞ **Box 5.5 (continued)**

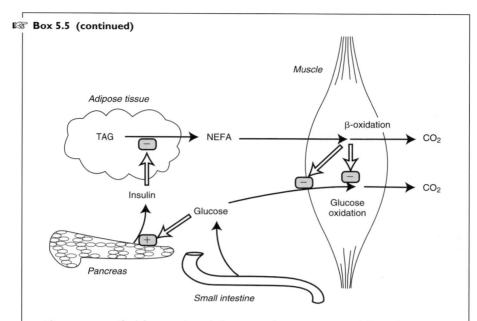

oxidize non-esterified fatty acids and glucose at the rates expected from their concentrations in plasma; there is no mechanism for disposing of excess ATP, and it would clearly be wasteful of energy and of precious carbohydrate. Then the operation of the glucose–fatty acid cycle leads to an impairment of glucose uptake and metabolism, with the net effect that glucose uptake by muscle is reduced compared with that expected at given concentrations of insulin and glucose in the plasma. It appears that insulin does not stimulate glucose uptake as normal, and this is known as *insulin resistance*. Insulin resistance, perhaps better termed 'reduction in sensitivity to insulin', is a common alteration and will be covered in detail later (see Sections 9.2.3 and 10.3.4).

5.5.1   The post-absorptive state: waking up

Plasma concentrations of glucose and insulin are at their lowest in the normal 24 h cycle, and plasma non-esterified fatty acid levels at their highest. Glucose enters the blood from the breakdown of liver glycogen and from hepatic gluconeogenesis. Of this glucose, a large portion is taken up by the brain and completely oxidized; some is taken up by red blood cells and other obligatorily glycolytic tissues, which return the carbon to the liver in the form of lactate to be recycled through gluconeogenesis. Skeletal muscle uses very little glucose, because the glucose and insulin concentrations are low, and also because concentrations of non-esterified fatty acids are high and the glucose–fatty acid cycle operates. There is net breakdown of protein in muscle, mainly because of the low insulin concentration. Some of the amino acids released — especially the branched-chain amino acids — are oxidized in the muscle and their amino groups transferred to pyruvate (resulting from muscle

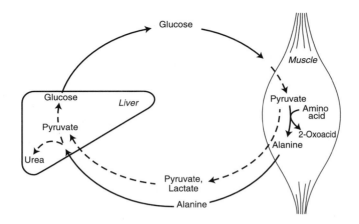

**Figure 5.17 The glucose–alanine cycle operates in parallel with the Cori cycle
(glucose–lactate cycle)**
Muscle is shown, but adipose tissue also participates, and a number of tissues, e.g. red blood
cells, take part in the glucose–lactate cycle.

glycogen breakdown as well as the small amount of glucose uptake) to form
alanine; this is taken up by the liver as a substrate for gluconeogenesis.

Liberation of fatty acids from adipose tissue is high because of the lack of
restraint of hormone-sensitive lipase by insulin. These non-esterified fatty
acids become the preferred fuel for muscle. In the liver, fatty acids are taken up
and the low insulin/glucagon ratio leads them into oxidation rather than esterification. The ATP formed is used to drive gluconeogenesis among other
metabolic processes. Fatty acid oxidation is accompanied, as usual, by ketone
body formation although the blood ketone body concentration is not high
enough to make ketone bodies a major fuel for any tissue. The ketone bodies
are taken up and oxidized by a number of tissues, including muscle, brain and
adipose tissue.

5.5.2   Breakfast goes down

Here we will follow two divergent stories, beginning with a lazy day on
holiday — plenty of food and not much exercise. Breakfast is a substantial
meal with carbohydrate, protein and plenty of fat. The time-course over which
these nutrients are absorbed and enter the circulation differs: glucose and
amino acids enter the portal vein and then the general circulation (via the liver)
within about 15–30 min, although after a good meal the plasma glucose concentration will remain somewhat elevated for another 3–4 h. As the glucose
concentration in the portal vein rises, so glucose uptake into hepatocytes
increases, thus 'damping down' the increase in glucose concentration in the
general circulation. Nevertheless, the pancreas responds rapidly to the
increasing glucose concentration, and plasma insulin concentrations rise in
parallel with those of glucose. Glucagon secretion into the portal vein may also
be somewhat decreased.

Under the influence of the increasing glucose concentration and the insulin/glucagon ratio, hepatic glycogen metabolism switches from breakdown to synthesis. Much of the incoming glucose remains within the liver. The liver also extracts many of the amino acids arriving in the portal vein, although leaving the branched-chain amino acids which enter the general circulation.

The increasing glucose and insulin concentrations act on adipose tissue to reduce the release of non-esterified fatty acids. Because the uptake of non-esterified fatty acids by tissues is driven mostly by the plasma concentration, it decreases as the plasma concentration falls, reaching its lowest at about 1–2 h after a meal.

The declining plasma non-esterified fatty acid concentration removes the drive for muscle to oxidize fatty acids; instead, glucose uptake is stimulated by the increasing glucose and insulin concentrations. Thus skeletal muscle switches to glucose uptake, glycolysis increases, the output of lactate and pyruvate increase, and glucose oxidation increases. Glycogen synthesis is stimulated by insulin. Muscle also takes up amino acids, particularly the branched-chain amino acids, which it may use as an oxidative fuel; however, net protein synthesis is also stimulated in this state.

Increased glucose uptake by a number of tissues leads to increased lactate release into the bloodstream. Hepatic gluconeogenesis is maintained through the increased substrate supply; lactate channelled through gluconeogenesis leads to production of glucose 6-phosphate which is directed into glycogen synthesis rather than glucose release.

Thus the metabolic picture within the first 1–4 h after a meal reflects an intense switch to glucose utilization, and particularly to glucose storage as glycogen. The body's fat stores are conserved by suppression of fatty acid release. The body is in 'storage and conservation mode'.

This is reinforced towards the end of the period by the arrival of chylomicron-triacylglycerol. At the same time, lipoprotein lipase in adipose tissue has been increasing in activity, stimulated by the insulin response. Thus the drive is for esterification and storage of fatty acids as triacylglycerol in adipocytes.

At around 4 h after the meal, intense storage of carbohydrate has been occurring for some time and fat storage is now getting into full swing. But this is a holiday, and we are not going to sit around and let ourselves get back into a post-absorptive state — it's surely time for lunch, or at least coffee and a snack!

5.5.3 Another meal follows

Insulin-stimulated processes become 'primed' by previous insulin stimulation. The probable explanation is that cellular metabolism is influenced by insulin which has left the plasma compartment and found its way to receptors on cell membranes. The effect of a second meal following on the heels of breakfast will be to considerably reinforce the pattern of substrate storage. The events described for the first meal will occur again but are likely to do so to a greater extent: the plasma non-esterified fatty acid concentration will remain suppressed, glycogen synthesis in liver and muscle will continue with little lag, and storage of triacylglycerol in adipose tissue may be almost continuous, one plasma triacylglycerol peak merging into another. It is not difficult to imagine how the body's energy stores will be increased by such events.

Suppose now that the second meal, whether elevenses or an early lunch, is followed not so many hours later by yet more food: there will hardly be a break in the storage of nutrients in the tissues. We can well see that the body's energy stores will end the day in a considerably more replete state than that in which they started.

5.5.4   An energetic day

Now contrast this with a different sort of day: one in which more widely spaced meals are interspersed with some activity, requiring the use of metabolic fuels. The aim is to show how the overall storage of energy is regulated in such a way that the body's immediate needs are met, and any surplus stored; there is integration not just between different modes of substrate storage, but also between substrate storage and utilization. Some specific details of metabolism in exercise have not yet been covered; this will be done in Chapter 7.

First, imagine that the subject for this 'thought experiment' is sufficiently health-conscious to eat a mainly carbohydrate breakfast: cereals and semi-skimmed milk, perhaps, but no bacon and eggs. Such a breakfast is also likely to be lower in energy content than a high-fat breakfast.

The disposition of glucose and amino acids will be much as described earlier, although there may be a sharper peak in glucose (and hence insulin) concentration, depending upon the amount and type of carbohydrate eaten. Release of non-esterified fatty acids from adipose tissue will be suppressed, leading to preservation of the adipose tissue triacylglycerol store.

About an hour after this breakfast, our health-conscious subject sets out for some exercise: nothing strenuous, perhaps a swim or brisk walk for an hour, or even cycling to work. What effects will this have on substrate flow? Clearly the skeletal muscles will require more substrate to produce the energy required. For relatively gentle exercise, the mechanisms involved in supplying this are basically those which have already been presented, but they are accompanied by some physiological changes: increased activity of the sympathetic nervous system increases the heart rate and strength of pumping, and blood flow through the exercising muscles increases, delivering more substrate. This in itself leads the exercising muscle to take up more glucose from the plasma. In addition, depending on how strenuous the exercise is, sympathetic nervous activity and increased adrenaline in plasma may gently switch on fat mobilization in adipose tissue. Thus the rise in plasma glucose concentration following the meal is diminished (or the decline from the peak concentration is accelerated), and the correspondingly lower glucose concentrations are accompanied by lower insulin concentrations and less conservation of fat stores.

Any suppression of glucagon secretion by the high glucose concentration is somewhat relieved, and glucagon concentrations may rise a little, stimulated also by the sympathetic nervous system (this will be discussed in more detail in Chapter 6). The general 'hormonal tone' is changed from one of high insulin/glucagon ratio and intense substrate storage, to one in which substrate storage is lessened and substrate is diverted instead to the working muscle.

It is probably unnecessary to labour the point by following our health-conscious subject much further. A low-fat lunch will be imposed upon a metabolic regulation system much less primed for storage. An afternoon walk will divert yet more substrate into oxidation rather than storage. The net result at the end of the day is that less substrate will have been stored, and more oxidized. This is not in the least bit surprising: the *first law of thermodynamics* (the law of *conservation of energy*) tells us that if more substrate has been oxidized, less can have been stored. But the laws of thermodynamics do not enable us to see how the body achieves this, diverting substrates into different pathways and between tissues to maximize the amount stored when nutrients are available, while making energy available for activity as required.

5.6   Recap: metabolic control in a physiological setting

The term 'somewhat' has been used fairly liberally in Section 5.5. This was deliberate. The hormonal regulation of metabolism is not 'on or off'; it is mostly achieved by subtle, gradual changes. An analogy was used earlier to describe control of the plasma glucose concentration by insulin, likening the glucose concentration to the temperature in a water bath which triggers a thermostat to switch a heater (the insulin concentration) on or off. By now it should be clear that a much better analogy is that of a *proportional control* system. A different kind of thermostat regulates the flow of current through the heater depending on the departure of the water temperature from the desired temperature — the 'set-point'. The more the temperature falls below the set-point, the greater the current through the heater. As the temperature rises to the set point, the current diminishes to just that required to balance heat loss. If the temperature rises above the set-point, the current is further reduced in proportion to the amount of rise. Similarly, insulin and other hormones do not change in an 'all or none' fashion; their concentrations are regulated in a continuous manner to achieve extremely precise control of energy metabolism.

Suggestions for further reading

Glucose, fatty acid and ketone body turnover

Balasse, E.O. & Féry, F. (1989) Ketone body production and disposal: effects of fasting, diabetes, and exercise. *Diabetes Metab. Rev.* **5**, 247–270

Bonadonna, R.C., Groop, L.C., Zych, K., Shank, M. & DeFronzo, R.A. (1990) Dose-dependent effect of insulin on plasma free fatty acid turnover and oxidation in humans. *Am. J. Physiol.* **259**, E736–E750

Sugden, M.C., Holness, M.J. & Palmer, T.N. (1989) Fuel selection and carbon flux during the starved-to-fed transition. *Biochem. J.* **263**, 313–323. (This is a useful review on integrated metabolism, particularly on the regulation of pyruvate dehydrogenase and its role.)

Rizza, R.A., Mandarino, L.J. & Gerich, J.E. (1981) Dose-response characteristics for effects of insulin on production and utilization of glucose in man. *Am. J. Physiol.* **240**, E630–E639

Waldhäusal, W.K. & Bratusch-Marrain, P. (1987) Factors regulating the disposal of an oral glucose load in normal, diabetic, and obese subjects. *Diabetes Metab. Rev.* **3**, 79–109

Protein and amino acid metabolism

Abumrad, N.N., Williams, P., Frexes-Steed, M., *et al.* (1989) Inter-organ metabolism of amino acids *in vivo*. *Diabetes Metab. Rev.* **5**, 213–226

Chang, T.W. & Goldberg, A.L. (1978) The metabolic fates of amino acids and the formation of glutamine in skeletal muscle. *J. Biol. Chem.* **253**, 3685–3695. (This and the reference by Palmer *et al.* (1985) below show some of the evidence which has led to our present understanding of amino acid metabolism, particularly the relationships between muscle and liver.)

Christensen, H.N. (1990) Role of amino acid transport and countertransport in nutrition and metabolism. *Physiol. Rev.* **70**, 43–77

Krebs, H.A. (1972) Some aspects of the regulation of fuel supply in omnivorous animals. *Adv. Enz. Reg.* **10**, 397–420. [This paper by Hans Krebs is old but not out-of-date: it indicates clearly how a physiological problem (why the body tends to oxidize excess dietary protein) can be analysed by the application of biochemical knowledge (mainly the kinetic characteristics of the enzymes involved).]

Lund, P. & Williamson, D.H. (1985) Inter-tissue nitrogen fluxes. *Br. Med Bull.* **41**, 251–256

Palmer, T.N., Caldecomt, M.A., Snell, K. & Sugden, M.C. (1985) Alanine and inter-organ relationships in branched-chain amino and 2-oxo acid metabolism. *Biosci. Rep.* **5**, 1015–1033

Sugden, P.H. & Fuller, S.J. (1991) Regulation of protein turnover in skeletal and cardiac muscle. *Biochem. J.* **273**, 21–37

Glutamine metabolism

Abumrad, N.N., Kim, S. & Moling, P.E. (1995) Regulation of glutamine metabolism: role of hormones and cytokines. *Proc. Nutr. Soc.* **54**, 525–533

Calder, P.C. (1994) Glutamine and the immune system. *Clin. Nutr.* **13**, 2–8

Krebs, H.A. (1980) Glutamine metabolism in the animal body. In *Glutamine: Metabolism, Enzymology, and Regulation* (Mora, J. & Palacios, R., eds), pp. 319–329, Academic Press, New York

Integration of metabolism in the fasting and fed states

Elia, M., Folmer, P., Schlatmann, A., Goren, A. & Austin, S. (1988) Carbohydrate, fat, and protein metabolism in muscle and in the whole body after mixed meal ingestion. *Metabolism* **37**, 542–551

Elia, M., Schlatmann, A., Goren, A. & Austin, S. (1989) Amino acid metabolism in muscle and in the whole body of man before and after ingestion of a single mixed meal. *Am. J. Clin. Nutr.* **49**, 1203–1210

The nervous system and metabolism

6.1 Outline of the nervous system as it relates to metabolism

6.1.1 The nerve cell

Nerve cells, also known as *neurons*, have a number of distinctive properties. They may be very long and thin (spinal cord to toe length, for instance). They are very long-lived (in many cases the lifetime of an individual) but cannot divide by mitosis; hence, if a nerve cell is destroyed, it cannot be replaced by cell division. They have a very high rate of metabolism, and require glucose and oxygen to support this; if deprived of oxygen for more than a few minutes they will die.

All nerve cells have a *cell body*, an enlarged part in which are found the nucleus and all the biosynthetic apparatus of the cell (including rough endoplasmic reticulum), from which extend various projections. The *dendrites* are multiple-branched extensions from the cell body, which are involved in receiving information from the environment and other nerve cells. The *axon* is a long, slender, usually unbranched projection, which extends from the cell body to the point where the nerve cell will exert its effects. At the distal (far) end the axon may branch, extending several 'feet' to the target tissue or organ (Figure 6.1).

At the end of each 'foot' of the axon, contact is made with another neuron or with another type of cell through the structure known as a *synapse*. The synapse is formed by a swelling on the end of the axon facing, across a small space known as the *synaptic cleft*, a specialized receptor area on the cell that will receive the signal. There are two sorts of synapse. *Electrical synapses* occur between two neurons; ion channels effectively connect the cytoplasm of the two cells, and the electrical signal that is transmitted along one continues

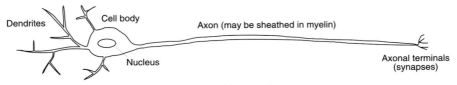

Figure 6.1   Basic structure of a nerve cell (neuron)

almost without interruption along the next. However, more relevant for the regulation of metabolism are the *chemical synapses*. At a chemical synapse, vesicles which contain a *neurotransmitter* are stored within the swelling at the end of the axon. There are a great many neurotransmitters used by different neurons, but of particular relevance are *acetylcholine* and *noradrenaline* (Figure 6.2). When an electrical impulse arrives, the neurotransmitter is released into the synaptic cleft, and acts on receptors on the target cell. The nature of a nerve impulse, and the events occurring at a synapse, are discussed in Box 6.1 and Box 6.2.

There are different forms of synapse, as discussed in Box 6.2. The synapse may be with another neuron. Alternatively, it may be with a muscle cell, in which case it is called a *neuromuscular junction*, or with an endocrine cell, in which case it is sometimes known as a *neuroglandular junction*. The neuro-muscular junction is a specialized structure, activation of which leads to muscle contraction. It will be considered in more detail later (Section 6.2.2.3).

A nerve, in the anatomical sense, is a specialized structure containing a number of axons and associated supporting cells, together with fine blood vessels.

6.1.2   The wiring diagram

There are a great many neurons in the body, which perform a wide variety of functions, although the nervous system as a whole is highly integrated and also interacts with many other body systems. However, the nervous system can be subdivided according to the general function of different groups of neurons.

The term *central nervous system* (CNS) refers to the brain and spinal cord. The *peripheral nervous system* refers to other parts of the nervous system, mainly nerves which run to and from the spinal cord (*spinal nerves*) and to and

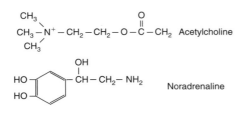

Figure 6.2   The structures of two important neurotransmitters

Acetylcholine is the neurotransmitter in the parasympathetic nervous system, in parts of the sympathetic nervous system and in the somatic nervous system which is responsible for activating muscle contrac-tion. Noradrenaline is the neurotransmitter in the peripheral parts of the sympathetic nervous system. The route of synthesis of noradrenaline was given in Figure 4.9.

from the brain (*cranial nerves*). This is a structural definition. There is also a functional classification, as listed below.

1. The *autonomic (involuntary) nervous system* is a system of nerves which carries impulses from the CNS to other organs and tissues. This part of the nervous system cannot be controlled voluntarily, hence its name. It controls functions such as heart rate, some aspects of digestive function, and some aspects of hormone secretion and of metabolism. The autonomic nervous system can be subdivided.

    *   The *sympathetic nervous system* acts as though 'sympathetic' to the body's needs: it speeds up the heart when we are excited or exercising, for instance.

    *   The *parasympathetic nervous system* appears in many ways to counter the sympathetic system: for instance, it slows the heart.

2. The *somatic (voluntary) nervous system* is the system of nerves which runs from the CNS to the skeletal muscles, causing them to contract. We can activate specific parts of it voluntarily (e.g. lift a hand).

3. The *afferent nervous system* refers to those nerves which conduct signals from tissues and organs back to the CNS. This includes, for instance, pain receptors, chemoreceptors which monitor the pH of the blood, and receptors which monitor the presence of digestion products in the intestinal tract; some examples connected with digestion were discussed in Chapter 2.

4. The *enteric nervous system* regulates gastrointestinal function. This is closely connected with both the sympathetic and the parasympathetic nervous systems, but also functions to some extent autonomously; local 'circuits' enable one part of the intestinal tract to regulate the function of another without the involvement of the CNS. It is highly complex, and will not be considered further here.

6.2   Basic physiology of the nervous system

The operation of the nervous system is highly integrated: there are interconnections between neurons so that one affects the functioning of another (in either an *excitatory* or *inhibitory* way), local 'feedback loops' and other interactions. In a simple way, the brain is the controlling centre and, for the most part, nervous signals travel either towards the brain (*afferent signals*) or away from the brain (*efferent signals*). The brain is the great integrating centre. It receives signals from receptors all over the body: *mechanical* — pressure, stretch etc.; *chemical* — pH, presence of food in the gastrointestinal tract etc.;

Box 6.1 The membrane potential and nerve impulses

An axon is a prolongation of a cell (see Figure 6.1). As in all cells, the cytoplasmic K^+ concentration (about 150 mmol/l) is considerably greater than that outside (in the interstitial fluid and plasma — about 5 mmol/l). The nerve cell membrane is selectively permeable to K^+ ions, which therefore diffuse out down their concentration gradient. But since only K^+ ions can do this, they take with them positive charge — leaving the interior of the cell with a negative charge relative to the outside. This is known as the *resting membrane potential*. It can be measured with a voltmeter in a large nerve, and is about −70 mV. (The negative sign is conventional, implying that the inside is negatively charged with respect to the outside.) Na^+ ions have the opposite distribution: they are present at higher concentration outside (about 150 mmol/l) than inside (about 15 mmol/l). However, the membrane is less permeable to Na^+ ions than to K^+ ions, so the potential difference is maintained. In addition, nerve cell membranes contain the Na^+/K^+-exchanging ATPase (discussed in Section 2.3.1), which pumps out three Na^+ ions in exchange for two K^+ ions from outside (and uses ATP for this). This further maintains the resting energy potential (since there is a net outward movement of positive charge).

The above is true for most cells. However, nerve cells and skeletal muscle cells have the characteristic of *excitable membranes*. They possess proteins in the membrane which are *voltage-gated sodium channels*: they have pores which can be opened to allow Na^+ ions to pass through, but these pores are normally closed by the negative membrane potential. An *action potential* is started by depolarization of the membrane (the negative membrane potential is lost) in a specific area. This allows the opening of voltage-gated sodium channels in adjacent parts of the membrane, so that Na^+ ions can flow in (down their concentration gradient), thus depolarizing yet more of the membrane. Thus this depolarization spreads like a wave (the *nerve impulse*) along the length of the axon. It passes any one point very rapidly: as Na^+ ions flow in and the local membrane potential falls to zero (or becomes positive) the entry of further Na^+ ions is restricted, K^+ ions again leak out and the normal resting membrane potential is re-established after about 2 ms.

'*noxious*' — pain, damage; and *special senses* — vision, hearing, smell etc. It collates and integrates these, and sends out signals via the autonomic and somatic branches of the nervous system to regulate bodily function appropriately. The nature of the afferent (incoming) nervous system is largely outside the scope of this book, although we have met some examples. We begin with a look at the organization of the brain.

6.2.1 The brain

The brain is composed of a great many cell types, organized in a highly structured manner, and it has a relatively high rate of blood, and therefore nutrient, supply (Section 3.3). Of the many cell types found in the brain,

---

Box 6.2 Synaptic transmission

A *synapse* is where an axon makes contact with another cell. When an action potential (see Box 6.1) reaches the *synaptic terminal* (or axonal terminal), it leads to opening of *voltage-gated calcium channels*, which allow extracellular Ca^{2+} ions to enter the cell; these lead (as in other secretory cells) to exocytosis of the secretory vesicles containing the neurotransmitter. Exocytosis involves the granules — each of which is surrounded by a phospholipid membrane — fusing with the synaptic membrane and discharging their contents into the space outside, the *synaptic cleft*.

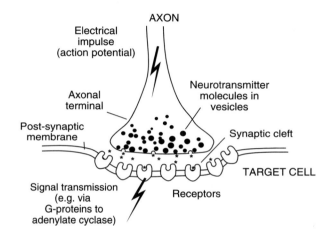

The neurotransmitter molecules can then diffuse across the narrow gap of the synaptic cleft and bind to specific receptors on the target cell membrane. Events then depend upon the nature of the target cell. It may be another neuron, in which case binding of the neurotransmitter will open ion channels and begin the passage of an action potential along the new neuron. If it is a skeletal muscle cell, the result will be increased permeability to Na^+ ions, depolarization spreading across the membrane, and the opening of Ca^{2+} channels which allow Ca^{2+} ions to enter the intracellular space; it is these Ca^{2+} ions which trigger muscle contraction. On the other hand, the target cell may not be another excitable cell. If the neurotransmitter is noradrenaline, the target cell may have β-adrenergic receptors; binding of noradrenaline to these will activate (through the G-protein system) adenylate cyclase and raise the cellular level of cyclic AMP.

---

neurons are outnumbered approximately nine times by other cells, generally referred to as *glial* cells (from the Greek for glue). These glial cells perform many functions of mechanical support and electrical 'insulation', protection against infection and repair of damage. The most abundant type, the *astrocytes* (so-called because of their star shape, with multiple radiating projections), probably act as intermediaries between the capillaries and the neurons, thus regulating the supply of nutrients and also the extracellular ionic environment.

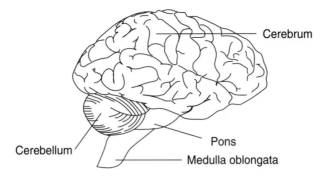

Figure 6.3   The human brain and its main components

The brain contains both complete neurons and the cell bodies of neurons which extend into the spinal cord and beyond. It is organized into a number of relatively discrete structural parts (Figure 6.3). The two *cerebral hemispheres* are the most prominent parts. They are actually roughly quarter spheres, together making up about one hemisphere, but the terminology is unlikely to change. The outer layer, which is a few millimetres thick, contains many cell bodies and is referred to (from its appearance when fixed with alcohol for microscopy) as *grey matter*; it forms the *cerebral cortex* and is responsible for many higher functions, including receipt of information from the special senses, and motor control (control of muscles). Although only 2–4 mm thick, the cerebral cortex occupies a surprisingly large proportion of brain volume (around 40%) because of the many convolutions of the brain surface — hence it also has a large surface area. Underlying the cortex is the *cerebral white matter* (again from its appearance when fixed with alcohol). The white matter is largely composed of myelinated fibres grouped into large bundles and is responsible for transmission within the brain. Among the white matter are found a number of local regions of grey matter, known as *nuclei*, where there are further groups of cell bodies. These nuclei have names and their functions are becoming clear, but more detailed description is beyond the scope of this book. Within the cerebral hemispheres is the central core of the brain, the *diencephalon*, a structure composed of three parts: the *thalamus*, underneath which is the *hypothalamus* with the *epithalamus* behind.

6.2.1.1   The hypothalamus

The hypothalamus is the region of the brain of most interest with respect to metabolic regulation. It is an integrating centre, and it receives and sends out information. It receives information from other brain areas, but in addition the hypothalamus itself contains important sensors. It monitors the concentration of glucose in the blood, and initiates appropriate responses to maintain this close to a constant level of around 4–5 mmol/l. (This includes both autonomic responses, e.g. initiation of glycogen breakdown in response to a fall in blood glucose concentration, and regulation of dietary intake by control of appetite.) The hypothalamus also senses fluid balance by monitoring the osmolarity of the blood, and initiates appropriate measures to maintain an optimal level (via regulation of thirst and control of water excretion by the kidneys). It has a temperature-sensitive region, which monitors the temperature of blood flowing through it, and responds as necessary to maintain the required body temperature. This includes elevation of the body temperature when appropriate during infection.

The hypothalamus controls drives such as thirst and appetite by signalling to other brain areas. It regulates other bodily functions in two main ways. (i) It is responsible for most of the output of the sympathetic nervous system; signals from the hypothalamus are transmitted via other brain centres to the sympathetic tracts within the spinal cord, and thus to tissues and organs within the body. (ii) It regulates the secretion of hormones by the pituitary gland. (Connections between the hypothalamus and pituitary gland were discussed in Section 4.3.) The term *neuroendocrine system* is often used to describe the combination of nervous and hormonal systems of regulation, and the hypothalamus is at the centre of this combination.

6.2.1.2 The cerebellum and brain stem

Other parts of the brain act as further regulatory centres, and as 'relay stations'. The *cerebellum* has important functions in coordinating movement; disorders of cerebellar function can lead to uncoordinated movements, trembling etc. The *brain stem* is the connection between higher centres of the brain and the spinal cord. In some ways it is analogous to a primitive brain, and regulates very basic functions such as heart rate, breathing and blood pressure in a 'preprogrammed', automatic manner. Thus if the spinal cord is severed from the brain stem, these vital functions cease. On the other hand, if the brain stem remains intact after severe injury to other parts of the brain, the victim can enter a state of primitive existence in which consciousness is absent but life can be maintained so long as food is provided.

6.2.2 The autonomic nervous system
6.2.2.1 The sympathetic nervous system

The nerves of the sympathetic nervous system are carried in the spinal cord in discrete bundles known as the *sympathetic trunks*. There are synapses between neurons arranged 'in series' (one follows another), and the cell bodies of the neurons which eventually emerge from the spine are located in the thoracic and lumbar regions of the spine (the back of the chest and the lower back). Their axons emerge from between vertebrae and reach out towards other parts of the body. At this stage the sympathetic nerves mostly make chemical synapses with other cells, using the neurotransmitter acetylcholine. Only one branch of the sympathetic nervous system reaches its target tissue directly: that controlling the *adrenal medulla* (discussed in Section 4.5.2). Thus the nerves regulating the adrenal medulla liberate acetylcholine to cause it, in turn, to release the hormone *adrenaline* into the blood. However, most branches of the sympathetic nervous system emerge from the spinal cord and then meet groups of cell bodies, located near the spine, called *sympathetic ganglia* (each one is called a *ganglion*). The ganglia are relay stations. The terminals of the sympathetic nerves synapse with new neurons. The fibres that emerge from the spinal cord, the *preganglionic fibres*, liberate acetylcholine, and this excites the new fibres to transmit impulses. However, the neurotransmitter used by these new *postganglionic fibres* is not (for the most part) acetylcholine but noradrenaline. Noradrenaline is usually regarded as the characteristic neurotransmitter of the sympathetic nervous system, although you will see that this applies only to transmission of signals to the target tissues. Noradrenaline can interact with receptors on other tissues, and these receptors are broadly classified as α- or β-adrenergic receptors (see Section 4.5.2).

There are some exceptions to this rule. For instance, the sympathetic nervous system regulates sweat secretion via *cholinergic* fibres (i.e. using acetylcholine as their transmitter). In addition, the sympathetic nervous system has cholinergic fibres that innervate the blood vessels in skeletal muscle to cause relaxation of the vessels. The significance of this will be considered in more detail later (Section 7.4.5). But most aspects of metabolism which it regulates are mediated by *adrenergic* impulses (i.e. liberation of noradrenaline).

6.2.2.2 The parasympathetic nervous system

The parasympathetic nerves do not, for the most part, run in the spinal cord. Those fibres that regulate functions in the head and face — e.g. salivary secretion, contraction of the pupils of the eyes — are cranial nerves. The most important branch of the parasympathetic nervous system from the point of view of metabolic regulation is a large nerve called the *vagus nerve* (from the Latin *vagus* for wandering, since it 'wanders' around the body). The vagus is also a cranial nerve; i.e. it emerges directly from the brain and a branch runs down the neck close to the carotid artery. It divides and its branches run to various organs, particularly the heart and stomach, other parts of the digestive tract and the pancreas. (The importance of parasympathetic regulation of the production of saliva and gastric secretions was discussed in Chapter 2.)

The neurotransmitter of the parasympathetic nervous system is acetylcholine. Thus blockers of cholinergic transmission block its effects. One of the classic blockers is the substance *atropine* found in the deadly nightshade plant, *Atropa belladonna*. We saw in Chapter 2 that the parasympathetic nervous system stimulates the flow of saliva, and one of the effects of low doses of atropine is a dry mouth. The parasympathetic nerves usually contract the muscles that control the size of the pupil of the eye; when this action is inhibited, the pupil dilates and becomes unresponsive to light. Eye-drops containing extracts of deadly nightshade were used by the Greeks and Romans to produce 'beautiful ladies' — hence the name *belladonna* for the plant.

Larger doses of atropine block the normal restraining effect of the parasympathetic system on the heart rate; hence the heart speeds up.

6.2.2.3   The somatic nervous system

The nerves of the somatic nervous system (except those which supply the muscles of the head, neck and face) run down the spinal cord, and emerge again between the vertebrae. They do not form further synapses, but run directly to the muscles that they stimulate. Their neurotransmitter is acetylcholine. The nerve terminals meet the muscle cells at specialized structures known as neuromuscular junctions (Figure 6.4). Here, acetylcholine is released when the nerve is activated. The flattened, branching end of the axon is known as the *end-plate*; it makes contact with a receptive area on the muscle cell membrane (the sarcolemma) called the *sole-plate*. We will look in more detail at the effects of activation of the motor neurons which supply skeletal muscle in Section 7.4.3.

6.2.3   Neurotransmitters and receptors

There are an enormous number of neurotransmitters, including amino acids and derivatives, amines, peptides and acetylcholine. Much of the diversity of transmitters occurs within the CNS, and also within the enteric nervous system. With regard to metabolic regulation, we will consider mainly adrenergic and cholinergic transmission.

6.2.3.1   Adrenergic transmission

The pathway for synthesis of noradrenaline and adrenaline was shown in Figure 4.9; adrenaline is one biosynthetic step beyond noradrenaline. Dopamine is also a neurotransmitter in the CNS. The sympathetic nerve terminals release noradrenaline, although a small amount of dopamine (present in the secretory vesicles) is co-secreted. The adrenal medulla is, in effect, a

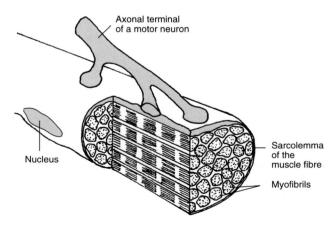

Figure 6.4   The neuromuscular junction

modification of a postganglionic neuron — it is, as we have seen, stimulated by a (cholinergic) preganglionic fibre, and has evolved to secrete the hormone adrenaline into the bloodstream rather than noradrenaline into a synaptic cleft.

Adrenaline and noradrenaline are thus similar in structure, and they act through the same receptors in a molecular sense, but it is probable that some receptors (for instance, those on the receiving side of a synaptic cleft) will only be exposed to noradrenaline, whereas others closer to the circulation will respond to adrenaline carried in the blood. After noradrenaline has been liberated into the synaptic cleft, it is rapidly taken up again, both back into the synaptic terminal (and thus recycled) and into other tissues. However, a proportion escapes re-uptake and enters the extracellular fluid, and thence the plasma. The concentration of noradrenaline in the plasma is, in fact, usually higher than that of adrenaline, although it is only there through this spillover effect. The concentration of noradrenaline in plasma gives an indication of the overall activity of the sympathetic nervous system in the body. (This concept can even be refined. It is possible to show release of noradrenaline from the muscle of the forearm, for instance, by measurement of the concentrations in the artery supplying, and in a vein draining, this muscle. It has been shown that noradrenaline release correlates with the activity of the sympathetic nerves that supply this muscle, measured by micro-electrodes applied to the nerves.)

The two broad subtypes of adrenergic receptors (α and β), and the subdivisions of these receptors, were discussed in connection with adrenaline action in Section 4.5.2 and Table 4.1.

6.2.3.2 Cholinergic transmission

Acetylcholine (see Figure 6.2) is synthesized from acetyl-CoA and choline. After its release from cholinergic nerve endings, acetylcholine is rapidly degraded (into choline and acetate) by the enzyme *acetylcholinesterase* (EC 3.1.1.7), which is present on the postsynaptic membrane. The choline is taken up again by the nerve terminal for synthesis of more acetylcholine. A large group of pesticides, the *organophosphorus esters*, act by binding to the enzyme acetylcholinesterase and thus causing excessive accumulation of acetylcholine. They are, of course, toxic to humans by exactly the same mechanism, and lead to muscle paralysis, and eventually death from respiratory paralysis. The effects can be reversed to some extent with atropine.

Recognition that there are two main types of cholinergic receptor was one of the early triumphs of experimental pharmacology. In 1914, Dale showed that there were some actions of acetylcholine which could be mimicked by administration of *muscarine*, the active component of the poisonous mushroom *Amanita muscaria*; these effects were abolished by small doses of atropine. They correspond roughly to the effects of the parasympathetic nervous system. Other effects of acetylcholine were apparent after blockade with muscarine, and these were similar to the effects of *nicotine* (the active component of tobacco). The effects produced by nicotine include stimulation

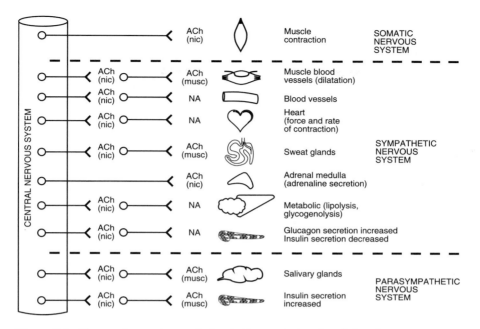

Figure 6.5 **Types of neurotransmission in the central and peripheral nervous systems**
Abbreviations used: ACh, cholinergic transmission; nic, a nicotinic receptor; musc, a muscarinic receptor; NA, noradrenaline. Based loosely on Rang & Dale (1991).

of the contraction of skeletal muscle, and the release of adrenaline from the adrenal medulla. We now recognize that these effects are mediated through two specific types of acetylcholine receptor: the *muscarinic receptor* and the *nicotinic receptor*. Both nicotinic and muscarinic receptors have since been further subdivided on the basis of cloning of homologous receptor proteins. Cholinergic synapses within the central nervous system are nicotinic; outside the central nervous system they are mostly muscarinic at target organs, unless they are preganglionic fibres.

The function of the two types of receptor, together with noradrenaline, in the central and peripheral nervous systems is illustrated in Figure 6.5.

6.3 Major effects of adrenergic stimulation

6.3.1 Stimuli for activation of the sympathetic nervous system and adrenal medulla

The sympathetic nervous system affects many bodily functions. It would clearly be a very inefficient means of control if the whole system had to be activated at once, but this is not so: particular branches of the sympathetic nervous system are activated specifically under different conditions. This could make a complete description of sympathetic activation very complex, but for the most part it is still reasonable to think of the general effects of the whole system. Not only does the whole of the sympathetic nervous system tend to respond as one, but also the secretion of adrenaline from the adrenal medulla (which is, effectively, an extension of the sympathetic nervous system) tends to occur under the same conditions. This makes some generalizations possible.

The activity of the sympathetic nervous system is constantly altering, and is, in fact, changing in specific branches, regulating physiological functions such as heart rate and blood pressure; however, overall (as reflected by the concentration of noradrenaline in the plasma) it is relatively constant during normal daily life. The secretion of adrenaline is similarly relatively constant during everyday life. When a 'stress' hits the system, on the other hand, the adrenal medulla springs into action, and there is a more general activation of the sympathetic nervous system.

The stimuli for activation of the sympathetic nervous system are generally those of 'stress' in the most general sense. This was first described clearly by the American physiologist Walter B. Cannon, whose book, *Bodily Changes in Pain, Hunger, Fear and Rage*, published in 1915 summarized the role of adrenaline and of the sympathetic nervous system in stress states.

For instance, the effects of the sympathetic nervous system on the circulatory system are brought into play by a fall in blood pressure. This may happen quite often. Think for a moment of the hydrostatic pressure of a column of blood about 2 m high. Then contemplate the fact that when you get out of bed and stand up, the pressure of blood available to perfuse your brain is going to drop rapidly and dramatically. This is an immediate stimulus to the sympathetic nervous system to maintain blood pressure, which it does, as we shall see in more detail below, by effects both on the heart and the blood vessels. Most people are familiar with a feeling of faintness on standing up too quickly, particularly on a hot day when blood volume may be depleted by sweating. (It is the author's personal opinion that this is one reason why there is a human tendency to like lying in bed and put off getting up — it is clearly safer for the brain to stay in bed!) The brain receives the information that blood pressure is beginning to fall from receptors in the great vessels, collates this in the hypothalamus and causes the appropriate responses to be set in motion.

Another type of stress is exercise. Even gentle exercise (running for the bus, for instance) requires both circulatory and metabolic adjustments. More substrate needs to be made available for energy production, and blood flow and oxygen delivery need to be increased. The only component over which we have voluntary control is the decision to cause our muscles to contract in a particular way. The necessary adjustments that follow are looked after by the sympathetic nervous system, triggered by changes in the circulation. For example, diversion of the blood to the muscles, brought about by local metabolic changes, will tend to cause a fall in blood pressure — the sympathetic nervous system will counteract this — and an increase in the acidity of the blood, caused by lactic acid production, will trigger an increased depth of breathing via chemoreceptors and activation of the sympathetic nervous system.

A more severe stress, rarely met in everyday life but commonly studied in laboratories (because it is a reproducible test of responses to stress, unlike, for instance, trying to frighten someone), is a rapid lowering of the concentration of glucose in the blood to produce the state of *hypoglycaemia*. Experimentally, this is brought about by injection of insulin. Outside the laboratory it can occur in certain metabolic diseases, in which gluconeogenesis or glycogenolysis are impaired, or in people with diabetes who have injected too much insulin. Glucose receptors in the hypothalamus relay the information that more glucose is needed, and there is activation both of the sympathetic nervous system generally and of adrenaline secretion from the adrenal medulla (Figure 6.6). We will see shortly how these responses act to restore a normal glucose concentration.

Note that I have emphasized a rapid lowering of glucose concentration. The slow, gentle fall which occurs during early starvation (e.g. fasting overnight) is probably not a stimulus for the sympathetic nervous system. The direct role of the sympathetic nervous system and of adrenaline in metabolic regulation is most important in acute stress situations rather than normal everyday fluctuations. On the other hand, the sympathetic nervous system is active continuously, maintaining bodily functions such as blood pressure. These specific actions of the sympathetic nervous system do, of course, also affect metabolism indirectly; if blood flow to the brain is reduced, it cannot metabolize at a normal rate.

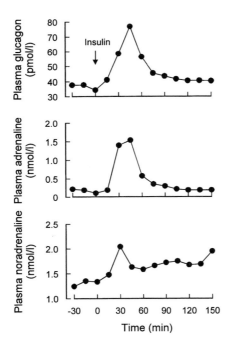

Figure 6.6 Plasma glucagon, adrenaline and noradrenaline concentrations in response to rapid lowering of the blood glucose concentration (by injection of insulin)
Based on Gerich et al. (1979); reproduced with permission from the American Physiological Society.

More dramatic stress states, such as physical injury or severe infection, are very potent stimuli for activation of the sympathetic nervous system and of adrenaline secretion from the adrenal medulla. The stimuli reaching the brain are multiple. The special senses may alert the brain to danger (you may see a bus about to hit you, for example). Loss of blood reduces the circulating blood volume; this is sensed through pressure receptors and is a particularly potent stimulus for adrenaline secretion. Lack of blood volume leads to impaired oxygen delivery and hence anaerobic glycolysis; the resulting acidity in the blood is detected by *chemoreceptors* and relayed to the brain. There are also afferent (incoming) impulses arriving in the nerves responding to pain, tissue damage etc. All these afferent signals are integrated in the hypothalamus, and appropriate activation of the sympathetic nervous system and adrenal medulla is set in motion from there. It is probably in such extreme situations that the sympathetic nervous system and adrenal medulla play their most vital roles.

It should now be appreciated that the sympathetic nervous system can influence metabolism in both direct and indirect ways. The indirect ways include changes in the circulatory system and effects on hormone secretion, which we will consider next.

6.3.2   Circulatory effects of adrenergic activation

Activation of β_1-receptors in the heart increases both the force of contraction and the rate of beating; thus the rate of delivery of blood to the rest of the body (the *cardiac output*) is increased. This is probably an effect of noradrenaline released from sympathetic nerve endings rather than of adrenaline, except at very high adrenaline concentrations (e.g. in severe stress).

In the blood vessels, the resistance of particular blood vessels (the diameter of the lumen) is regulated by smooth muscle in the walls. These smooth muscles are regulated by the sympathetic nervous system. For the most part, this is achieved through α_1- and α_2-receptors which bring about contraction of the muscle and *vasoconstriction* (narrowing of the vessels). This has two effects: in the body as a whole blood pressure will be increased, since the heart is pumping blood through narrower channels; in specific organs and tissues, this is a means of selectively increasing or decreasing blood flow under different conditions. In fact, in most tissues there is continuous *vasomotor tone*; the sympathetic fibres are active continuously, under the influence of the *medulla oblongata* in the brain stem (the very primitive part of the brain). Variations in flow are brought about by relaxation of this tone, or further constriction.

In skeletal muscle, it was mentioned earlier that the smooth muscle of the blood vessels is innervated by cholinergic sympathetic fibres. Activation of these fibres leads to *vasodilatation* (opening up of the vessels with a consequent increase in blood flow).

6.3.3 Metabolic effects of catecholamines

Adrenaline and noradrenaline are, chemically, both amines derived from the catechol nucleus, and the term *catecholamines* is often used to describe them both (see Figure 4.9). The catecholamines have indirect effects on metabolism that are mediated through 'physiological' changes — heart rate, blood flow etc. — and through changes in hormone secretion, as well as direct effects in some tissues.

6.3.3.1 Glycogenolysis

In the liver, the catecholamines stimulate glycogen breakdown (*glycogenolysis*) through β_2 (adenylate cyclase-linked) receptors and the cascade mechanism discussed earlier (see Box 3.2). In addition, they can activate glycogenolysis through a second mechanism, via the α_1 (phospholipase C-linked) receptors. (This was mentioned in Chapter 4. The means by which elevation of intracellular Ca^{2+} concentrations stimulates glycogenolysis will be dealt with later; see Figure 7.7.) The degradation of glycogen, via glucose 1-phosphate, leads to production of glucose which can be released into the bloodstream. This is a major response to hypoglycaemia and leads to rapid restoration of the glucose concentration provided there is adequate glycogen stored in the liver. There is much experimental evidence that the liver is supplied with sympathetic nerves that can activate glycogenolysis directly, although adrenaline from the adrenal medulla is also released under such conditions and will certainly play a role. In humans, it has been very difficult to show directly that the sympathetic nerves are involved, but people whose adrenal glands have been removed can respond fairly normally to glucose deprivation, implying that at least in that situation the sympathetic nerves to the liver can play a role (see Brodows *et al.* 1974, 1975).

In skeletal muscle, the catecholamines are undoubtedly important for stimulation of glycogenolysis; but they are not by themselves sufficient to activate it. The activation of skeletal muscle glycogen breakdown is intimately linked with the stimulation of muscle contraction, which, as we have seen, is brought about by the cholinergic fibres of the somatic nervous system. (The links between contraction and glycogenolysis will be fully discussed in Chapter 7; see Figure 7.7.) Glycogenolysis seems to be 'primed' by catecholamines, perhaps released in response to anticipation of exercise. Circulating adrenaline is likely to be more important in this respect than noradrenaline from sympathetic nerve terminals, since the main (possibly the only) sympathetic supply to muscle is to the smooth muscle of the blood vessels and is responsible for regulation of blood flow.

6.3.3.2 Lipolysis

Human fat cells have both α_2- and β_1-adrenergic receptors. There are also β_3 ('atypical') receptors, although their role is unclear at present.

The α_2-receptors are linked to adenylate cyclase, via inhibitory G_i-proteins, and reduce its activity. The β_1-receptors are linked to the enzyme through G_s-proteins and stimulate its activity. Activation of adenylate cyclase will increase the cellular concentration of cyclic AMP and activate the enzyme hormone-sensitive lipase (see Figure 3.11), bringing about a breakdown of the triacylglycerol stores and the release of non-esterified fatty acids into the plasma.

There is usually a balance between stimulatory and inhibitory effects, and in normal sedentary daily life it is probable that regulation of hormone-sensitive lipase by insulin predominates. However, in response to any kind of stress, including exercise, there is activation of the β_1-receptors so that lipolysis is stimulated. Blockade of the β-receptors with the β-antagonist propranolol reduces, or may completely suppress, the liberation of non-esterified fatty acids into the plasma in response to exercise (Figure 6.7). Activation of hormone-sensitive lipase can be brought about purely by mental stress. Stimulation of lipolysis is an important feature of the response to physical stress such as surgical operations or injury. It is not certain to what extent the direct innervation of adipose tissue is involved, or whether circulating adrenaline plays the major role. But, as with glycogenolysis, people without adrenal glands can raise their plasma non-esterified fatty acid concentration in response to lack of glucose, so the sympathetic nerves must play a role in that situation.

Not only is the rate of lipolysis regulated by the nervous system, but also the rate of blood flow through adipose tissue. This can have indirect effects on the release of non-esterified fatty acids. In very severe stress states, typified by physical injury with major blood loss, α-adrenergic effects predominate in the blood vessels of adipose tissue and cause them to constrict. Presumably the

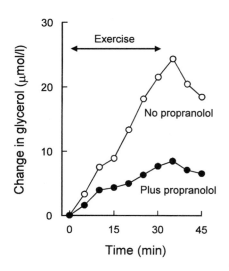

Figure 6.7 Propranolol (a β-adrenergic blocker) inhibits lipolysis in response to exercise
The figure shows changes in the concentration of glycerol (released in fat mobilization) in the interstitial fluid in adipose tissue, measured with a small probe. During exercise (0–30 min) the glycerol concentration rises, indicating lipolysis: when propranolol is introduced (via the probe) the rise is inhibited. In separate experiments, when phentolamine (an α-adrenergic blocker) was introduced, glycerol release was not affected. Based on Arner *et al.* (1990) with permission from The Society for Clinical Investigation and the authors.

body is trying to preserve blood for more vital organs and tissues. This reduces the ability of adipose tissue to liberate fatty acids into the plasma, since the binding sites on the albumin become saturated, and fatty acids may accumulate within the tissue. Thus after moderately severe injuries or during surgical operations the level of non-esterified fatty acids in the plasma is usually very high, but after very severe injuries the level may be relatively normal. Although there is no doubt that lipolysis is activated, the fatty acids are unable to leave the adipose tissue as rapidly as they are released from triacylglycerol (Table 6.1). The same phenomenon may come into play to some extent during strenuous exercise (see Chapter 7).

6.4   Effects of the autonomic nervous system on hormone secretion

The pancreatic islets have both α- and β-adrenergic receptors, and are innervated by sympathetic nerves. They also receive fibres of the parasympathetic nervous system. These nerves regulate the secretion of both insulin and glucagon, as summarized in Table 6.2. These influences on pancreatic hormone secretion probably operate at the level of 'fine tuning' in normal daily life, and it is not easy to demonstrate their role. In rodents, there is undoubtedly a normal adrenergic restraint on insulin secretion, since the plasma insulin concentration rises if the adrenal medullae are removed. In humans, the effects of

Table 6.1 Plasma glycerol and non-esterified fatty acid (NEFA) concentrations after physical injury

Measurement	Non-injured (after overnight fast)	Minor injuries	Moderate injuries	Severe injuries
Plasma NEFA (μmol/l)	400	740	910	680
Plasma glycerol (μmol/l)	50	90	110	140
Plasma adrenaline (nmol/l)	0.4	1.0		13
Plasma noradrenaline (nmol/l)	2.1	3.4		13

Minor injuries included single arm bone fractures; moderate injuries included single leg bone fractures and combined injuries; severe injuries were life-threatening multiple injuries. All injured patients were studied within 12 h of injury; they were in a variety of nutritional states. The plasma glycerol concentration may be taken as an indication of the rate of lipolysis: it increases consistently with increasing severity of injury. The plasma NEFA concentration, on the other hand, is not as high as expected after severe injuries (despite very high catecholamine concentrations) because of constriction of the blood flow through adipose tissue. The same phenomenon occurs during exercise, although not to such a marked extent. (Sources: Frayn, 1982, 1986; Coppack et al., 1990.)

Table 6.2 Adrenergic and parasympathetic effects on hormone secretion from the pancreas

Input	Insulin secretion	Glucagon secretion
α-Adrenergic	Suppresses (dominant effect)	Suppresses
β-Adrenergic	Increases (only seen if α-effects blocked)	Increases
Parasympathetic	Increases	Increases

Sources: Robertson & Porte (1973); Bloom *et al.* (1974); Humphrey *et al.* (1975*a*), (1975*b*); Brunicardi *et al.* (1987).

adrenergic blocking drugs in the whole body are very difficult to interpret because they cause such widespread changes in both circulation and metabolism. The effects of the parasympathetic innervation of the pancreatic islets are undoubtedly important. They mediate the 'cephalic phase' of insulin secretion in response to the sight or smell of food (Section 2.2.1). Also, in patients whose vagus nerve is cut at surgery to reduce gastric acid secretion (a former treatment for gastric ulcers), insulin secretion in response to a glucose drink is impaired, as is glucagon secretion in response to hypoglycaemia.

However, the effects of the nervous system (particularly adrenergic influences) on pancreatic hormone secretion become of great importance in stress situations such as strenuous exercise or physical injury. In these situations, there is β-adrenergically mediated stimulation of glucagon secretion, and α-adrenergic suppression of insulin secretion. These mechanisms reinforce the mobilization of fuel stores (glycogen and triacylglycerol) and, in the case of physical injury, reinforce the resultant *hyperglycaemia* (elevation of the blood glucose concentration). During strenuous exercise, glucose utilization by exercising muscle is increased greatly by insulin-independent mechanisms, so these effects may be seen as a means of maximizing the availability of energy-providing substrates to the muscles without compromising glucose utilization. (Metabolism during exercise will be discussed in Chapter 7.)

6.5   Summary

The nervous system may affect metabolism in three major ways: (i) direct effects on metabolically active tissues (e.g. stimulation of lipolysis), and on the digestive system (e.g. stimulation of salivary flow, gastric acid secretion); (ii) indirect effects mediated through changes in hormone secretion (especially modulation of insulin and glucagon release); and (iii) indirect effects through other bodily systems, particularly the circulatory system (e.g. changes in cardiac output and distribution of blood flow to different organs and tissues).

The indirect effects are operative continuously, thus maintaining normal operation of the body. The importance of the direct effects of the nervous system on metabolism in everyday life is probably a matter of 'fine tuning', but becomes more apparent in acutely stressful situations, such as exercise, mental stress or physical injury. The adrenal medulla works in many ways like an extension of the sympathetic nervous system (which it is, anatomically), and it is often difficult to distinguish effects of noradrenaline released at sympathetic nerve terminals from those of circulating adrenaline.

Suggestions for further reading

Catecholamines and metabolism

Clutter, W.E., Rizza, R.A., Gerich, J.E. & Cryer, P.E. (1988) Regulation of metabolism by sympathochromaffin catecholamines. *Diabetes Metab. Rev.* **4**, 1–15. (Chromaffin granules are secretory granules which contain catecholamines.)

Esler, M., Jennings, G., Lambert, G., Meredith, I., Horne, M. & Eisenhofer, G. (1990) Overflow of catecholamine neurotransmitters to the circulation: source, fate, and functions. *Physiol. Rev.* **70**, 963–985

Exton, J.H. (1985) Mechanisms involved in α-adrenergic phenomena. *Am. J. Physiol.* **248**, E633–E647

Nicoll, R.A., Malenka, R.C. & Kauer, J.A. (1990) Functional comparison of neurotransmitter receptor subtypes in mammalian central nervous system. *Physiol. Rev.* **70**, 513–565

Catecholamines and the endocrine pancreas

Porte, D., Jr & Robertson, R.P. (1973) Control of insulin secretion by catecholamines, stress, and the sympathetic nervous system. *Fed. Proc.* **32**, 1792–1796

Hypoglycaemia and the counter-regulatory response

Amiel, S. (1991) Glucose counter-regulation in health and disease: current concepts in hypoglycaemia recognition and response. *Q. J. Med.* **80**, 707–727

Cryer, P.E. (1993) Glucose counterregulation: prevention and correction of hypoglycemia in humans. *Am. J. Physiol.* **264**, E149–E155

7

Coping with some extreme situations

7.1   Situations in which the body needs to call on its fuel stores

So far, we have looked mainly at how the body stores nutrients when they are in excess, and releases them when required during a normal daily cycle. At the end of each day the body's fuel stores end up in more or less the same state as they started. Much of this regulation is achieved through the levels of substrates in the plasma (e.g. the plasma glucose concentration rising as carbohydrate is absorbed from the intestine), and modulation of the secretion of the pancreatic hormones, insulin and glucagon.

However, there are a number of situations in which the body needs to mobilize stored fuels more rapidly, or to a greater extent. These situations include exercise, when the requirement for energy is suddenly increased, and starvation, when continued existence depends upon the use of stored fuels. This chapter will contrast the means by which fuel mobilization is brought about in these two states. In starvation, the mechanisms seem to be largely extensions of the normal daily pattern, and mediated through gradual changes in plasma substrate and hormone concentrations, whereas in the more sudden situation of exercise, more vigorous changes in metabolic regulation take place, and the role of the nervous system, particularly the sympathetic, comes into prominence. Body fuels are also mobilized rapidly in stress states, such as mental stress (e.g. fear or sitting an examination), and, more extreme, physical injury or severe infection. In these states, the role of the sympathetic nervous system and adrenal medulla may become dominant.

7.2   The body's fuel stores

7.2.1   Carbohydrate

The amount of free glucose in the circulation and extracellular fluid is small (see Section 5.1), about 12 g in all. If we were able to use all of this without replenishing it, it would support the metabolism of the brain for about 2 h. Clearly, this is not adequate even to keep us alive overnight, and hence we have stores of carbohydrate. We looked in Chapter 1 (Section 1.2.2.1) at the osmotic problems that would arise if free glucose were stored in cells, and why we store our carbohydrate in polymeric form as glycogen. Only two tissues, skeletal muscle and liver, have stores of glycogen that are significant in relation to the needs of the whole body, although most tissues have a small store for 'local' use. Approximately 40% of the human body is skeletal muscle — say 25 kg on average. A typical concentration of glycogen in skeletal muscle is around 15 g/kg of wet weight, i.e. each kilogram of muscle in its normal, hydrated state contains ~15 g of glycogen; thus the total muscle glycogen store is ~350–400 g.[1] This is not available directly as glucose to enter the circulation, since muscle lacks glucose-6-phosphatase (EC 3.1.3.9), although it can be exported to the liver as lactate, pyruvate and/or alanine (see Chapter 5; Figure 5.17) for formation of glucose. In contrast, the liver glycogen store is more directly available as glucose, and undoubtedly plays the major role of a 'buffer' for changing hour-to-hour requirements. A typical liver glycogen concentration is ~50–80 g/kg of wet weight, and varies during the day. The liver weighs ~1–1.5 kg, so the total liver glycogen store is ~50–120 g. You will see immediately that this is not far from '24 hours' worth' for the brain. Thus our carbohydrate stores are sufficient to enable us to ride out periods of a day or so without food.

7.2.2   Fat

On the other hand, our fat stores are usually larger by one to two orders of magnitude. This should not surprise us. We saw in Chapter 1 (Section 1.2.2.2) the considerable advantage, in weight terms, of storing excess energy in the form of hydrophobic triacylglycerol molecules, in the lipid droplets of adipocytes. A typical figure for body fat content is about 15–30% of body weight. Thus an average fat store is of the order of 10–20 kg. The energy content of fat is around 37 kJ/g, so we store the equivalent of around 500 MJ in the form of fat. A typical daily energy expenditure (to be discussed further in Chapter 10) is around 10 MJ, so we store sufficient energy for about 50 days of life or more; as we shall see, one of the prominent aspects of the metabolic adaptation to starvation is that daily metabolic rate (energy expenditure) is

---

[1]*This is very variable, and can be expanded considerably under certain conditions, such as high carbohydrate intake after exercise.*

reduced. This accords well with recorded times for survival of starvation victims of up to 60 days for people who were initially normal. A few obese people have starved, voluntarily, for therapeutic reasons for considerably longer periods. (They were closely monitored medically, and given the necessary vitamin and mineral supplements.)

However, storage of most of our energy reserves in the form of fat poses a biochemical problem, since some tissues and organs require glucose and cannot oxidize fatty acids. Fatty acids cannot be converted to glucose in mammals because acetyl-CoA formed from fatty acids is oxidized completely to CO_2 in the tricarboxylic acid cycle and is therefore unable to contribute to the gluconeogenic pathway. Only the glycerol component of triacylglycerol can form glucose, and this is a minor contributor in terms of numbers of carbon atoms. As we shall see, one strategy adopted during starvation is an increased conversion of fatty acids into water-soluble intermediates, the *ketone bodies*, which can be used by tissues which normally require glucose, particularly the brain.

7.2.3 Amino acids

The body contains around 20% by weight of protein — around 10–15 kg. Amino acids can be oxidized to provide energy, or converted to glucose and fatty acids, which can then be oxidized. Amino acids, when completely oxidized in a calorimeter, liberate around 24 kJ/g. This is not a realistic figure for metabolic oxidation, since urea is formed, which itself has a certain energy content; amino acid catabolism to CO_2 and urea liberates about 17 kJ/g. Thus about 200 MJ of biological energy is present in the body in the form of protein; however, we must be careful in interpreting this as an energy store. Animals do not produce any specific protein purely for storage of amino acids; all proteins have some other function — as structural components, enzymes etc. Thus the body's content of protein is only available as an energy store at the expense of loss of some functional protein. In fact, in the metabolic adaptation to starvation, the body protein is conserved so far as is consistent with the body's metabolic requirements; protein is not utilized as an energy reserve in the same way that carbohydrate and fat are.

Of the 10–15 kg of protein in the body, about 5 kg is in skeletal muscle. This appears to be the main source of supply when amino acids are required. There is some loss from other organs and tissues, but presumably they are relatively 'spared' because of their vital functions. It appears that the body can only tolerate a loss of about half of its muscle protein. After this, the respiratory muscles become so weakened that chest infection and pneumonia may set in (probably assisted by impaired immune function as a result of malnutrition) and death follows.

The body's fuel reserves are summarized in Table 7.1.

Table 7.1 The body's fuel stores

Fuel	Amount (typical in 65 kg person)	Energy equivalent	Days supply if the only energy source
Carbohydrate			
Free glucose	12 g	0.2 MJ	0.02 = 30 min
Glycogen	450 g	7.65 MJ	0.77 = 18 h
Fat			
Triacylglycerol	15 kg	550 MJ	55
Protein	12.5 kg*	210 MJ	21

The numbers on this table should be taken as rough estimates only. They are discussed further in the text. Assumptions: energy produced by biological oxidation is 17 kJ/g for carbohydrate and protein, 37 kJ/g for fat; energy expenditure is 10 MJ/day.

*As discussed in the text, not all the body protein can be utilized, so the numbers for protein are notional only.

7.3   Starvation

The response to absolute deprivation of food proceeds in a number of stages, leading ultimately to death; but the manner in which metabolism adapts, to postpone that final end-point as long as possible, illustrates a number of important points about the integration of metabolic regulation in the whole body. Starvation has, undoubtedly, always been a threat to humans and other animals, and the metabolic responses which minimize its impact have evolved throughout the development of all living things. Because this response has evolved so directly to counteract the threat posed by lack of food, it is tempting to look on it as 'purposeful', and indeed it helps considerably in understanding it if we think in terms of the body's 'strategy'. Nevertheless, bear in mind that the use of a term such as strategy does not imply anything other than a response that has evolved because it is beneficial.

There are distinctions between absolute starvation and partial starvation or undernutrition. We will consider absolute starvation, as this provides the clearest illustration of metabolic adaptation. Figure 7.1 shows a scheme for looking at the different phases of total starvation.

7.3.1   The early phase

We have already looked at the pattern of metabolism in very-short-term starvation (Section 5.5.1), namely the *post-absorptive state* after overnight fast. A gentle decrease in the concentration of glucose in the plasma led to a small decrease in the ratio of insulin/glucagon, stimulation of hepatic glycogenolysis and liberation of fatty acids from adipose depots. The availability of fatty acids in the plasma leads tissues such as muscle to use fat — and spare glucose — as their major metabolic fuel.

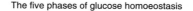

The five phases of glucose homoeostasis

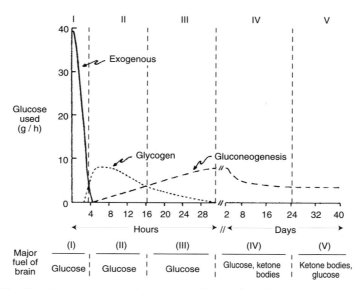

Figure 7.1   The phases of starvation, assessed from the point of view of glucose metabolism
Reproduced from Ruderman (1975) with permission from Annual Reviews Inc.

The post-absorptive state leads into the *gluconeogenic phase*, which lasts until the second or third day of absolute starvation. Liver glycogen stores are virtually depleted within 24 h (Figure 7.2), and, therefore, gluconeogenesis must come into operation to supply the requirements of the brain and other glucose-requiring tissues (e.g. erythrocytes). The main signal for this will again be the change in insulin/glucagon ratio. The concentration of another important hormonal stimulator of gluconeogenesis, cortisol, does not change systematically in starvation. In addition, the supply of substrate for gluconeogenesis will increase over this period, as net proteolysis in muscle — resulting from the falling insulin concentration — leads to release of amino acids, mainly alanine and glutamine; the latter is partially converted to alanine in the intestine (see Section 5.3.2.3), and thus the liver receives an increased supply of this amino acid. Increasing lipolysis in adipose tissue releases glycerol, which is also a substrate for gluconeogenesis.

Gluconeogenesis in this early stage of starvation is, therefore, proceeding largely at the expense of muscle protein, a situation which is clearly not good for survival. Studies of experimental underfeeding of volunteers have shown that muscle function is impaired with surprisingly small degrees of undernutrition. Not all amino acid carbons can be converted into alanine and glutamine, and some are oxidized, representing an irreversible loss from the body's stores. Around 1.75 g of muscle protein must be broken down to provide each gram of glucose, since not all amino acids can be converted to glucose, and, with the

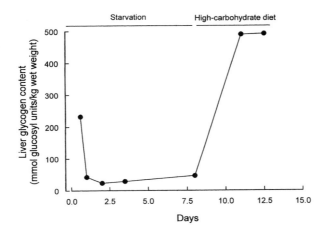

Figure 7.2   Liver glycogen concentrations in normal human volunteers after overnight fast, during 2–10 days total starvation, and after re-feeding with a carbohydrate-rich diet
The 'basal' value already includes the effects of 12–14 h without food; a sample was not taken in the fed state. The samples were obtained with a fine needle inserted through the rib cage. Based on Nilsson & Hultman (1973).

brain requiring around 100–120 g of glucose per day, the rate of muscle protein breakdown could be rapid. If no other adaptations took place, this would require the breakdown of around 150 g of protein per day. (Some glucose is, of course, provided from glycerol.) The body's store of protein in muscle would be rapidly depleted. This is avoided by a series of inter-related adaptations to starvation, which are summarized in Table 7.2.

The sparing of the body's protein stores is brought about gradually. The excretion of nitrogen in the urine, a measure of the irreversible loss of amino acids, decreases steadily from the start of starvation (Figure 7.3). At first sight, this seems to contradict the idea of increased gluconeogenesis from amino acids in the early phase of starvation; however, this is not a fair picture. We should think in terms of *nitrogen balance*. Nitrogen balance is the difference between total nitrogen intake, and total nitrogen loss. Some nitrogen is lost in

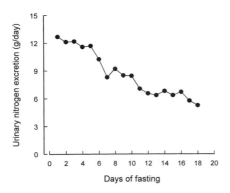

Figure 7.3   Rate of urinary nitrogen excretion in five obese subjects during starvation
Based on Owen *et al.* (1990); reproduced with permission from Baillière Tindall.

Table 7.2 Metabolic adaptations which lead to sparing of muscle protein in starvation

---

1. Ketogenesis increases; brain begins to use significant quantities of ketone bodies. Therefore, the need for glucose production is decreased.
2. Gluconeogenesis is stimulated, so other precursors are used maximally (e.g. lactate recycled).
3. As lipolysis increases, glycerol becomes an increasingly important substrate for gluconeogenesis.
4. Metabolic rate is decreased, thus lessening demand for energy generally.
5. Ketone bodies may exert a restraining influence on muscle protein breakdown (discussed in text).

---

faeces and shed skin cells, but most is lost in the urine in the form of urea and ammonia, and represents the catabolism of amino acids. During normal life, we are approximately in nitrogen balance on a day-to-day basis; the amount of nitrogen we take in is equal to the amount we lose, and the body store of nitrogen (mainly in amino acids and protein) stays roughly constant. At the start of starvation, nitrogen intake falls suddenly to zero, but nitrogen excretion continues at about the same level as before. Suddenly, therefore, there is a net loss of the body's protein stores. Nitrogen excretion then declines steadily, representing the sparing that is necessary for starvation to be prolonged beyond a week or two.

7.3.2   The period of adaptation to starvation

The changes listed in Table 7.2 come into place gradually over the first three weeks or so of total starvation; this is the period of adaptation. Beyond three weeks, the body has adapted as far as it can, and a kind of steady state is reached.

7.3.2.1 Hormonal changes

The onset of starvation is marked by a decrease in the level of the active thyroid hormone tri-iodothyronine (T_3) in the blood (Figure 7.4). It is not clear what causes this, although the mechanism is in part a shift towards production of an inactive form, reverse-T_3 (Figure 7.4). The effect of the fall in T_3 concentration is to reduce overall metabolic rate, and to reduce the rate of proteolysis in muscle. The reduction in overall metabolic rate leads to a decrease in the rate of depletion of the body's fuels stores. However, it is unlikely that the metabolism of the brain, usually the largest glucose consumer, is reduced significantly, so the need for glucose is still present; it is reduced, however, by the mechanisms described below.

Both the sympathetic nervous system and the adrenal medulla play some role during starvation. However, although starvation is a state in which fuel mobilization is required, the adrenergic systems play a much lesser role than in other, more stress-driven states (such as exercise). There is some activation of both sympathetic nervous system and adrenaline secretion during the first week or so of starvation. These changes would normally cause an elevation in overall metabolic rate; this is not seen, since it is outweighed by the reduction in T_3 concentration. On the other hand, the adrenergic systems are probably important in stimulation of lipolysis in adipose tissue. This latter will be reinforced by the continuing reduction in insulin concentration. Therefore, the plasma non-esterified fatty acid concentration rises during the adaptation period (Figure 7.5).

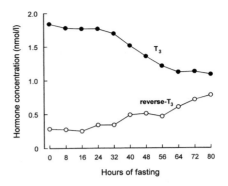

Figure 7.4   Serum concentrations of T_3 and reverse-T_3 during early starvation in normal volunteers
Based on Gardner et al. (1979).

7.3.2.2   Adaptation of fatty acid, ketone body and glucose metabolism

The elevation in plasma non-esterified fatty acid concentration leads to a number of adaptations. Skeletal muscle will use non-esterified fatty acids almost entirely in preference to glucose for its energy production. In the liver, the rate of fatty acid esterification, usually stimulated by insulin, will decrease; fatty acids will be diverted into oxidation (glucagon stimulates this pathway). This diversion is mediated in part by a decrease in hepatic malonyl-CoA concentration, a result of the decrease in insulin concentration (see Figure 3.3). Increased oxidation of fatty acids leads to increased production of the ketone bodies, 3-hydroxybutyrate and acetoacetate (see Figure 3.3). These can be used as an oxidative fuel by many tissues, at a rate which simply depends on their

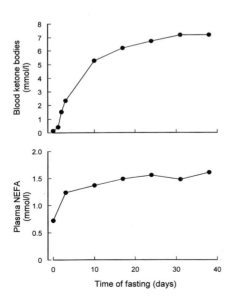

Figure 7.5   Concentrations of non-esterified fatty acids (NEFA) and ketone bodies (the sum of acetoacetate and 3-hydroxybutyrate) in blood in obese subjects during starvation
Based on Owen et al. (1990); reproduced with permission from Baillière Tindall.

concentration in the blood. Most importantly, they can be used by the brain, which begins to use a fuel derived from the fat stores in preference to glucose. By the end of the third week of starvation, blood ketone body concentrations may reach 6–7 mmol/l, compared with <0.2 mmol/l normally (Figure 7.5). At this stage, ketone body oxidation can account for approximately two-thirds of the oxygen consumption of the brain. Thus about 70–80 g of glucose per day is spared oxidation.

The body's need to form new glucose from amino acids is also reduced by the stimulation of gluconeogenesis in the liver, which enables glucose to be efficiently recycled. Glycolytic cells and tissues such as erythrocytes and the renal medulla will still need to use glucose. (They cannot use ketone bodies since they do not have the oxidative capacity.) Glycolysis in these tissues, however, leads to the release of lactate which is returned to the liver and avidly reconverted into glucose. Thus the glucose which must be used by these tissues is recycled. Energy for this process comes from the increased oxidation of fatty acids in the liver, forming the NADH necessary to drive gluconeogenesis (so that, in effect, the glycolytic tissues 'run' on energy derived from the fat stores).

7.3.2.3   Sparing of muscle protein

By these mechanisms, the need to produce glucose from muscle protein is reduced, and the loss of nitrogen in the urine decreases. However, with the insulin concentration decreasing, the net stimulus would seem to be for increasing muscle protein breakdown. How is the sparing of muscle protein brought about?

The possible role of the decreasing T_3 concentration has been mentioned: T_3 usually has the effect of stimulating muscle proteolysis (see Section 5.3.3; Figure 5.16). Another possibility is that the increase in plasma adrenaline concentration may be involved. Adrenergic drugs have an anabolic effect on muscle (see Section 5.3.3), although this effect is not clearly understood and the receptors by which it is mediated have not been delineated.

The other possible mediator is the increase in blood ketone body concentration. Some experimental studies show that this leads to a reduction in the net breakdown of muscle protein. There is a possible mechanism. The branched-chain amino acids are catabolized in muscle by transamination, followed by the action of the branched-chain 2-oxo-acid dehydrogenase complex (see Section 5.3.2.2). This enzyme complex has many similarities with pyruvate dehydrogenase. Like pyruvate dehydrogenase, its activity is inhibited by phosphorylation in response to a high acetyl-CoA/CoASH ratio. In other words, if the muscle is plentifully supplied with other substrates for oxidation (such as fatty acids and ketone bodies, in starvation) then the oxidation of the branched-chain amino acids will be suppressed.

However, the fall in nitrogen loss in starvation may be another facet of the general slowing down of metabolism. In this case no specific mechanism need be postulated. This has been discussed by Henry *et al.* (1988), who argue that conventional understanding of the response to starvation is heavily biased, since it is based largely on obese subjects undergoing starvation for the purpose of weight reduction.

7.3.2.4 Kidney metabolism

During this period of starvation, there are marked changes in the metabolic pattern of the kidney which will be briefly discussed. The concentrations of lipid-derived fuels — non-esterified fatty acids and ketone bodies — are high in the plasma, as shown in Figure 7.5. These are biological acids. Therefore, the production of hydrogen ions increases and the pH of the blood tends to fall. To counter this, the body must excrete excess hydrogen ions. In Section 5.3.2.3 one means for achieving this was mentioned: the kidney can excrete ammonia, which carries with it one hydrogen ion, since it will be in the form of NH_4^+. The ammonia may be derived from the action of glutaminase on glutamine, and glutamate dehydrogenase on glutamate, in the kidney (see Section 5.3.2.3). The renal uptake of glutamine increases in starvation to provide a means for excretion of excess hydrogen ions[2]. Glutamine metabolism in the kidney can lead to glucose production, especially during starvation when the kidney can become an important gluconeogenic tissue. Thus again we see the efficiency of metabolism: a metabolic process (ammonia excretion) necessary to regulate blood pH is coupled with the conversion of a muscle-derived amino acid to glucose.

7.3.3   The period of adapted starvation

From about three weeks of total starvation onwards, the body appears to be fully adapted to starvation and there is a kind of steady state, in which there is gradual depletion of the body's protein mass (minimized by the mechanisms discussed earlier), and steady depletion of the fat stores. Ketone body concentrations in the blood reach about 6–8 mmol/l, and ketone bodies provide about two-thirds of the metabolic requirement of the brain. Other tissues that require glucose (e.g. erythrocytes, renal medulla) produce lactate which is efficiently recycled, using energy derived from fatty acid oxidation. Thus the rate of irreversible loss of glucose is minimized. The major fuel flows in this state are summarized in Figure 7.6.

The pattern of metabolism is governed by the physico-chemical features of fat and carbohydrate outlined in Chapter 1, so that fat — the most energy-dense fuel store — constitutes the major long-term fuel reserve, and metabolism is geared to derive the maximum proportion of energy from fat oxidation. The changes which bring about this metabolic adaptation are

---

[2]*The role of the kidney in maintenance of blood pH has been challenged: for another viewpoint see Atkinson & Bourke (1987).*

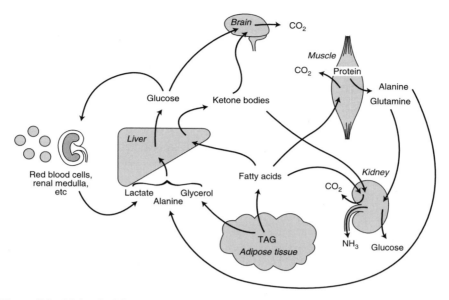

Figure 7.6 Major fuel flows in prolonged starvation
Protein (especially that in muscle) is the only long-term source of glucose (with a contribution from glycerol). The complete oxidation of glucose is reduced by the production of ketone bodies which serve as an alternative fuel, e.g. for the brain. Those tissues which must use glucose (e.g. red blood cells, renal medulla) produce lactate which is recycled in gluconeogenesis. The major source of fuel for oxidation is thus adipose tissue triacylglycerol (TAG), providing fuel in the form of non-esterified fatty acids and (via the liver) ketone bodies.

mediated in a gradual way by changing concentrations of substrates in the blood, and by the almost automatic responses of the endocrine system: insulin secretion decreases as the plasma glucose concentration falls, while glucagon secretion increases. The central nervous system is involved in these responses, with a change in thyroid hormone secretion (via the hypothalamic–pituitary system) and mild activation of the adrenal medulla and sympathetic nervous system. However, the involvement of the central nervous system is very much less than in situations such as exercise and trauma.

The adapted state may come to an end with re-feeding. Otherwise it will continue, usually until weakness of the respiratory muscles leads to inability to clear the lungs properly, and pneumonia sets in and leads to death. There is some evidence that survival is determined by the size of the fat stores: when the fat stores are depleted as far as they can be, there is a sudden additional loss of protein and death follows quickly.

Nevertheless, it is worth pondering the ability of the metabolic pattern to adapt to such an extreme situation. We began our tour of metabolic regulation by looking at the changes that occur during normal daily life, with food coming in regularly three times a day. Most of us in the Western world are not used to missing a meal, let alone a day's food: the fact that the body could survive for around two months without any food intake is a clear illustration of the coordinated regulation of metabolism which not only underpins our daily lives, but also allows us to continue in some very extreme situations.

7.4   Exercise

Total starvation is a very extreme situation in one sense. On the other hand, as stressed in the earlier part of this chapter, it involves a relatively gradual adaptation. The flux through any particular metabolic pathway changes over a period of days or even weeks. Exercise represents another type of extreme situation, but one which demands rapid adaptation. In sprinting, for instance, the net flux through the glycolytic pathway in muscle increases at least 1000-fold between the starting blocks and the track, i.e. probably in less than 1 s. In strenuous endurance exercise, such as cross-country skiing or elite marathon running, the rate of whole-body energy expenditure increases by about 18-fold over the resting level. This involves major changes in the transport of substrates through the blood, which could not be achieved without coordinated physiological changes, in the circulatory and respiratory systems, and metabolic changes.

7.4.1   Types of exercise

It is convenient to think of two extreme types of exercise: *anaerobic* and *aerobic*.

Anaerobic exercise is typified by sprinting or weight-lifting; it is of short duration, but may involve great strength. It is dominated by the activity of the fast-twitch (Type II) muscle fibres.

For those with an understanding of physics, this can be confusing. Work is done when a force acts through a distance. Thus, apart from the initial snatch, it is not obvious that a weight lifter is doing any work in a physical sense when he or she holds a weight aloft for any length of time; and yet we all know that this is tiring. The key to this lies in understanding that muscle contraction is only maintained by continued small contractions of individual muscles fibres; there has to be continued stimulation of the muscle by the somatic nerves and continued ATP production within the muscle to maintain a contraction. A closely related term which may help to understand this is *isometric contraction* (isometric meaning equal length): the muscle maintains a contraction without changing its length. In true isometric exercises the muscles are tensed against a resistance. Again no obvious outside work is done, but it certainly requires energy! The key feature of anaerobic exercise is rapid generation of energy over a short period. Energy is generated too rapidly for the diffusion into the muscle of substrates, including O_2, from the blood, and this is achieved by utilization of the muscle's own energy stores, phosphocreatine and glycogen.

Aerobic exercise involves prolonged exercise but at a lower intensity than can be achieved anaerobically. It is typified by long-distance running or swimming, or cross-country skiing. Here, the duration is such that it could not be maintained solely from the fuels stored within muscle: the fuel stores in the rest of the body (fat in adipose tissue and liver glycogen) must be used. Hence, these substrates must be brought to the muscle in the blood, and there are necessary adjustments to the circulatory system. The muscle fibres involved are predominantly the oxidative, Type I fibres. It is called aerobic because, to maximize efficiency, substrates (fatty acids and glucose) are completely oxidized.

7.4.2   Intensity of exercise

It will be useful to have an idea of the intensity of exercise in a quantitative sense. There are a number of terms and physical concepts which are related to this discussion. They are summarized in Table 7.3.

Force relates to the strength of a muscle contraction, for example. In physical terms, force is defined as that which tends to cause a body to accelerate. It is measured in newtons (N). Force may not cause a body to accelerate if it is opposed by an equal and opposite force. For instance, when we hold an object against the pull of gravity, we exert a force on it. The force necessary to hold it steady will be equal to the mass of the object in kilograms multiplied by the acceleration due to gravity, about 9.8 m/s². A convenient way of getting a feel for one newton is that it is (roughly) the force needed to hold an average apple against gravity.

Work is done on an object when a force acts on it over a distance. An example is lifting something through a height. The work done is the product of

Table 7.3 Units related to energy and work

Name	Brief definition	Units	Abbreviation	Notes
Force	That which tends to cause a body to accelerate	newton $(kg \cdot m/s^2)$	N	One newton is about the force needed to hold an apple against gravity
Work	Product of distance moved and the force exerted	joule $(kg \cdot m^2/s^2)$	J	In dietary terms, it is useful to use kJ $(= 10^3 \, J)$ and MJ $(= 10^6 \, J)$
Energy	Capacity to do work	joule	J	
Power	Rate of doing work	watt (J/s)	W	

Note that joules have replaced calories (1 cal = 4.18 J). Because calories are small (when dealing with nutrition) it used to be more common to use kilocalories (kcal; these were often abbreviated to Cal). Beware of confusion caused by this if you consult older nutritional literature.

the distance moved (in metres) and the force exerted (which is, in turn, the mass of the object in kilograms multiplied by the acceleration due to gravity). This refers to the *external work* performed. It does not depend on the rate at which the object is moved. This is because the object is being given *energy* (in this case, potential energy), and the gain in the object's potential energy is the same when it moves from the floor to the shelf (for instance) however fast it is moved. Energy can also be described as the capacity to perform work: we could then lower the object down with a string over a pulley and make it do some work in return (turn a clock, for instance). Energy and work are both measured in joules: one joule is the work done when a force of one newton acts over a distance of one metre.

It is not so obvious why external work is done when we move ourselves through a distance horizontally: if we had frictionless roller skates (and no air resistance), we would expend no energy to keep going at a constant speed. In reality, we have to contend with friction against the air and loss of energy when our feet strike the ground. Running is not an efficient means of movement compared with wheels.

The rate of doing work is measured in energy units per unit of time (joules per second, or watts). This is called *power* or *power output*. Lifting an object against gravity is a convenient way of estimating power output, and a useful practical exercise is to run as fast as possible up a flight of stairs, through a known height, and calculate the external work done against gravity (this is independent of the speed), and the power output (the work done divided by the time). An example calculation is given in Box 7.1.

However, the external work done is not the same as the energy expended by the person doing the work. The body is like any other machine which uses a fuel to produce external work. (The analogy with a petrol engine is obvious.) It is not fully efficient: some of the energy it uses from its store will be converted, not into external work, but into *heat*. As a rough approximation, the human body is about 25% efficient: of the energy it uses from its fuel stores, about 25% is converted to external work, and 75% into heat. The rate of using our fuel stores is measured as *energy expenditure* by the whole body. We can assess this in two ways.

If we can measure the rate of heat production by the body, and add to this the rate of doing external work, then we can assess energy expenditure directly. This requires a form of *calorimeter*, or instrument for measuring heat. A *direct calorimeter* is a room-sized chamber with temperature sensors in its walls to detect heat production. If the external work is done on an exercise bicycle by turning the pedals against friction, heat is produced, and the external work done will be included in the total heat produced.

A direct calorimeter is a sophisticated piece of equipment, and there are not many in the world. A simpler method for measuring the total energy expenditure is *indirect calorimetry*. Energy expenditure is assessed by the consumption of O_2 and, in more sophisticated systems, by the production of CO_2.

Box 7.1 Measurement of power by climbing stairs

A volunteer runs up a flight of stairs and is timed with a stopwatch; the vertical height climbed is measured.

For example, the results are:
- the runner has a body mass (including clothing) of 70 kg;
- the vertical height climbed is 2.5 m;
- the time taken is 2 s.

The potential energy gained = mass (kg) $\times$ g $\times$ height (m), where g is the acceleration due to gravity ($9.8 m/s^2$)

$$= (70 \times 9.8 \times 2.5) J$$

$$= 1715 J$$

The rate of doing external work (power) = total work done/time taken

$$= 1715/2 J/s$$

$$= 858 J/s \text{ (or 858 W)}$$

Notes:

1. A power output of 858 W would count as extremely heavy work on the scheme outlined in the text (where 200 W is regarded as 'heavy'); but the classification given in the text refers to sustained exercise, whereas much greater power output is feasible over a short time. In fact, power output measured over a very short time (a few seconds) is effectively a measure of the rate at which phosphocreatine can be used.

2. A more accurate measure of short-term anaerobic power output is to time the subject over a shorter distance — for instance, to use electronic switch-pads under two stairs perhaps separated by 1 m vertically.

3. You should realize that the calculation is an approximation. For instance, it ignores work done against friction of shoe on floor, etc. Nevertheless, in this situation by far the majority of work done will be the work against gravity, and it is a fairly good approximation.

This is feasible because the body as a whole derives energy from the complete oxidation of substrates, excreting only water, CO_2 and urea. The principle of indirect calorimetry will be described in detail in Chapter 10 (Box 10.1).

Thus there are two ways of expressing the rate of working. We may measure it as external work done, usually referred to as power or power output, and measured in watts.

Typical gradings of exercise are: 65 W, light exercise; 130 W, moderate exercise; 200 W, heavy exercise. These refer to rates of doing external work.

Alternatively, we may measure the rate of whole-body energy expenditure, which includes external work done and heat produced. This may also be measured in watts, although it is very convenient to relate it to the body's resting rate of energy expenditure. The unit MET (abbreviated from metabolic rate) has been coined for this measure. Some typical rates of energy expenditure expressed in this way are given in Table 7.4.

This enables us to answer a simple question which is often asked. We are about to walk up a mountain. We start by eating a confectionery bar to give us the energy. Is it enough energy — or might we end up fatter than we started? The approximate calculation is given in Box 7.2.

7.4.3 Metabolic regulation during anaerobic exercise

Exercise begins in the brain. We decide to contract our muscles in that particular way which will move us forwards, upwards, backwards or whatever. The appropriate somatic nerves are activated, and electrical impulses travel towards the muscle(s) to be contracted. On arrival of the impulse at the nerve terminal, acetylcholine is liberated and attaches to the nicotinic receptors at the sole-plate (see Section 6.2.2.3 and Figure 6.4). The binding of acetylcholine to these receptors sets a number of events in motion, described in Box 7.3. ATP is hydrolysed as the muscle contracts. It must be replaced rapidly or the muscle would run out of energy; the amount of ATP present in skeletal muscle is sufficient for about 1 s of maximal effort.

Initially, the utilization of ATP is 'buffered' by the phosphocreatine system (see Figure 3.5). But the amount of phosphocreatine is relatively small — it would sustain intense sprinting for about 4 s. The phosphagen store

Table 7.4 Energy expenditure during various activities

Activity	Energy expenditure (metabolic rate) (MET)
Resting (not asleep)	1.0
Sleeping	0.9
Light housework (e.g. sweeping floor)	2.5
Walking steadily (3 miles/h or 5 km/h)	3.5
Heavy housework (e.g. washing car, mopping floor)	4.5
Dancing	3–7
Swimming	6–11
Jogging	10–12
Squash	12
Marathon running	18

One MET is defined as the normal resting metabolic rate (i.e. whole-body energy expenditure); it is about 4.8 kJ/min for a man of average size, and 3.8 kJ/min for a woman of average size. Note that 4.8 kJ/min is 4800/60 = 80 W (about the heat output of a light bulb). Remember that the figures given are for total energy expenditure by the body; the amount of external work done will be about one-quarter of this (since the body as a machine has an efficiency of about 25%). The figures in this table are, of course, approximations only. The data are taken from Newsholme & Leech (1983) and Ainsworth *et al.* (1992).

Box 7.2 Does a confectionery bar provide enough energy to climb a mountain?

Let's start with the pleasant bit: a 65 g Mars Bar provides 1230 kJ (294 kcal) of energy (if oxidized completely).

Now for the climb: let's suppose

• we are going to climb 1000 m (3000 ft)

• our body mass (with clothing, boots, rucksack containing a picnic for the top, etc.) is 75 kg.

The external work done (against gravity) in reaching the summit is:

$$\text{force} \times \text{height gained}$$

$$= \text{mass (kg)} \times g \text{ (m/s}^2) \times \text{height gained (m)}, \text{ where } g \text{ is the acceleration due to gravity}$$

$$= (75 \times 9.8 \times 1000) \text{ J}$$

$$= 735000 \text{ J (or 735 kJ)}$$

But the body is only about 25% efficient in converting chemical energy into external work. Therefore, the total energy expenditure is about four times this, or ~3000 kJ (~3 MJ).

Thus we are permitted to stop halfway and eat another Mars Bar!

Note that the bar should not really be necessary; our fat stores (see Table 7.1) can provide typically about 540 MJ, enough for nearly 200 mountains without eating any more!

(phosphocreatine + ATP) must be replenished, and this occurs initially by glycogen breakdown and glycolysis.

Much has been written about the rapid increase in the flux through the glycolytic pathway in muscle at the start of exercise. It may increase by something like 1000-fold. However, it is clear that the flux cannot increase unless there is substrate to sustain it, and in rapid, intense exercise this substrate is glucose 6-phosphate produced by glycogen breakdown, rather than glucose taken up from the plasma. Therefore, there must be a mechanism for coordinated stimulation of glycogenolysis and muscle contraction.

There are two aspects to this coordinated control. The first is that the elevation of sarcoplasmic Ca^{2+} concentration (Box 7.3) also activates glycogen phosphorylase (Figure 7.7). The second is that glycogen phosphorylase cannot act unless the concentration of its co-substrate, inorganic phosphate (P_i), increases. This happens through the splitting of ATP in muscle contraction (Figure 7.7). Since the ATP concentration is kept 'topped up' by phosphocreatine, this P_i really comes from phosphocreatine. Thus glycogen breakdown

Box 7.3 Events occurring in skeletal muscle on receipt of a somatic nerve impulse

The structure of the end of the nerve (the *end-plate*) and the receptive area (the *sole-plate*) on the muscle cell membrane (the *sarcolemma*) is shown in Figure 6.4. On arrival of an impulse, acetylcholine is liberated into the synaptic cleft and binds to nicotinic receptors in the sole-plate. This causes opening of Na^+ channels and depolarization of the sarcolemma (see Box 6.1 for a description of these processes). The depolarization spreads across the sarcolemma as an *action potential*. It is relayed to invaginations of the sarcolemma which form tubes running into the muscle cell, the *T-tubules* (T for transverse). The arrival of the action potential causes the release into the muscle cell cytoplasm (the *sarcoplasm*) of Ca^{2+} ions from stores in the *sarcoplasmic reticulum*, a system of membranes within the cell. Thus the sarcoplasmic Ca^{2+} concentration is rapidly elevated throughout the cell.

An increase in the concentration of Ca^{2+} causes contraction by binding to troponin C, a component of the *thin filaments* of muscle, and, via a conformation change, by allowing the myosin heads (part of the *thick filaments*) to bind actin. Thin and thick filaments move (slide) relative to one another to cause contraction. (Details are given in more specialized books.) The hydrolysis of ATP to ADP and P_i by the actomyosin ATPase provides energy for this process. Therefore, contraction and the hydrolysis of ATP are intimately linked.

These steps are shown diagrammatically below:

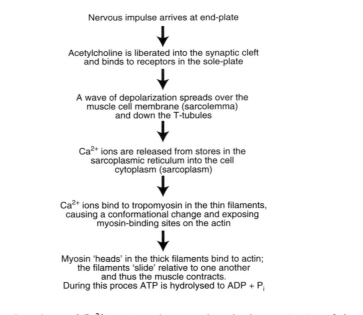

Nervous impulse arrives at end-plate

↓

Acetylcholine is liberated into the synaptic cleft
and binds to receptors in the sole-plate

↓

A wave of depolarization spreads over the
muscle cell membrane (sarcolemma)
and down the T-tubules

↓

Ca^{2+} ions are released from stores in the
sarcoplasmic reticulum into the cell
cytoplasm (sarcoplasm)

↓

Ca^{2+} ions bind to tropomyosin in the thin filaments,
causing a conformational change and exposing
myosin-binding sites on the actin

↓

Myosin 'heads' in the thick filaments bind to actin;
the filaments 'slide' relative to one another
and thus the muscle contracts.
During this proces ATP is hydrolysed to ADP + P_i

In addition, the release of Ca^{2+} ions into the sarcoplasm leads to activation of glycogen breakdown, as shown in Figure 7.7.

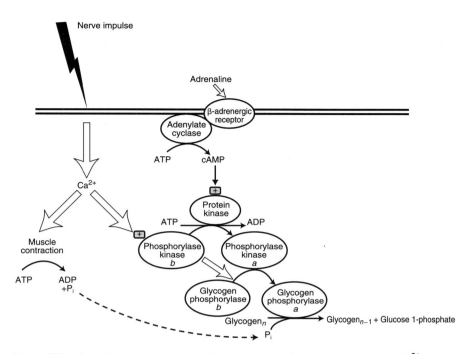

Figure 7.7   Coordinated regulation of glycogenolysis and contraction by Ca^{2+} ions in skeletal muscle
Elevation of the concentration of Ca^{2+} ions in the sarcoplasm occurs in response to the arrival of a nerve impulse (see Box 7.3) and is responsible for the initiation of contraction. The figure also shows the activation of phosphorylase by adrenaline (as in liver). It has been suggested that the anticipation of exercise may 'prime' the system by an increase in adrenaline. Glycogen cannot be broken down until there is an increase in the concentration of inorganic phosphate (P$_i$) — which is released as soon as contraction begins. The regulation of glycogen breakdown by Ca^{2+} ions is not confined to muscle; it can also occur in liver, and accounts for activation of glycogenolysis by catecholamines acting via α_1 receptors. However, the physiological significance is not known.

and muscle contraction are intimately connected within the muscle: there is no need for rapid stimulation by hormones.

The increased flux through glycolysis, now that substrate is available, requires alterations in enzyme activity which are brought about by interconnected changes in the levels of metabolites within the cell, discussed in Box 7.4. Nevertheless, the rate of change of glycolytic flux is so great that it seems unlikely that it can be accounted for solely by rapid changes in the concentrations of enzyme effectors, and this has led to the idea that the sensitivity of metabolic regulation of this pathway may be increased by the existence of substrate cycles (see Box 7.4).

During intense exercise, energy is thus derived very rapidly from anaerobic glycolysis. There is no need for increased delivery of other substrates or oxygen in the plasma. Anaerobic glycolysis produces lactic acid which, at physiological pH, will be in the form of lactate ions and hydrogen ions. Thus the local hydrogen ion concentration in the muscle increases. This

Box 7.4 Activation of the pathway of glycolysis at the start of anaerobic exercise

At the start of anaerobic exercise, the net flux through the glycolytic pathway increases about 1000-fold. The link between contraction and glycogen breakdown is explained in the text and Figure 7.7. Nevertheless, the enzymes of the pathway itself must be activated to allow this increase in flux. Regulation of the enzyme phosphofructokinase (PFK) is best understood and will be discussed here as an illustration.

Allosteric regulation

Regulation by fructose 2,6-bisphosphate, important in the liver, is probably not a major factor in exercising muscle. However, a number of intermediates act as allosteric effectors of PFK. These include:

Activators	Inhibitors
AMP	ATP
P_i	Citrate*
Fructose 1,6-bisphosphate	Phosphocreatine*
Fructose 6-phosphate	
NH_3	

*These potentiate the inhibitory effect of ATP.

During contraction, ATP is hydrolysed to ADP and P_i. It is partially replenished by phosphocreatine (see Figure 3.5). The following associated reactions occur:

Reaction	Effect
ATP $\longrightarrow$ ADP + P_i (associated with contraction)	ATP↓, P_i↑
2ADP $\longrightarrow$ ATP + AMP (adenylate kinase)	AMP↑
PCr + ADP $\longrightarrow$ Cr + ATP (creatine kinase)	PCr↓↓
AMP + H_2O $\longrightarrow$ IMP + NH_3 (AMP deaminase)	NH_3↑

Abbreviations used: PCr, phosphocreatine; Cr, creatine; IMP, inosine monophosphate.

Thus the changes in allosteric effectors all act to activate PFK.   ☞

may be one cause of fatigue. A local fall in pH may have a number of effects which tend to cause lessening of the force of muscle contractions. These include effects on the interaction between myosin and actin, on the binding of Ca^{2+} to troponin, and on the enzyme phosphofructokinase, an important regulatory enzyme in glycolysis which is inhibited at low pH.

The ability to perform this type of exercise depends largely on the bulk of the glycolytic, type II fibres, which can be increased through training (see Section 7.4.9). Certain interventions may aid performance. Recently there has been considerable interest in dietary supplementation with creatine in amounts

---

☞ Box 7.4 (continued)

Substrate cycling

It is difficult to envisage that an enzyme can alter its activity by a factor of 1000 in less than 1 second. For this reason, it has been proposed that the sensitivity of control may be increased by the existence of a substrate cycle between fructose 6-phosphate (F 6-P) and fructose 1,6-bisphosphate (F 1,6-P_2). The reverse reaction is catalysed by fructose 1,6-bisphosphatase (FBPase).

The concept may be illustrated as follows:

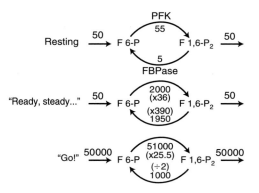

(Top) The flux through PFK is 55 arbitrary units and the reverse flux 5 units, giving a net flux along the pathway of 50 units. On the starting blocks, anticipation (perhaps mediated via stress hormones) leads to a 36-fold activation of PFK and a 390-fold activation of FBPase (these are reasonable changes since they need not be instantaneous); the net flux (50 units) along the pathway remains unchanged. On the starting gun, an almost instantaneous 25.5-fold activation of PFK and halving of FBPase activity leads to a 1000-fold change in net flux through the pathway. The numbers illustrate the potential for increased sensitivity of metabolic control arising through substrate cycling, but are not based on physiological measurements.

This box and the figure are based largely on Newsholme & Leech (1983); reproduced with permission from John Wiley. Quantitative estimates of the extent of substrate cycling *in vivo* are given in Newsholme & Challis (1992).

---

of 5 g/day. This has been shown to improve anaerobic performance, probably by increasing the amount of phosphocreatine in the muscles. Another intervention that has shown some success in experimental situations is ingestion of large amounts of sodium bicarbonate ($NaHCO_3$), which acts as a buffer to minimize hydrogen ion accumulation and thus postpones fatigue.

7.4.4 Metabolic regulation during aerobic exercise

In Section 7.4.1, anaerobic and aerobic exercise are described as the two extreme forms of exercise. Many forms of exercise consist of a combination of the two. Tennis and soccer require moments of intense power output (serving, kicking), accompanied by endurance performance (running about the court or pitch for 90 min or more). In running events, the 100 m sprint is virtually completely anaerobic: it is said that the elite sprinter has no need to draw breath during it. (Most of us would doubtless need several breaths.) The 400 m is a combination of anaerobic and aerobic exercise, and with increasing distance, the aerobic component becomes more dominant. The marathon run (42.2 km, 26.2 miles) is often taken as an example of almost pure aerobic exercise.

The characteristic of aerobic exercise is that it can be sustained for long periods. This means that stored fuels other than those in the muscles must be used, and must be completely oxidized so that partial breakdown products such as lactic acid do not build up. Complete oxidation of substrates also gives a much higher energy yield than partial breakdown: for instance, complete oxidation of 1 molecule of glucose gives rise to 38 molecules of ATP, whereas anaerobic glycolysis to 2 molecules of lactate gives rise to 3 molecules of ATP (net). Not surprisingly, the muscle fibres most involved in aerobic exercise are the more oxidative, slow-twitch, Type I fibres (see Section 3.4.2). For these muscles to produce external work at a high rate over a long period, they must be supplied with substrates (including O_2), and the products of metabolism, such as CO_2, must be removed, at a sufficiently high rate. This necessitates coordinated changes in the circulatory system.

The major fuels used in aerobic exercise vary with the intensity and the duration of the exercise. Carbohydrate tends to predominate early on; fat becomes more important later as glycogen stores are depleted. The amount of glucose present in the circulation and the extracellular fluid is small and cannot be depleted without harmful effects. Therefore, the carbohydrate used during endurance exercise comes from glycogen stores in exercising skeletal muscle and the liver. In principle, it might also come from gluconeogenesis: exercising muscles always produce some lactic acid, even in aerobic exercise, and this should be a good substrate for hepatic gluconeogenesis. In fact, gluconeogenesis seems to be restricted during exercise, perhaps because blood flow to the liver is restricted as blood is diverted to other organs and tissues (mainly skeletal muscle, as discussed below). The use of different fuels at different intensities of exercise is illustrated in Figure 7.8.

The contribution of fat to muscular work shows some odd characteristics. If we set out to design an 'exercise system' using our knowledge of metabolism gained so far, we might think that as large a proportion as possible of the energy for exercise should be generated by oxidation of fat. We have far more energy stored as fat than as carbohydrate, and there is not the same need to 'preserve' it for the functioning of organs such as the brain. In addition, fat is a very 'light' way of storing a lot of energy. However, a number of studies have shown that oxidation of fat can only support around 60% of the maximal aerobic power output. The evidence is briefly this. In ultra-endurance athletes

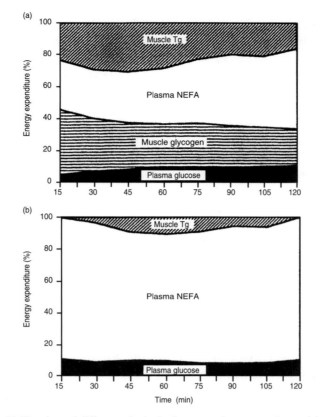

Figure 7.8   Utilization of different fuels during exercise at two intensities
The intensities of exercise are judged by oxygen consumption, in relation to the maximal rate of oxygen consumption for the individual ($\dot{V}O_2$max). Panel (a) shows exercise at 65% $\dot{V}O_2$max; 2 h at 65% $\dot{V}O_2$max is relatively heavy exercise. Panel (b) shows exercise at 25% $\dot{V}O_2$max; 2 h at 25% $\dot{V}O_2$max is relatively light. (An elite marathon runner would maintain about 85% of $\dot{V}O_2$max. for 2 h 10 min.) The figure shows the relative contribution to energy expenditure (total energy expenditure is taken in each case to be 100%, although it is 65/25 or 2.6 times greater in the top panel). The data were obtained by a combination of indirect calorimetry and use of isotopic tracers to measure the whole-body turnover of glucose, glycerol and fatty acids. Abbreviations used: NEFA, non-esterified fatty acids; Tg, triacylglycerol. Reproduced from Romijn *et al.* (1993) with permission from The American Physiological Society.

(e.g. 24 h runners), power output drops with time to about 50% of maximal aerobic power, at about the same time as the glycogen stores would be expected to be depleted. In less-well-trained subjects, it also appears that fat oxidation contributes a maximum of about 60% of muscle oxygen consumption.

Therefore, the maintenance of maximal aerobic power output requires that carbohydrate is oxidized as well as fat. Since this carbohydrate comes from the glycogen stores, the time for which maximal aerobic power can be sustained depends on the amount of glycogen stored initially. Depletion of the glycogen stores leads to a sudden feeling of fatigue, described by marathon runners as 'hitting the wall'. The Swedish physician Jonas Bergström, and a Swedish physiologist, Eric Hultman, showed this directly during the 1960s. They measured the content of glycogen in small muscle biopsies, taken with a special needle, in a group of athletes who were each studied on two or three occasions, after consuming different diets. The different diets (mixed; low-carbohydrate; high-carbohydrate) produced different initial concentrations of muscle glycogen, and it was found that the time to exhaustion, when working at 75% of maximal aerobic power, correlated with the initial muscle glycogen concentration (Figure 7.9). This observation has led to the development of methods for boosting the muscle glycogen stores for endurance runners (*glycogen loading*).

Having looked at the overall pattern of fuel utilization during aerobic exercise, we shall now consider in more detail the regulation of the utilization of individual fuels, and how the delivery of energy is regulated by the hormonal and nervous systems.

7.4.5   Nervous system and cardiovascular responses during aerobic exercise

Two components of the nervous system are intimately involved with metabolic regulation during aerobic exercise.

The somatic nervous system carries the stimuli for contraction of the appropriate muscles, and the arrival of a nervous impulse at the end-plate triggers both contraction and a coordinated activation of glycogen breakdown. This is true just as much during aerobic exercise, and there appears to be 'obligatory' breakdown of muscle glycogen associated with muscle contrac-

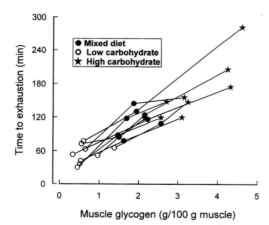

Figure 7.9   Relationship between initial glycogen concentration in the quadriceps muscle and maximal work time (until exhaustion) in nine different subjects who followed different diets before each test
The greater the initial glycogen concentration, the longer the ability to sustain exercise. Redrawn from Bergström *et al.* (1967); with permission from Acta Physiol. Scand.

tion, even if there are plentiful substrates in the blood (e.g. if the athlete has eaten well beforehand).

The sympathetic nervous system, accompanied by adrenaline secretion from the adrenal medulla, brings about the necessary changes in the cardiovascular system and the mobilization of stored fuels, glycogen and triacylglycerol.

An important part of the physiological response during endurance exercise is an increase in cardiac output (both the rate and force of heart contraction increase), and in the delivery of blood to skeletal muscle. The increase in cardiac output is mediated mainly by the sympathetic nervous system, acting on β-adrenergic receptors in the heart. An increase in cardiac output in itself might cause an increase in muscle blood flow, but there is an additional specific dilatation of the blood vessels in the muscle, brought about by cholinergic impulses from the sympathetic nerves (discussed in Section 6.3.2 and Figure 6.5). As we saw in Chapter 6, muscle is unusual in that activation of the sympathetic nervous system causes vasodilatation; in other organs (e.g. skin, kidneys and abdominal organs) blood flow is restricted by sympathetic activation. Thus yet more blood is diverted to the muscles. Blood flow to the exercising muscles is also increased by local effects of the products of metabolism: in particular, hydrogen ions (produced as lactic acid) cause relaxation of the blood vessels. Thus a number of factors operate to bring more blood to the working muscles, allowing the delivery of more substrates (including O_2), and also the removal of more of the products of metabolism (lactic acid and CO_2 in particular) (Figure 7.10).

Increased delivery of O_2 to the muscles and removal of CO_2 from the body requires increased depth and rate of breathing. This is brought about mainly by the fall in blood pH (increase in H^+ ion concentration) that occurs as lactic acid and CO_2 are produced. The change in pH is sensed by receptors in the brain stem (see Section 6.2.1.2) which trigger changes in respiration.

7.4.6   Other hormonal responses during aerobic exercise

The sympathetic nervous system and adrenaline bring about the mobilization of stored fuels (discussed in detail later). Other hormones respond to aerobic exercise, and are involved in the regulation of fuel availability. Growth hormone and cortisol are both secreted in response to exercise, rising gradually in concentration in the plasma over the first 30 min to 1 h (Figure 7.11). These are relatively slow responses and are likely to be involved particularly in the release of stored fuels during prolonged exercise. The plasma glucose concentration may rise or fall during exercise (discussed below), but the insulin concentration falls somewhat during endurance exercise (Figure 7.12). This represents α-adrenergic inhibition of its secretion from the pancreas, brought about by the increased concentration of circulating adrenaline. Glucagon secretion may increase, although this is not a major change except with very strenuous, prolonged exercise. The increase in adrenaline, glucagon, growth hormone and cortisol concentrations is a typical 'stress' response.

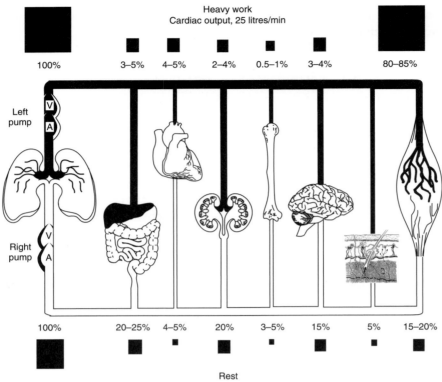

Figure 7.10 Schematic drawing of the distribution of blood flow between various organs and tissues at rest (bottom) and during strenuous exercise (top)
Distribution is shown by the area of the black squares. Adipose tissue is not shown, but accounts for about 5–10% of cardiac output at rest, about 1% during exercise. Reproduced from Åstrand & Rodahl (1977) with permission from McGraw-Hill Inc and the authors.

The way in which the somatic and sympathetic nervous systems coordinate physiological and metabolic changes during endurance exercise is illustrated in Figure 7.13.

7.4.7 Carbohydrate metabolism during endurance exercise

Oxidation of glucose provides a major source of energy for the working muscles during aerobic exercise. During aerobic exercise at a high rate (e.g. 80–90% of maximal oxygen consumption, typical of an elite marathon runner) the rate of energy expenditure is around 80–90 kJ/min. The proportion of this supplied by glucose oxidation varies according to the preceding diet and other factors, but 50% might be a reasonable working figure (i.e. 40–45 kJ/min from glucose). Oxidation of 1 g of glucose releases 17 kJ, so that 42.5/17 or about 2.5 g of glucose must be oxidized each minute.

The amount of glucose available in the blood and extracellular space is around 12 g (see Section 5.1). Therefore, even if it could all be used without

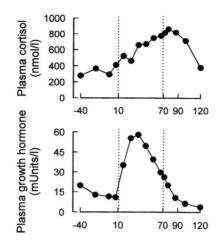

Figure 7.11 Plasma concentrations of cortisol (top panel) and growth hormone (lower panel) during aerobic exercise at about 60% of maximal aerobic power
The exercise, on a bicycle, began with a 'warm-up' (shown as 0–10 min) and then carried on for 60 min (until 70 min on the X-axis). Based on Hodgetts *et al.* (1991); with permission from The American Physiological Society.

adverse consequences, this would support high-intensity aerobic exercise for only a few minutes. The liver glycogen store is around 100 g (see Section 7.2.1). Therefore, this could support exercise for less than 1 h. The total store of muscle glycogen may be around 300–400 g. The utilization of muscle glycogen is more extensive in the muscles that are used for the exercise than in others, so not all the whole-body store of muscle glycogen may be used. Remember that these are all 'ball-park' figures. You will note that the total store of glycogen in liver and muscle could support glucose oxidation at a rate of 2.5 g/min for something over 2 h. This is about the time taken for an elite runner to finish the marathon: when the glycogen store is depleted, the rate of energy expenditure will drop and performance will suffer. The marathon is about the longest event that can be undertaken at such a high percentage of maximal oxygen consumption.

Hepatic gluconeogenesis has been ignored here; it probably does not make a large contribution, since hepatic blood flow may be decreased during exercise as the blood is diverted to working muscles. Moreover, much of the gluconeogenesis that occurs will be from lactate, released by the working muscles from their glycogen stores. Therefore, this is only part of the complete pathway for oxidation of those glycogen stores.

What are the factors responsible for mobilization of the glycogen stores? In the working muscles, the effects of neural activation of contraction probably predominate, since the glycogen concentration in non-working muscles falls much less, if at all. This has been demonstrated in subjects performing one-legged exercise on a modified exercise bicycle; the glycogen content of the exercised leg falls, whereas that of the other leg does not change

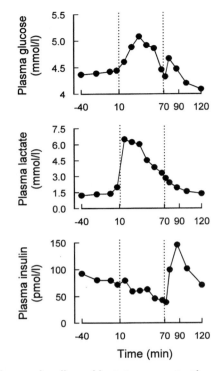

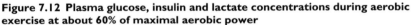

Figure 7.12 Plasma glucose, insulin and lactate concentrations during aerobic exercise at about 60% of maximal aerobic power
The protocol was the same as in Figure 7.11. Note how the plasma insulin concentration (bottom panel) falls during exercise, despite a rise in the plasma glucose concentration (top panel). The plasma lactate concentration is also shown (middle panel); it increases at the beginning of exercise and then subsides. Based on Hodgetts *et al.* (1991); with permission from The American Physiological Society.

(Figure 7.14). As discussed earlier, the stimulation of contraction is intimately linked with the stimulation of glycogen breakdown. An elevation in the concentration of adrenaline may also contribute, potentiating the effect of somatic nerve stimulation; it is not a stimulus on its own, however, as evidenced by the one-legged exercise experiment, in which both legs are exposed to the same adrenaline concentration.

In the liver, the stimulus for glycogen breakdown is not entirely clear. Glucagon would be the obvious signal but, as noted earlier, its concentration is not always elevated. However, it should be remembered that when the concentration of glucagon is measured in 'peripheral blood' it may not reflect the concentration reaching the liver in the portal vein, so that there may be some increase in glucagon secretion. In addition, the concentration of glucose may rise or fall somewhat — largely depending on the nutritional state of the subject — but the plasma insulin concentration falls gently during sustained exercise (Figure 7.12), probably representing the effects of increased adrenergic

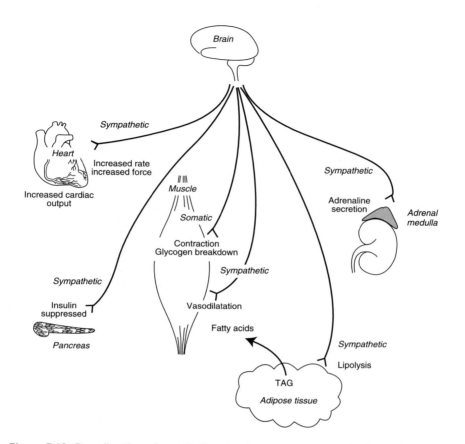

Figure 7.13 Coordination of metabolism by the nervous system during endurance exercise

Adrenaline secreted from the adrenal medulla may be responsible, or may reinforce the effects of the sympathetic nerves, for increased lipolysis and for suppression of insulin secretion.

stimulation to the pancreas (via sympathetic nerves or plasma adrenaline). Therefore, the glucagon/insulin ratio reaching the liver will undoubtedly rise, favouring glycogen breakdown. There may, in addition, be some direct effect of activation of the sympathetic innervation of the liver; this is very difficult to test in humans.

Note that the comment that the plasma glucose concentration may not change much during endurance exercise does not mean that there are no changes in glucose utilization: the concentration of glucose in the plasma merely represents the balance between glucose production and glucose utilization, whereas the turnover of glucose in plasma increases several-fold during endurance exercise (see Romijn *et al.*, 1993).

One other aspect of glycogen mobilization is worthy of mention. You will recall that glycogen, a hydrophilic molecule, is stored in hydrated form with about three times its own weight of water. When glycogen is mobilized, that water is released. Therefore, as well as providing the store of carbohydrate,

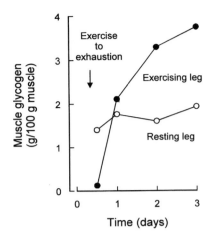

Figure 7.14 Glycogen concentrations in leg muscle during one-legged exercise (cycling on a specially-adapted bicycle) in the exercising leg (●) and the non-exercising leg (○)
Average of two subjects. Based on Bergström & Hultman (1966).

glycogen also contributes to the water necessary for endurance exercise, helping to replace that lost as sweat, etc. If 300 g of glycogen are mobilized in all, this could mean almost 1 litre of water.

7.4.8   Fat metabolism during endurance exercise

The activity of muscle hexokinase is sufficient, in principle, for all the energy for sustained aerobic exercise to be derived from uptake of plasma glucose. In fact, as we have seen, this would reduce the length of time during which the exercise can be sustained at the highest rate. Simultaneous oxidation of glucose and fatty acids, therefore, produces the longest possible period of sustained high-intensity exercise. The availability of fatty acids to the muscles also reduces the rate of glucose oxidation via the glucose–fatty acid cycle (see Section 5.4.1.2). There is experimental evidence to show that increasing the availability of fatty acids leads to sparing of glycogen, thus, at least in principle, allowing high-intensity exercise to be continued for longer[3].

The fatty acids oxidized during endurance exercise come from two main sources: triacylglycerol stored in adipose tissue and triacylglycerol stored in the muscles themselves. The latter is difficult to study and the factors which

---

[3]*The availability of fatty acids may be increased experimentally as follows. The subject or animal is either fed a high-fat meal or given a triacylglycerol emulsion into a vein. Then heparin (an anticoagulant) is given. This displaces lipoprotein lipase bound to capillary endothelial cells into the bloodstream where it acts rapidly on the circulating triacylglycerol to release fatty acids into the plasma. Examples of such studies in exercise are given by Costill et al. (1977) and Dyck et al. (1993).*

control its utilization are not clear. Nevertheless, the muscle triacylglycerol concentration falls during intense, long-lasting exercise. The regulation of fat mobilization from adipose tissue is better understood. The main stimulus for this to increase during exercise is adrenergic: blockade of β-adrenergic receptors in adipose tissue with the drug propranolol prevents the increase in lipolysis during exercise (see Figure 6.7). It is not certain whether the main stimulus is circulating adrenaline or activation of the sympathetic nerves. The adrenergic stimulation of lipolysis may be reinforced by the slight fall in insulin concentration (thus relieving the normal suppression of lipolysis by insulin). In sustained exercise (longer than, say, 30–60 min) then the increases in plasma growth hormone and cortisol concentrations (Figure 7.11) may potentiate the adrenergic stimulation of lipolysis, perhaps by an increase in the amount of enzyme (hormone-sensitive lipase) present.

The fatty acids liberated in adipose tissue are transported bound to plasma albumin for uptake and oxidation in muscle. It may be a step in this pathway that limits the rate at which fatty acids can be oxidized, leading to the restriction of the contribution of fatty acid oxidation to about 60% of the maximal sustainable rate of energy expenditure. The evidence, from experiments in which the availability of fatty acids in the plasma is increased, suggests the following. In moderate-intensity exercise, up to about 65% of the maximal aerobic power, increased availability of fatty acids increases the rate of fat oxidation, implying that the normal limitation on their oxidation is at the level of release from adipose tissue. However, in higher intensity exercise (an elite marathon runner maintains 80–85% of maximal aerobic power), the increased availability of fatty acids leads to very little increase in fat oxidation; it appears that the rate of fatty acid utilization by muscle is limited (see Romijn et al., 1995).

There is some information as to why these steps may be rate-controlling. The release of non-esterified fatty acids into the plasma depends upon the availability of albumin. If the blood flow through adipose tissue is restricted, there may be insufficient albumin available to carry away all the fatty acids formed in lipolysis. Non-esterified fatty acids may then accumulate in the tissue, as described in the case of physical trauma (Section 6.3.3.2 and Table 6.1). To some extent this may cause an increase in their re-esterification to form triacylglycerol, but it also appears that they accumulate as such. There is evidence for this: when exercise stops, there is a sudden release of fatty acids into the general circulation not accompanied by the expected 1 mol of glycerol for each 3 mol of fatty acids. It is not, perhaps, surprising that blood flow through adipose tissue should be restricted. We have already seen that a high sympathetic activity or circulating adrenaline concentration can restrict blood flow through many tissues by α-adrenergic effects on the blood vessels, and during exercise this occurs as part of the redistribution of blood to the working muscles. Adipose tissue is affected in just this way.

At higher intensities of exercise, the muscles are unable to oxidize more fatty acids even if they are available in the plasma. The reason may be this.

Table 7.5	Changes that occur with endurance training

Cardiovascular and whole-body
  Increased cardiac output, and ability to increase this during exercise
  Improved respiratory function
  Increased lean body mass (mainly muscle bulk)
  Decreased body fat
  Increased bone strength

Structural changes in muscle
  Increased density of capillaries
  Increased number of mitochondria
  Increased size of mitochondria
  Increased myoglobin concentration

Metabolic changes in muscle
  Increased expression of GLUT4
  Increased sensitivity to insulin
  Increased activity of lipoprotein lipase
  Increased activity of oxidative enzymes in mitochondria (tricarboxylic acid cycle and
  β-oxidation)
  Increased glycogen synthase activity

Based in part on Åstrand & Rodahl (1977) and on Holloszy & Booth (1976).

Glucose metabolism in muscle proceeds at a high rate, as we have seen. Acetyl-CoA is produced, via the action of pyruvate dehydrogenase, but will primarily be oxidized in the tricarboxylic acid cycle. However, the high concentration may cause some increase in flux through the pathway of *de novo* lipogenesis, thus increasing the concentration of the next intermediate in that pathway, malonyl-CoA. As was discussed in Section 3.2.2.2, malonyl-CoA inhibits the entry of fatty acids into the mitochondrion for oxidation. Thus glucose oxidation proceeding at a high rate may limit the muscles' ability to oxidize fat.

Thus fat metabolism during high-intensity endurance exercise does not follow the rules we might expect on the basis of everything we know about human metabolism. The contribution of fatty acids is limited and the availability of glycogen limits the time for which high-intensity exercise can be maintained. We may speculate that perhaps the ability to run at high intensity — above about 65% of maximal aerobic power — for long periods was not important in terms of the evolution of *Homo sapiens*. Maybe the ability to sprint, to escape from a predator, was more important.

7.4.9 The effects of training

Exercise training has a number of effects, which cannot be discussed at length in this book. In the case of anaerobic exercise (such as weight-lifting or sprinting) the changes brought about by training are largely increased muscle bulk and strength. The increase in muscle bulk is mainly the result of muscle *hypertrophy* rather than *hyperplasia*: i.e. muscle cells become bigger rather than increasing in number. A weight-lifter, sprinter or high-jumper may have a higher proportion of Type II fibres than a long-distance runner (see Figure 3.7), but this is not primarily a result of training; it appears to be genetically determined. Rather, he or she is a weight-lifter or sprinter *because* he or she has a high proportion of Type II fibres.

The changes that occur with endurance training are rather more varied. They are listed in Table 7.5. They concern increased ability to deliver O_2 and other substrates to the working muscle, and increased ability within the muscle to utilize substrates. The activity of glycogen synthase is usually found to be increased, whereas that of glycogen phosphorylase is not; presumably the activity of the latter is not usually rate-controlling for generation of power in endurance exercise.

Suggestions for further reading

Starvation: 'classic' papers

Cahill, G.F., Herrera, M.G., Morgan, A.P., *et al.* (1966) Hormone–fuel inter-relationships during fasting. *J. Clin. Invest.* **45**, 1751–1769

Cahill, G.F.J. (1976) Starvation in man. *Clin. Endocrinol. Metab.* **5**, 397–415

(These two papers by Cahill review the classic studies of human starvation on which much of our present knowledge is based. For references to specific organs, see Chapter 3.)

Starvation: reviews

Henry, C.J.K. (1990) Body mass index and the limits of human survival. *Eur. J. Clin. Nutr.* **44**, 329–335

Owen, O.E., Tappy, L., Mozzoli, M.A. & Smalley, K.J. (1990) Acute starvation. In *The Metabolic and Molecular Basis of Acquired Disease* (Cohen, R.D., Lewis, B., Alberti, K.G.M.M. & Denman, A.M., eds.), pp. 550–570, Baillière Tindall, London

Exercise: skeletal muscle physiology and biochemistry

Booth, F.W. & Thomason, D.B. (1991) Molecular and cellular adaptation of muscle in response to exercise: perspectives of various models. *Physiol. Rev.* **71**, 541–585

Geeves, M.A. (1991) The dynamics of actin and myosin association and the crossbridge model of muscle contraction. *Biochem. J.* **274**, 1–14

Rayment, I. & Holden, H.M. (1994) The three-dimensional structure of a molecular motor. *Trends Biochem. Sci.* **19**, 129–134

Stanley, W.C. & Connett, R.J. (1991) Regulation of muscle carbohydrate metabolism during exercise. *FASEB J.* **5**, 2155–2159

Exercise: fuel supply and metabolism

Bergström, J. & Hultman, E. (1972) Nutrition for maximal sports performance. *J. Am. Med. Assoc.* **221**, 999–1006. (This old paper reviews much of the classic data on muscle glycogen and exercise.)

Dyck, D.J., Putman, C.T., Heigenhauser, G.J.F., Hultman, E. & Spriet, L.L. (1993) Regulation of fat–carbohydrate interaction in skeletal muscle during intense aerobic cycling. *Am. J. Physiol.* **265**, E852–E859

Spurway, N.C. (1992) Aerobic exercise, anaerobic exercise and the lactate threshold. *Br. Med. Bull.* **48**, 569–591

8

Lipoprotein metabolism

8.1   Introduction

The major energy store of the body is a hydrophobic compound, triacylglycerol, for reasons discussed in earlier chapters. Other hydrophobic molecules play important roles in cellular function, particularly cholesterol and its esters (cholesteryl esters). Therefore, mechanisms for transporting these non-water-soluble lipid species in the blood have evolved.

Non-esterified fatty acids are carried in the plasma bound to albumin. Some fat-soluble micronutrients and regulators of metabolism — e.g. fat-soluble vitamins and steroid hormones — are transported in the plasma by specific carrier proteins, such as the *cortisol-binding globulin* which carries cortisol. The transport of both triacylglycerol and cholesterol occurs in specialized structures known as *lipoproteins*. Because triacylglycerol and cholesterol are carried by the same system, their metabolism is closely interrelated.

Lipoproteins are particles with a highly hydrophobic lipid core and a relatively hydrophilic outer surface. A typical lipoprotein particle (Figure 8.1) consists of a core of triacylglycerol and cholesteryl ester, with an outer surface layer of phospholipid and free cholesterol. [As discussed in Section 1.2.1.1, cholesteryl esters are highly hydrophobic. By comparison, free (unesterified) cholesterol has amphipathic properties because of its hydroxyl group.] Each particle has associated with it one or more protein molecules, the *apolipoproteins*, which have hydrophobic domains, which 'dip into' the core and anchor the protein to the particle, and hydrophilic domains which are exposed at the surface.

Lipoproteins consist of a heterogeneous group of particles with different lipid and protein compositions, and different sizes. They have traditionally been separated into groups, or fractions, on the basis of either electrophoretic mobility or flotation in an ultracentrifuge. The latter technique has given rise to a much-used classification system, which will be used here. The fractions isolated in the ultracentrifuge also have some functional distinction. However, the distinctions are not absolute, and each ultracentrifugal fraction may consist of a range of particles with somewhat different functions.

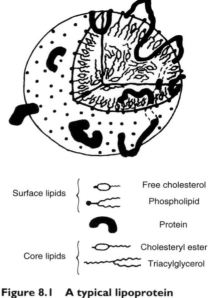

The characteristics of the major lipoprotein fractions are listed in Table 8.1. Chylomicron and very-low-density lipoprotein (VLDL) particles are relatively rich in triacyl-glycerol and are often referred to as the triacylglycerol-rich lipoproteins; they are mainly concerned with delivery of triacylglycerol to tissues. The smaller low-density lipoprotein (LDL) and high-density lipoprotein (HDL) particles are more involved with transport of cholesterol to and from cells. The major apolipo-proteins involved in lipoprotein

Figure 8.1   A typical lipoprotein particle
Reproduced from Durrington (1989) with permission from Butterworth–Heinemann.

metabolism are listed in Box 8.1, and some important plasma enzymes associated with the lipoproteins are listed in Box 8.2.

8.2   Pathways of lipoprotein metabolism

8.2.1   Chylomicron metabolism: the exogenous pathway

The metabolism of chylomicrons is often called the *exogenous pathway* of lipoprotein metabolism. Exogenous means 'from outside the body', and this pathway transports dietary fat. The pathway is summarized in Figure 8.2. Triacylglycerol and cholesterol are absorbed and re-esterified in the cells of the intestinal wall, and secreted as chylomicron particles, via the lymphatics, into the circulation (see Figure 2.6). The newly secreted chylomicron particles consist of a core of cholesteryl ester and triacylglycerol, with a surface of un-esterified cholesterol and phospholipid, and the apolipoproteins B48 and A1.

In the circulation, chylomicrons interact with other particles, and some of the smaller apolipoproteins are passed from one particle to another, probably by passive diffusion down concentration gradients. In particular, chylomicrons rapidly acquire apolipoprotein C2, which makes them substrates for lipopro-tein lipase as they pass through capillaries of tissues that express this enzyme, such as adipose tissue and muscle. The triacylglycerol is thus hydrolysed, and the particles shrink. They may pass through a number of capillary beds, and

Table 8.1 Characteristics of the major lipoprotein classes

Fraction	Density range (g/ml)	Diameter (nm)	Major lipids	Major apolipoproteins	Composition (percentage by weight)			
					Protein	TAG	Cholesterol	PL
Chylomicrons	<0.950	80–1000	Dietary TAG	B48, A1, A2, C, E	1	90	5	4
VLDL	0.950–1.006	30–80	Endogenous TAG (from liver)	B100, C, E	10	65	13	13
LDL	1.019–1.063	20–22	Cholesterol and cholesteryl ester	B100	20	10	45	23
HDL	1.063–1.090	9–15	Cholesteryl ester and PL	A1, A2, C, E	50	2	18	30

Abbreviations used: HDL, high-density lipoprotein; LDL, low-density lipoprotein; PL, phospholipid; TAG, triacylglycerol; VLDL, very-low-density lipoprotein.

Notes. (1) There are other fractions and sub-fractions not distinguished here: for instance, between VLDL and LDL there is an intermediate-density lipoprotein (IDL) fraction; its half-life is short and its concentration normally low. (2) The proportions shown are approximate only and vary within each major class. (3) Apolipoprotein C refers to the presence of apolipoproteins C1, C2 and C3; these are usually found together.

Box 8.1   The major apolipoproteins involved in lipoprotein metabolism

Apolipoproteins A1, A2

These apolipoproteins are not related except in that they often occur together in lipoprotein fractions. A1 is the better characterized. It has a relative molecular mass (M_r) of 28 000 (243 amino acids) and it has two major functions. It is an activator of the enzyme lecithin–cholesterol acyl transferase (LCAT; see Box 8.2). In addition, its amino acid sequence contains six repeated 22 amino acid sequences, which fold into α-helices with strong polar and non-polar faces. Thus it has amphipathic properties which enable it to bind very strongly to various lipid classes including phospholipids and cholesterol. This property may give it a special role in interacting with cell membranes and 'collecting' cholesterol from the cells. It is produced in the cells of the small intestine and the liver.

Apolipoprotein B

This is a large protein found in chylomicrons, VLDL and LDL. There are two isoforms: apolipoprotein B100 and apolipoprotein B48. The former contains 4536 amino acids $(M_r\ 513 000)$. Apolipoprotein B48 is the N-terminal 2152 amino acids of this $(M_r\ 241 000)$, i.e. it represents about 48% of the apolipoprotein B100 molecule (and hence their names). Apolipoprotein B48 is produced from the same gene as Apolipoprotein B100, by editing of the messenger RNA to introduce a stop codon. Apolipoprotein B48 is produced in intestinal cells and incorporated into chylomicrons, whereas B100 is produced in the liver and incorporated into VLDL. Since LDL particles are produced from VLDL (discussed in the text), these particles also contain B100. There is just one molecule of apolipoprotein B (B100 or B48) per particle: it wraps around the particle, and its hydrophobic regions 'dip down' into the core to anchor it. It functions as a receptor ligand (discussed below).

Apolipoproteins C1, C2 and C3

Like the apolipoproteins A, these are not structurally related, but are often found together. Apolipoprotein C2 is the best understood. It is a protein of M_r 8900 with 78 amino acids. It is an essential activator of lipoprotein lipase (discussed in Sections 3.6.2.1 and 5.2.2.2). Thus lipoprotein lipase can only act on the triacylglycerol in particles that contain apolipoprotein C2. It is produced in the liver.

Apolipoprotein E

This is a protein of M_r 34 000 (299 amino acids), which exists in three major isoforms (E2, E3 and E4). Each person carries two alleles: an individual may be E2/E3, E3/E3 etc. Apolipoprotein E functions as a receptor ligand. The different isoforms have different affinities for the receptor and contribute to the variation in lipoprotein concentrations found within any population. Apolipoprotein E is found in association with the triacylglycerol-rich particles, chylomicrons and VLDL, and also in HDL. It is synthesized in many tissues, but the major source of apolipoprotein E in the plasma is probably the liver.

Box 8.2 Some important enzymes involved in lipoprotein metabolism

Lipoprotein lipase

This enzyme is found in a number of tissues outside the liver, particularly adipose tissue, skeletal muscle and heart muscle. Its role in lipid metabolism has already been discussed (in Sections 3.6.2.1 and 5.2.2.2). It is synthesized within the cells of the tissue (e.g. the adipocytes) and exported to the capillaries, where it is attached to the endothelial cells. Here it is bound (non-covalently) to highly negatively charged glycos-aminoglycan chains, such as heparan sulphate. Lipoprotein lipase acts on lipoprotein particles passing through the capillaries by hydrolysing triacylglycerol molecules to release non-esterified fatty acids which may be taken up into the tissue for esterification (and hence storage, mainly in adipose tissue) or oxidation (in muscle). It will only do this if the particles contain apolipoprotein C2 (see Box 8.1). Lipoprotein lipase activity in adipose tissue is stimulated by insulin, over a relatively long time-course (a few hours). In muscle it is slightly suppressed by insulin but its activity is increased by exercise (both acutely and by training).

Hepatic lipase

This enzyme is structurally related to lipoprotein lipase, but has a number of different characteristics. It does not require apolipoprotein C2 for activity, and it is present in the liver. It is more active against the smaller triacylglycerol-rich particles, whereas lipoprotein lipase is more active against the larger; the significance of this will be discussed below. In addition, it will hydrolyse both triacylglycerol and cholesteryl esters.

Lecithin–cholesterol acyltransferase

This enzyme comes from the liver and is found in the plasma. It associates with particles containing apolipoprotein A1 (which activates it). It transfers a fatty acid from position 2 of the phospholipid lecithin to unesterified cholesterol, thus forming a cholesteryl ester (see Figure 1.6 for the structures of these species).

---

lose more triacylglycerol each time. At the same time they lose some surface coat, by dissociating some unesterified cholesterol and phospholipid, and some apolipoproteins, which are taken up by other particles such as HDL.

The 'slimmed down' chylomicron particles are known as *chylomicron remnants*. They are relatively enriched in cholesteryl ester, since they have lost their triacylglycerol, and are potentially harmful (as discussed in Section 8.4.3). When they reach a certain size they become ligands for a receptor in the liver. The nature of this receptor is uncertain but it may be the α2-macroglobulin receptor — this is currently an area of intense research. Thus dietary triacylglycerol is delivered to the tissues, some unesterified cholesterol enters the HDL fraction, and some cholesteryl ester is delivered, in the remnant particles, to the liver.

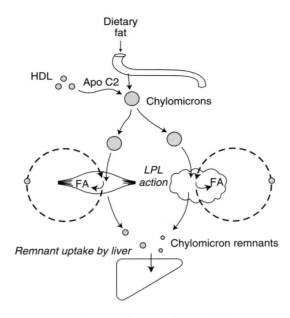

Figure 8.2   The exogenous pathway of lipoprotein metabolism
The dashed lines show that particles may pass through several cycles of hydrolysis by lipoprotein
lipase in capillary beds, shrinking each time eventually to produce a chylomicron remnant particle
that is taken up by specific receptors in the liver. Abbreviations used: Apo, apolipoprotein; FA,
fatty acids; LPL, lipoprotein lipase.

8.2.2   VLDL and LDL metabolism

8.2.2.1   VLDL metabolism: the endogenous pathway

In contrast with the metabolism of chylomicrons, the *endogenous pathway* of
lipoprotein metabolism distributes triacylglycerol from the liver to other
tissues. It is summarized in Figure 8.3. VLDL particles, secreted by the liver,
contain triacylglycerol, cholesteryl ester, apolipoprotein B100 and small
amounts of apolipoproteins E and C. They have a surface coat, like all lipoprotein particles, of phospholipids and unesterified cholesterol. The content of
apolipoproteins E and C rapidly increases in the plasma, by transfer from
other lipoproteins, mainly HDL.

VLDL particles are substrates for lipoprotein lipase in capillary beds, and
deliver triacylglycerol from the liver to other tissues. This is a means of distrib-
uting lipid energy to the tissues. Hydrolysis of the triacylglycerol core by
lipoprotein lipase leads to redundant surface material which is passed to other
particles, again mainly those of the HDL fraction. The cholesteryl ester-
enriched particles that result have two possible fates. (i) They may be taken up
directly by a receptor, in the liver and other tissues, which binds a homologous
region in apolipoprotein B100 and in apolipoprotein E. It is called the B/E
receptor or *LDL receptor*. Thus they deliver cholesteryl ester to tissues. (ii)
Alternatively, they may remain in the circulation, having shrunk through the

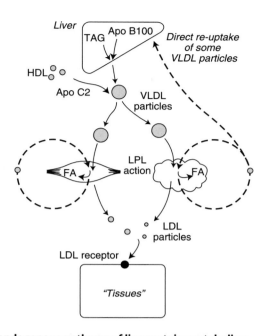

Figure 8.3   The endogenous pathway of lipoprotein metabolism
As in the exogenous pathway (Figure 8.2), particles may undergo several cycles of hydrolysis by
lipoprotein lipase (LPL) in capillary beds (dashed lines), forming smaller particles which may be
taken up directly by receptors in the liver; others remain in the circulation as LDL particles.
These are eventually removed by uptake into tissues via the B/E receptor or LDL receptor (see
Box 8.3).

action of lipoprotein lipase and hepatic lipase (which becomes more important
as the particles become smaller; see Box 8.2) until they have lost all surface
components, except apolipoprotein B100 and a shell of phospholipid and free
cholesterol, and have a core enriched in cholesteryl ester. In fact, they become
LDL particles. The LDL particle is therefore the 'VLDL remnant'.

8.2.2.2   LDL metabolism and regulation of cellular cholesterol content
LDL particles have a relatively long half-life in the circulation — about 3 days.
During this time they are relatively stable metabolically. They leave the circulation mainly through uptake into various tissues by the LDL receptor (Box
8.3), and deliver cholesterol to tissues.

The cellular content of cholesterol is thus increased in those tissues that
take up LDL particles. This has two effects. First, biosynthesis of cholesterol,
which can occur in all nucleated cells, is suppressed, primarily by suppression
of the enzyme *hydroxymethylglutaryl-CoA reductase* (HMG-CoA reductase;
EC 1.1.1.88). Secondly, synthesis of new LDL receptors is itself suppressed,
and the number of receptors expressed on the cell surface is reduced.
Therefore, the increase in cellular cholesterol content caused by uptake of
LDL-cholesterol by the LDL receptor is self-limiting (Box 8.3).

Box 8.3 The LDL receptor and regulation of cellular cholesterol content

The LDL receptor is a protein of M_r 120000 which spans the cell membrane; it has a short intracellular domain and a long extracellular domain, terminating in the ligand-binding N-terminus. It is expressed in most nucleated cells, but LDL uptake is particularly active in the liver and in some tissues which need cholesterol for particular biosynthetic purposes — e.g. the adrenal glands and ovaries, where it serves as a precursor for steroid hormone synthesis.

LDL particles bind to the receptor, which is then internalized by endocytosis. The cholesteryl ester contained in the LDL particle is hydrolysed in the lysosomes, thus liberating cholesterol, which forms part of the cellular cholesterol pool. This is used for incorporation into membranes (see Figure 1.5), for synthesis of steroid hormones, and, in the liver, for synthesis of bile acids and formation of VLDL. In addition, some is re-esterified to form cholesteryl esters, which can be removed from the cell by incorporation into HDL (see text).

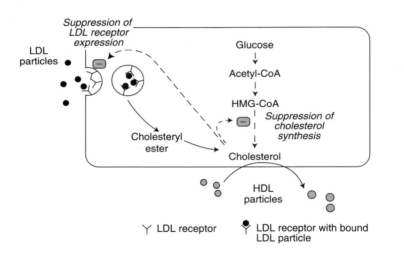

The cellular content of cholesterol is closely regulated, in two ways, described in more detail in the text: an increase in the cellular cholesterol pool (i) decreases the synthesis of LDL receptors, and (ii) suppresses cholesterol synthesis, primarily by repression of the synthesis of the regulatory enzyme HMG-CoA reductase.

There is an important variation on this theme. Some cells, particularly macrophages, express different receptors which take up LDL particles. One of these alternative receptors is known as the *scavenger receptor*. These receptors are not subject to down-regulation like the true LDL receptor, and, therefore, especially in people with a high plasma LDL-cholesterol concentration, the macrophages may become excessively cholesterol-laden. This can be the beginning of the process of *atherosclerosis*: deposition of fatty material in the arterial wall, which leads to narrowing of an artery and potential blockage.

8.2.3 HDL metabolism

Whereas LDL particles regulate the cholesterol content of cells by delivering cholesterol, HDL particles bring about the opposite process: the removal of cholesterol, which is transported to the liver for ultimate excretion.

8.2.3.1 HDL and reverse cholesterol transport

HDL particles begin their life as so-called discoidal HDL secreted by the liver. The discoidal particles consist mainly of phospholipid and apolipoprotein A1. They receive unesterified cholesterol which is released as 'excess surface material' during the action of lipoprotein lipase on the triacylglycerol-rich lipoproteins. They also pick up unesterified cholesterol by interaction with cells, possibly via a specific receptor, although this is still unclear. By this means, HDL particles remove cholesterol from cells. Unesterified cholesterol is esterified by the action of the plasma enzyme *lecithin–cholesterol acyltransferase* (LCAT; EC 2.3.1.43), which is activated by apolipoprotein A1. Thus the particles acquire a core of hydrophobic cholesteryl esters, and become spherical rather than discoidal.

The HDL fraction is not homogeneous. The spherical, relatively large cholesteryl ester-enriched particles are known as HDL_2. Their cholesteryl ester can be taken up by the liver by a number of mechanisms. There may be receptor-mediated uptake of large HDL particles which contain apolipoprotein E. In addition, there seems to be hepatic uptake of cholesteryl ester from the larger HDL particles, perhaps involving hydrolysis of cholesteryl ester by hepatic lipase. Some of the cholesteryl ester from larger HDL particles is also transferred to the triacylglycerol-rich lipoproteins (this mechanism is discussed further in Section 8.2.3.2). The smaller HDL particles that result are known as HDL_3 and are ready to accept further cholesterol from peripheral tissues.

Thus cholesterol is transferred from peripheral tissues to the liver, from where it can be excreted as cholesterol and as bile salts in the bile (see Box 2.1 and Box 8.4). This process of removal of cholesterol from the tissues, transport to the liver and ultimate excretion from the body is the opposite of the delivery of cholesterol by LDL: it is known as *reverse cholesterol transport* (Figure 8.4).

8.2.3.2 Cholesteryl ester-transfer protein

A circulating protein known as *cholesteryl ester-transfer protein* (CETP) catalyses the exchange of hydrophobic lipids, i.e. cholesteryl esters and triacylglycerol, between lipoprotein particles (Figure 8.5). They seem to exchange by facilitated diffusion along concentration gradients. When the plasma concen-

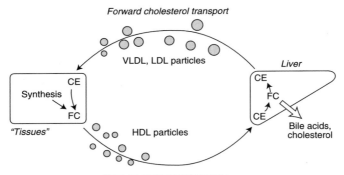

Figure 8.4   Forward and reverse cholesterol transport
Cholesterol is secreted by the liver in VLDL particles; these become LDL particles after hydrolysis of their triacylglycerol by lipoprotein lipase and hepatic lipase (see Figure 8.3) and are taken up by tissues. Cholesterol is removed from peripheral tissues by HDL particles. At first, it is in the form of free (unesterified) cholesterol (FC), but it is esterified by the action of lecithin–cholesterol acyltransferase (LCAT; Box 8.2), forming cholesteryl esters (CEs). This cholesterol is transferred to the liver and may be excreted in the bile. More detail of reverse cholesterol transport is shown in Figure 8.5.

tration of triacylglycerol is high, e.g. after a meal when triacylglycerol-laden chylomicrons are present, CETP will catalyse exchange of cholesteryl ester from HDL to chylomicrons, while triacylglycerol moves in the opposite direction. The cholesteryl esters remain with the chylomicron particle until it is taken up by the liver as a chylomicron remnant. The HDL has now become

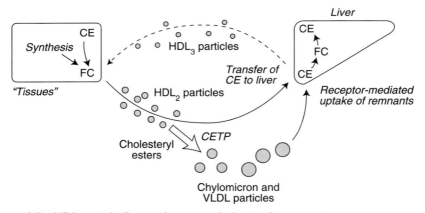

Figure 8.5   HDL metabolism and reverse cholesterol transport
Small HDL particles pick up free cholesterol (FC) from tissues. (Recent evidence suggests that this may be mediated by free apolipoprotein AI.) It is esterified by LCAT to form cholesteryl ester (CE), which makes the spherical, CE-enriched particles known as HDL$_2$. Some of the CEs may be exchanged for triacylglycerol with the triacylglycerol-rich lipoproteins, mediated by cholesteryl ester-transfer protein (CETP). HDL$_2$ particles deliver their CE to the liver and the smaller particles which result are known as HDL$_3$; they may then begin the cycle again. The triacylglycerol acquired through CETP action is removed by the action of hepatic lipase. The CE-enriched chylomicron remnants are taken up directly by receptors in the liver.

Box 8.4 Cholesterol homoeostasis in the body

The body pool of cholesterol is about 140 g. Of this, about 8 g is present in the plasma, mainly in LDL.

About 1 g of cholesterol enters the body pool each day, 400 mg from intestinal absorption and 600 mg from biosynthesis, i.e. there is <1% turnover per day of the body cholesterol pool. Note that this does not conflict with the figure of 1 g of cholesterol per day in the diet given in Table 2.1, since cholesterol absorption is incomplete.

There is a turnover of about 5 g of plasma cholesterol per day. Cholesterol enters the plasma in chylomicrons and VLDL particles, and from tissues into HDL, and leaves in the form of chylomicron-remnants, VLDL particles, LDL particles and by removal from HDL.

There is also turnover of cholesterol in the enterohepatic circulation (see Box 2.1). Bile salts, formed from cholesterol in the liver, are secreted in the bile and largely re-absorbed in the ileum. The total pool of 2.5–4 g of bile acids is recycled about twice with each meal, i.e. the turnover is rapid: about 18 g/day leaves in the bile and about 90% of this is reabsorbed. Cholesterol is also secreted in the bile, at a rate of about 1 g/day; of this, about one-half is re-absorbed and the remainder is lost in the faeces.

The enterohepatic circulation may be interrupted by a resin, such as *cholestyramine* or *cholestipol*, that binds the bile acids, prevents their re-absorption and leads to their excretion in faeces. More cholesterol is converted to bile acids to keep the total amount constant. If completely efficient, this treatment could lead to the loss of about 18 g of cholesterol each day — many times the normal turnover rate of the body cholesterol pool. It can thus help to lower the plasma cholesterol concentration. However, the powerful feedback control of cellular cholesterol content on HMG-CoA reductase will minimize its effect.

Data for this box taken from Newsholme & Leech (1983), Hunt & Groff (1990) and Lewis (1990).

---

enriched with triacylglycerol. This HDL-triacylglycerol can be hydrolysed by hepatic lipase to give smaller, cholesteryl ester-depleted HDL_3 particles which can then pick up further cholesterol from cells as outlined in the previous section.

In terms of defence against coronary heart disease this may sound like a beneficial process. Unfortunately, things are not so simple. Some species, such as the rat, do not have CETP activity, and do not suffer from atherosclerosis. Some families have been described in whom CETP is lacking; they have high HDL-cholesterol concentrations and appear to be protected against atherosclerosis. Probably the culprit is the cholesteryl ester-enriched chylomicron particle which results from CETP action. This will be considered again later.

8.3   Regulation of lipoprotein metabolism

The pathways of lipoprotein metabolism are regulated at many stages. Insulin plays a major role.

8.3.1   Insulin and triacylglycerol metabolism

Lipoprotein lipase is activated in adipose tissue by insulin (see Section 3.6.2.1). Thus, in the post-prandial period, clearance of the triacylglycerol-rich lipoproteins is increased, and this occurs at the peak of triacylglycerol concentration in plasma, a few hours after a fatty meal. The removal of chylomicron-triacylglycerol is a saturable process, and after a fat-rich meal it becomes saturated. Both chylomicrons and VLDL compete for hydrolysis by lipoprotein lipase, a process which has been termed the *common saturable removal mechanism*. For reasons that are not entirely clear, lipoprotein lipase acts preferentially on larger particles, so chylomicrons tend to 'win'. One corollary of this competition is that the rapidity of clearance of excess triacylglycerol from the plasma in the post-prandial period is dependent upon the subject's VLDL-triacylglycerol concentration: in someone with a low VLDL-triacylglycerol concentration, the clearance of triacylglycerol after a meal tends to be more rapid. Because of the competition between chylomicron-triacylglycerol and VLDL-triacylglycerol for hydrolysis by lipoprotein lipase, the VLDL-triacylglycerol concentration usually rises after a fatty meal.

It is probably beneficial to the individual to be able to clear excess triacylglycerol rapidly from the plasma after a meal (see Section 8.4.3). Thus it makes sense for the body not to add extra VLDL-triacylglycerol to the plasma in this period. A number of studies of hepatocytes *in vitro* have shown that insulin suppresses VLDL output in the short term. These studies are very difficult to perform *in vivo*, but it seems reasonable to suppose that hepatic VLDL-triacylglycerol secretion is suppressed by insulin in the post-prandial period. In addition, the rate of VLDL-triacylglycerol secretion depends strongly on the delivery of non-esterified fatty acids from the plasma as a substrate for triacylglycerol synthesis. These are taken up by hepatocytes and esterified for secretion as VLDL-triacylglycerol. As we saw in Chapter 5 (Figure 5.9), the concentration of non-esterified fatty acids in plasma falls after a meal owing to suppression of adipose tissue lipolysis by insulin. Therefore, VLDL-triacylglycerol secretion is again inhibited in this period.

8.3.2   Relationship between plasma triacylglycerol and HDL-
cholesterol concentrations

In studies of large numbers of individuals, an inverse relationship is usually observed between plasma triacylglycerol and HDL-cholesterol concentrations: the higher the subject's plasma triacylglycerol concentration, the lower tends to be the HDL-cholesterol concentration. We can now see how this inverse relationship is brought about.

Because hydrolysis of triacylglycerol-rich lipoproteins by lipoprotein lipase is accompanied by the transfer of cholesterol and other surface components into HDL, the HDL concentration can be increased by rapid lipoprotein lipase action in the post-prandial period. On the other hand, if removal of triacylglycerol is slow, then there will be increased opportunity for lipid exchange via the action of CETP. Thus HDL will become depleted of cholesteryl esters, and the triacylglycerol-rich lipoprotein remnants will become enriched with them. Again, the inverse relationship between plasma triacylglycerol and HDL-cholesterol concentrations will result.

8.3.3   Cholesterol homoeostasis

There is continuous turnover of the body's pool of about 140 g of cholesterol (free and esterified): see Box 8.4.

Insulin may regulate cholesterol turnover at a number of points. Insulin activates HMG-CoA reductase by reversible dephosphorylation and thus increases cholesterol synthesis; however, this effect is probably over-ridden by the control by cellular cholesterol content (see Section 8.2.2.2). Insulin also seems to stimulate expression of the LDL receptor; during insulin infusion, in an experimental situation, removal of LDL-cholesterol is increased, an effect which has been demonstrated in hepatocyte cultures *in vitro*. It is not known whether this occurs in all tissues or just in the liver. However, hormonal effects on cholesterol homoeostasis do not seem to be of major importance.

8.4   Disturbances of lipoprotein metabolism

8.4.1   Cholesterol and atherosclerosis

Lipoprotein metabolism has come to prominence because of its link with coronary heart disease. Coronary heart disease means a blockage — partial or complete — of one or more of the *coronary arteries* which supply blood to the muscular walls of the heart (the *myocardium*) (see Section 3.5). It arises initially because of the development of fatty deposits in the arterial wall (atherosclerosis), which may affect arteries anywhere in the body, and can lead to impaired blood supply to the limbs, for instance — a particular problem in heavy smokers. When it affects the blood supply to the heart the results can be fatal. At first, the restriction on blood supply to the myocardium may appear as chest pains (*angina*) during exercise, when the demand on the myocardium increases. Later, complete blockage may occur as the result of a blood clot at the site of the atherosclerotic lesion — this is a *coronary thrombosis*, or heart attack, or *myocardial infarction*. The region of myocardium supplied by the artery may necrose (die). More importantly in the short term, local disturbances to contraction of the heart can lead to disturbances in the electrical coordination of contraction, and the heart may go into uncoordinated fluttering (*ventricular fibrillation*) or complete stoppage (*asystole* or *cardiac arrest*). This is a serious situation with high mortality.

The fatty deposit is known as an *atherosclerotic plaque*. It is a complex structure, which involves proliferation of the smooth muscle cells of the arterial wall and connective tissue (collagen fibrils), and deposition of cholesterol-rich lipid. It is thought to begin as a smaller lesion called the *fatty streak*; this is a fatty deposit which is one of the earliest visible signs of the development of atherosclerosis. The fatty streak arises from the accumulation of so-called *foam cells*, macrophages which, under light microscopy, appear to be laden with foam from an accumulation of lipid, mainly cholesterol. Cholesterol accumulation is thus one of the first events in the development of atherosclerosis.

The link between cholesterol in the blood and coronary heart disease was recognized in part because the incidence of coronary heart disease varies widely from one country to another; in Finland, for instance, the incidence is almost ten times that in Japan. The average concentration of blood cholesterol also varies widely from country to country, and it varies almost exactly in parallel with the incidence of coronary heart disease (Figure 8.6). Within any one country, the incidence of coronary heart disease also varies with the plasma cholesterol concentration. These are epidemiological findings and we must be careful how we interpret them — perhaps a high plasma cholesterol concentration leads to the development of coronary heart disease, but it might be equally valid to suggest that people with coronary heart disease for some reason develop a high plasma cholesterol concentration. However, a number of long-term studies of the effects of lowering plasma cholesterol concentration in people at high risk of coronary heart disease have shown that lowering the cholesterol concentration reduces the risk of coronary heart disease.

8.4.2 Conditions which lead to elevation of lipid blood concentrations

The average concentration of blood cholesterol in the U.K. is about 6 mmol/l, of which the majority — around 4 mmol/l — is carried in the LDL fraction. The average concentration of triacylglycerol in the blood after an overnight fast is about 1–2 mmol/l. An elevated concentration of lipids in the blood is referred to as *hyperlipidaemia*. Usually this means an elevation of the cholesterol concentration, since there is more cholesterol than triacylglycerol. When it is necessary to distinguish the contribution of different lipids, elevation of the cholesterol concentration is known as *hypercholesterolaemia*, elevation of the triacylglycerol concentration as *hypertriglyceridaemia*. (Triacylglycerol has replaced the older term triglyceride, but physicians are not quite ready to battle with hypertriacylglycerolaemia.)

The blood lipid concentration may be elevated because of a genetic disposition (*primary hyperlipidaemia*) or because of environmental factors — diet, lifestyle, other diseases etc. (*secondary hyperlidaemia*). An alternative classification is based on the phenotype without consideration of the underlying cause, although often the underlying cause may be inferred from the phenotype (Table 8.2).

8.4.2.1 Primary hyperlipoproteinaemias

The most dramatic primary hyperlipidaemias are those known as *familial hypercholesterolaemia* (FH), a hereditary elevation of the blood cholesterol concentration, and Type I hyperlipoproteinaemia (Table 8.2) or *chylomicron-aemia syndrome*.

FH is manifested by a consistently raised blood cholesterol concentration, typically 8–10 mmol/l in people heterozygous for the disease, but closer to 15–20 mmol/l in people who are homozygous (i.e. who have two copies of the gene which causes it). The incidence of coronary heart disease in such people is very high unless they are adequately treated to lower the cholesterol concentration. This is another reason for believing that there is a direct cause-and-effect link between elevated blood cholesterol concentration and development of atherosclerosis. The defect in FH is in the amino acid sequence of the LDL receptor: the receptor does not bind LDL particles normally and they remain in the circulation. Recently, a few cases have been discovered in which a defect in the sequence of apolipoprotein B produces a very similar syndrome. Because lipoprotein cholesterol is not taken up into cells, the pathway of cholesterol synthesis is not repressed, and this adds to the problem. The preferred form of treatment is the use of drugs (the *statins*) which inhibit the pathway of cholesterol synthesis at the enzyme HMG-CoA reductase. A low-cholesterol diet also helps, as do substances (resins) which bind cholesterol and bile salts in the intestine, and prevent their re-absorption (see Box 8.4).

Type I hyperlipoproteinaemia is also an inherited condition, in which chylomicrons accumulate in the plasma, giving it a creamy appearance. The major abnormality, unlike in FH, is accumulation of triacylglycerol rather than cholesterol. The plasma triacylglycerol concentration may reach 50 or even 100 mmol/l. Interestingly, people with this condition are not at increased risk of coronary heart disease, and it is believed that hypertriglyceridaemia is not, in itself, a risk factor for coronary heart disease. People with hypertriglyceridaemia are at risk of inflammation of the pancreas (*pancreatitis*). This can be very serious: if the pancreatic juices, with their potent digestive enzymes, leak into the abdominal cavity, the results can be life-threatening. So the disease must be treated, but this can be done very effectively by means of a low-fat diet: without dietary fat, chylomicrons do not accumulate. The defect in type I hyperlipoproteinaemia is usually a deficiency in the enzyme lipoprotein lipase. The condition is usually only noticed in people who are homozygous for the defect; heterozygotes have sufficient lipoprotein lipase activity to remove chylomicrons relatively normally. In a few cases, the lipoprotein lipase is

Table 8.2 The classification of hyperlipidaemias according to phenotype

Type	Plasma cholesterol	Plasma triacylglycerol	Particles accumulating	Usual underlying defect
I	+	+++	Chylomicrons	Lipoprotein lipase deficiency, apolipoprotein CII deficiency
IIa	++	N	LDL	LDL receptor defect or LDL overproduction
IIb	++	++	VLDL, LDL	VLDL or LDL overproduction or impaired clearance
III	+	++	Chylomicron- and VLDL-remnants	Impaired remnant removal; may be due to particular isoform of apolipoprotein E, or apolipoprotein E deficiency
IV	N or +	++	VLDL	VLDL overproduction or clearance defect
V	+	+++	Chylomicrons, VLDL and remnants	Lipoprotein lipase defect (not complete absence) or apolipoprotein CII deficiency

This is known as the Fredrickson classification. N, normal; +, mildly raised; ++, moderately raised; +++, severely raised.

normal, but the sufferers lack apolipoprotein C2, the essential co-factor for lipoprotein lipase activity.

8.4.2.2 Secondary hyperlipoproteinaemias

Secondary hyperlipidaemias arise because of diet, bodily factors (e.g. obesity) or other diseases (e.g. diabetes mellitus). Here, we will look briefly only at the first of these. The effects of obesity and diabetes will be covered in the Chapters 9 and 10.

The average blood cholesterol concentration varies widely from country to country (see Figure 8.6). This might reflect racial genetic differences, but does not seem to. Japanese people who have moved to the U.S.A. have cholesterol concentrations and rates of coronary heart disease which are as high as, or even higher than, those of other Americans. Something in the Japanese lifestyle (in Japan) keeps the cholesterol concentration low, and the evidence suggests that this is a dietary factor (Box 8.5)

As Box 8.5 makes clear, dietary fatty acids play a much more important role in determining serum cholesterol concentration than does dietary cholesterol. The means by which individual fatty acids affect the plasma cholesterol concentration are not entirely clear, although two mechanisms are probably involved. (i) It appears that saturated fatty acids in the liver affect the distribution of hepatic cholesterol between unesterified and esterified forms. In the presence of saturated fatty acids, there is less conversion of unesterified

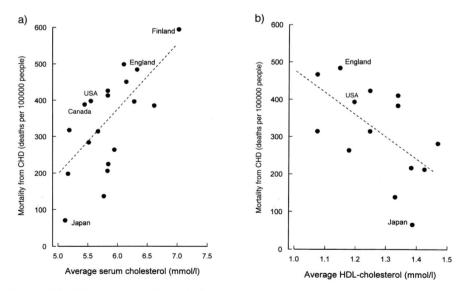

Figure 8.6 Cholesterol and heart disease
(a) The relationship between average serum cholesterol concentration and mortality from coronary heart disease in males in different countries. (b) The inverse relationship between average serum HDL-cholesterol concentration and mortality from coronary heart disease in males in different countries. The dashed lines are the regression lines. Based on Simons (1986).

Box 8.5 Dietary influences on the serum cholesterol concentration
Dietary cholesterol

The amount of dietary cholesterol is not a major factor which affects blood cholesterol concentration. We eat perhaps 1 g of cholesterol per day (see Table 2.1), whereas the amount of cholesterol in the body is approx. 140 g, of which about 8 g is in the plasma. In contrast, we eat several 'plasma's-worth' of glucose in a single meal (see Section 5.1). Cholesterol is not rapidly absorbed like glucose: it enters the plasma slowly, like triacylglycerol. Further, cholesterol intake leads to cholesterol entry into cells, which effectively suppresses cholesterol synthesis. For people with familial hypercholesterolaemia, a low-cholesterol diet will help, but for most people the blood cholesterol concentration is related far more closely to the dietary intake of saturated fatty acids.

Dietary fatty acids

The initial evidence for the role of saturated fatty acids in raising serum cholesterol concentrations was epidemiological: the wide differences in average plasma cholesterol concentration between different countries were found to relate to the average consumption of saturated fatty acids. More detailed studies since have shown that this is an over-generalization. Particular saturated fatty acids are worse 'culprits' than others: stearic acid ($C_{18:0}$) seems to be relatively inert, whereas palmitic acid ($C_{16:0}$) and myristic acid ($C_{14:0}$) raise the cholesterol concentration. Mono-unsaturated acids — of which oleic acid ($C_{18:1}$), found in olive oil, is the most common example in the diet — are relatively neutral, whereas polyunsaturated fatty acids, e.g. linoleic acid ($C_{18:2}$) and linolenic acid ($C_{18:3}$), have a cholesterol-lowering effect.

A change in the fatty acid content of the diet will produce a fairly predictable change in serum cholesterol concentration, and formulae have been derived to predict this e.g.: ☞

---

cholesterol to cholesteryl esters. Since it is the tissue unesterified cholesterol content that down-regulates LDL receptor expression, this change leads to decreased expression of hepatic LDL receptors, and thus an elevation of the plasma LDL concentration. (ii) Lipoprotein lipase has preferences for certain fatty acids at certain positions in triacylglycerol molecules. It acts more slowly on triacylglycerol molecules with a saturated fatty acid in the middle (C-2) position. Therefore, clearance of lipoprotein particles which contain saturated fatty acids may be impaired, and this may lead to direction of the lipoprotein particle remnants into different pathways or tissues than might have happened had they been cleared more rapidly. But this is not fully understood.

8.4.3   HDL-cholesterol, plasma triacylglycerol and coronary heart disease

In studies of large numbers of people, an inverse relationship has been observed between plasma triacylglycerol and HDL-cholesterol concentrations. It is also evident from such studies that, unlike LDL-cholesterol, elevated HDL-cholesterol concentrations are associated with decreased risk of

---

Box 8.5 (continued)

☞ Δ serum cholesterol = 0.026 × (2.16ΔS − 1.65ΔP + 6.66ΔC − 0.53)

where Δserum cholesterol represents the change in serum cholesterol concentration (mmol/l), ΔS the change in dietary saturated fatty acids (expressed as percentage of energy derived from them), ΔP the change in dietary polyunsaturated fatty acids, and ΔC the change in dietary cholesterol (in 100 mg/day). The factor 0.026 converts from mg/dl to mmol/l. (From Hegsted et al., 1965).

The important point is that dietary saturated fatty acids have a larger detrimental effect than the beneficial effect of polyunsaturated fatty acids (the factor for ΔS in the equation is greater than that for ΔP); hence the advice to change from dairy products such as butter, which contain a high proportion of saturated fatty acids, to spreads based on vegetable oils which contain more unsaturated fats.

A few points should be stressed. (i) Such a change alone may make an insignificant difference to coronary heart disease risk in any one individual, and other lifestyle factors (e.g. smoking, physical activity, body weight) may need to be modified as well to influence the risk. (ii) Many people are misled into thinking that spreads containing unsaturated fatty acids are less fattening than dairy products: this is not so. (iii) Recently another worry has emerged. Margarines are made by hardening unsaturated vegetable oils by the process of hydrogenation — reduction of some of the double bonds. (Remember from Chapter 2 that saturated fatty acids have higher melting points.) In this process, some of the double-bonds are converted to the *trans-* configuration rather than the usual *cis-*. There is now some evidence that *trans*-unsaturated fatty acids may themselves predispose to coronary heart disease.

---

coronary heart disease (Figure 8.6). Thus, because of the inverse relationship between plasma triacylglycerol and HDL-cholesterol concentrations, elevated plasma triacylglycerol concentrations are associated with increased risk of coronary heart disease. These relationships with coronary heart disease are not so clear-cut as those for LDL-cholesterol: for instance, people with extremely elevated plasma triacylglycerol concentrations in lipoprotein lipase deficiency do not have increased risk of coronary heart disease.

We have seen already (Section 8.2.3) how the inverse relationship between HDL-cholesterol and plasma triacylglycerol concentrations may be brought about. There are two lines of thought about their relationships with coronary heart disease risk. First, HDL-cholesterol may in itself be associated with protection against coronary heart disease. This may reflect the fact that it is a marker of the efficiency of reverse cholesterol transport, the removal of cholesterol from tissues. Alternatively, low HDL-cholesterol concentrations (and thus increased risk) may be a marker for some defect in the metabolism of the triacylglycerol-rich lipoproteins. One implication of this is that their remnant particles remain for longer in the circulation, while they are reduced to a sufficiently small size for receptor-mediated uptake. These remnants themselves may be taken up to initiate the formation of atherosclerotic lesions. In the case of VLDL, this is already clear since the VLDL remnant is the LDL particle. But the chylomicron remnant particle has attracted much suspicion, not least because one chylomicron particle may contain 30 times as many cholesterol molecules (free and unesterified) as a typical LDL particle (chylomicron, 60000; LDL particle, 2000).

The idea that chylomicron remnant particles have atherogenic potential explains neatly why people with lipoprotein lipase deficiency and enormously elevated plasma triacylglycerol concentrations are not at risk of coronary heart disease; if their particles are not metabolized at all, no smaller remnants will be produced. In this view, a 'sluggish' metabolism of the triacylglycerol-rich lipoproteins is worse than none at all. Such a condition may result from a genetic change in the lipoprotein lipase sequence, such that the enzyme is less effective than normal. Alternatively, it may reflect an increased concentration of VLDL-triacylglycerol which will prevent efficient clearance of chylomicron-triacylglycerol because of competition for lipoprotein lipase. This may result, in turn, from increased hepatic VLDL synthesis or impaired clearance. These are areas of current research.

Suggestions for further reading

General reviews of lipid and lipoprotein metabolism
Gurr, M.I. (1988) Lipid metabolism in man. *Proc. Nutr. Soc.* **47**, 277–285

Exogenous and endogenous pathways of lipoprotein metabolism
Sethi, S., Gibney, M.J. & Williams, C.M. (1993) Postprandial lipid metabolism. *Nutr. Res. Rev.* **6**, 161–183

Gibbons, G.F. (1990) Assembly and secretion of hepatic very-low-density lipoprotein. *Biochem. J.* **268**, 1–13

LDL metabolism, receptors and cholesterol homoeostasis
Dietschy, J.M., Turley, S.D. & Spady, D.K. (1993) Role of liver in the maintenance of cholesterol and low density lipoprotein homeostasis in different animal species, including humans. *J. Lipid Res.* **34**, 1637–1659

Fielding, C.J. (1992) Lipoprotein receptors, plasma cholesterol metabolism, and the regulation of cellular free cholesterol concentration. *FASEB J.* **6**, 3162–3168

Soutar, A.K. & Knight, B.L. (1990) Structure and regulation of the LDL-receptor and its gene. *Br. Med. Bull.* **46**, 891–916

HDL metabolism and cholesteryl ester-transfer protein

Swenson, T.L. (1991) The role of the cholesteryl ester transfer protein in lipoprotein metabolism. *Diabetes Metab. Rev.* **7**, 139–153

Tall, A.R. (1993) Plasma cholesteryl ester transfer protein. *J. Lipid Res.* **34**, 1255–1274

Tall, A.R. (1993) Plasma high-density lipoproteins: metabolism and relationship to atherogenesis. *J. Clin. Invest.* **86**, 379–384

Disorders of lipoprotein metabolism and atherosclerosis

Thompson, G.R. (1990) Primary hyperlipidaemia. *Br. Med. Bull.* **46**, 986–1004

Durrington, P.N. (1990) Secondary hyperlipidaemia. *Br. Med. Bull.* **46**, 1005–1024

Havel, R. (1994) McCollum Award Lecture, 1993: Triglyceride-rich lipoproteins and atherosclerosis: new perspectives. *Am. J. Clin. Nutr.* **59**, 795–799

9

Diabetes mellitus

9.1   Different types of diabetes

The disease *diabetes mellitus*, if untreated, is characterized by intense thirst and frequent urination; hence its name diabetes, from the Greek for syphon. The term mellitus means 'to do with honey', i.e. sweet. It refers to the fact that the urine is sticky and sweet with glucose. There is a completely different, and much rarer, disease called *diabetes insipidus*, which is also characterized by thirst and frequent urination, but the urine is insipid, i.e. watery and not sweet. Diabetes insipidus is caused by a failure of the *antidiuretic hormone* (*vaso-pressin*; see Section 4.3.2) to act, either because of a lack of the hormone, or because of a defect in its receptors in the kidney. Diabetes insipidus will not be considered further here.

Diabetes mellitus (which will be referred to simply as diabetes) can be divided into two types (Table 9.1). One form of the disease usually develops during childhood or adolescence. The sufferers tend to be on the thin side. (Note: most people with diabetes lead relatively normal lives and would not like the term 'sufferer'.) In this type of diabetes, lack of treatment leads to severe illness and the only effective treatment is injection of the hormone insulin. This is known as *insulin-dependent diabetes mellitus* (IDDM). The other, more common form of the disease usually starts later in life — from the mid-thirties onwards. Those who develop this form are very often overweight. This form is not life-threatening in the short term, even if not treated, and adequate treatment does not require use of insulin. But it is a mistake to think of this as a milder form of diabetes; as we shall see, the longer-term conse-quences of lack of treatment are just as severe as those of IDDM. This form is known as *non-insulin-dependent diabetes mellitus* (NIDDM).

Table 9.1 Different forms of diabetes mellitus

	Insulin-dependent diabetes mellitus	Non-insulin-dependent diabetes mellitus
Other names	Juvenile-onset diabetes; type I diabetes	Maturity-onset diabetes; type 2 diabetes
Defect	Auto-immune destruction of β-cells	Defective insulin secretion and insulin resistance
Age of onset (typical)	1–25 years	>40 years
Bodily physique (typical)	Lean (weight loss at diagnosis)	Obese
Prevalence (whole population)	0.5%	2%
Inheritance	~50%	~70–80%
Treatment	Insulin injections	Diet; drugs

9.2 History of the study of diabetes and clinical features

9.2.1 History of diabetes

Diabetes mellitus has been described since antiquity. The earliest known record is in an Egyptian papyrus dating from around 1500 BC. The Greek physician Aretaeus of Cappadocia named the disease in the first century AD and described the short and painful life of sufferers: "...it consists in the flesh and bones running together into urine; the patients are tortured with an unquenchable thirst; the whole body wastes away...". It is often claimed that the English physician, Thomas Willis, was the first to notice the sweet taste of the urine in 1679, but this fact is actually recorded in much earlier writings from the East. Indian medical writings, for instance, noted that ants find a particular interest in the urine of diabetics. The same writings also distinguished the two types of patient: young and thin, or older and overweight.

Important milestones in understanding the disease occurred in the nineteenth century: the discovery of the islets of Langerhans in the pancreas in 1869 (see Section 4.2.1), and the observation by Oskar Minkowski and Joseph von Mering in Strasbourg in 1889 that removal of a dog's pancreas led to diabetes. This was a chance observation, made while they investigated the role of the pancreas in fat absorption. Minkowski and von Mering also noted that if they attached a small piece of pancreas to the inside of the abdominal cavity, the dog did not develop diabetes; this led to the idea that the pancreas produced a substance that was essential for normal metabolism. The name insulin (from the Latin *insula*, meaning island) was given to this hypothetical substance by the English physiologist Edward Sharpey-Schafer in 1916. By that time, a link between diabetes and the destruction of the pancreatic islets was suspected. This was based partly on the observations of an American pathologist, Eugene Opie, at the turn of the century; Opie noticed that the islets were destroyed in the pancreas of patients who had died of diabetes. In 1921 in Toronto, Frederick Banting and Charles Best, a medical student assisting him, made an extract of pancreas which, when injected into a dog (called Marjorie) that had been made diabetic by removal of her pancreas, restored her to health. Production of this extract from the pancreases of cows and pigs was increased as rapidly as possible and it was soon made available (at first in small quantities) for treatment of human sufferers. The first person to be treated was a 14-year-old boy, Leonard Thompson. For such people it was a life-saving treatment (Figure 9.1).

9.2.2 Insulin-dependent diabetes mellitus

IDDM results from destruction of the insulin-secreting cells of the islets of Langerhans. This destruction is auto-immune in nature, i.e. it is brought about by the body's own natural defences, but directed against one of its own tissues. The liability to develop IDDM is to some extent inherited; however, among

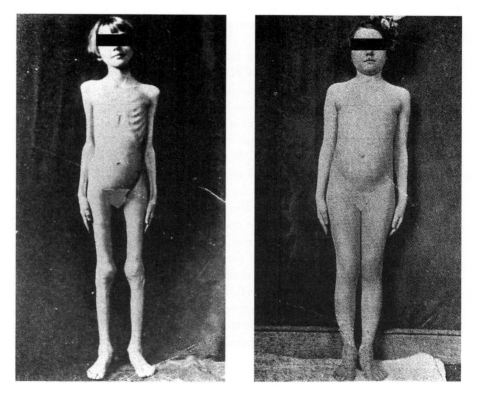

Figure 9.1   A patient with IDDM in the early days of insulin therapy, before (left) and after (right) treatment with insulin
Reproduced from Bliss (1983) with permission.

identical twins (who have the same genetic complement), if one has IDDM, only around 40% of their twins will have the disease.[1] Thus something in the environment must set the disease process in motion. There are a number of theories about what this trigger might be, including a belief that the trigger is a viral infection. Some people also believe that a traumatic episode can trigger the onset of diabetes. However, none of these theories has been proven. What is clear is that the metabolic changes in IDDM essentially represent a deficiency of insulin, and can largely be treated by injection of insulin. IDDM is not a very common disease; it is present in about 0.5% of the population in the U.K., and rather less in warmer parts of the world. However, the incidence of IDDM is increasing in some parts of the world, including the U.K. and particularly Scandinavia.

9.2.3   Non-insulin-dependent diabetes mellitus

NIDDM does not result so clearly from insulin deficiency. Defects in insulin secretion in people with NIDDM can be unmasked by laboratory tests: in particular, the initial phase of insulin secretion in response to a glucose load appears to be defective at an early stage in the disease. However, the prominent defect in NIDDM is not so much an absolute deficiency of insulin as a failure of insulin, at relatively normal concentrations, to exert its normal effects: this condition is known as *insulin resistance* (Figure 9.2).

Insulin resistance is a prominent feature of obesity. One very plausible hypothesis for the development of NIDDM is as follows. When people become obese, their tissues become resistant to the actions of insulin. Therefore, the concentration of glucose in the blood increases, initially only a little, and insulin is released in greater quantities from the pancreas. In obese subjects, the concentration of plasma insulin, and its response to a glucose load, are actually greater than normal. Some people can maintain this increased insulin secretion throughout their life and carry on as obese, but non-diabetic, individuals. In others, however, who are predisposed genetically, the ability of the islets to sustain high rates of insulin production begins to fail. Therefore, insulin levels fall: at first to less than necessary, so the glucose concentration rises somewhat; then to around normal, albeit with an elevated glucose concentration; and in the later stages of the disease to less than normal. Insulin resistance is still prominent. The result is frank, clinical diabetes. [This hypothesis for the development of NIDDM is explained fully in Felber *et al.* (1993).] However, because some pancreatic insulin secretion remains, these people do not usually need insulin for treatment. In those who manage to lose considerable amounts of weight (especially early in the disease) the diabetes

---

[1]*Figures vary from 36% to 54%. This is a difficult estimate to make because of bias in the selection of twins: if both are diabetic, they are more likely to register themselves for such a study. See Leslie* et al. *(1989) and Hitman & Niven (1989).*

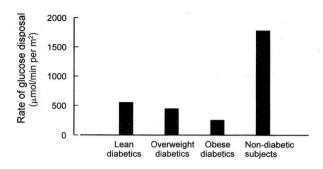

Figure 9.2   Rates of insulin-stimulated glucose disposal in non-diabetic controls, and in lean, overweight and obese people with NIDDM
Insulin was infused intravenously to produce the same plasma insulin concentration in all subjects. None of the diabetic subjects responds to the same extent as the controls — this is the phenomenon of insulin resistance. Of the diabetics, the more overweight are more severely affected. Based on Alberti et al. (1990); reproduced with permission from Baillière Tindall.

may revert almost to normal, and many people with NIDDM are managed on strict diet alone.

NIDDM is a more common disease than IDDM. It is present in about 2% of the population in the Western world, but its incidence increases steeply with age: in the over 70-year-old age group, for instance, the prevalence approaches 10%. NIDDM has a greater hereditary component than IDDM: among identical twins, if one twin has NIDDM, the chances are more than 90% that the other twin will have the disease. But, again, environment plays an important part. For instance, the incidence of NIDDM in people living in rural areas in the Indian sub-continent is low, but in Indians living in Britain the incidence is very high, and increasing: it is thought that some feature of the lifestyle here, probably related to diet and lack of exercise, leads to the development of the disease in a group who are genetically predisposed.

9.3   Alterations in metabolism in diabetes mellitus

It is important to draw a distinction here between the metabolic alterations that occur in untreated diabetes mellitus and those that occur in people with the disease nowadays, who usually receive treatment. The former are usually very severe and fatal. They may be studied in animal models of the disease in which drugs which are selectively toxic to the pancreatic islets are given to abolish or severely restrict insulin secretion.

It is a mistake to think, however, that people with treated diabetes are free from problems. It is now rare, at least in the developed world, for them to die from acute lack of insulin; however, their life expectancy is reduced, and their quality of life may be reduced by progressive onset of diabetic complications (Section 9.5).

9.3.1   Untreated IDDM

The metabolic picture in untreated IDDM, outlined in Figure 9.3, is of a *catabolic state*; i.e. one of breakdown of fuel stores and tissues. Lack of insulin leads to a net mobilization of glycogen. There is evidence that glucagon secretion is increased in this condition, perhaps because the general stress state leads to increased sympatho-adrenal activity. This, together with lack of insulin, leads to increased gluconeogenesis. Thus hepatic glucose production is increased. In addition, the supply of amino acid substrate for gluconeogenesis is increased because there is net breakdown of tissue protein, especially of the large amount in skeletal muscle. Glucose utilization in tissues in which it is normally activated by insulin, particularly skeletal muscle, is impaired or abolished. This is reinforced by increased availability of fatty acids (see later) for oxidation, which displace glucose as the oxidative fuel by the glucose–fatty acid cycle (see Section 5.4.1.2). Thus the concentration of glucose in the blood rises dramatically. The normal 'resting' concentration of around 5 mmol/l may increase to 10, 20 or even 50 mmol/l as the disease progresses. In addition, the change in blood glucose concentration when glucose or carbohydrate is

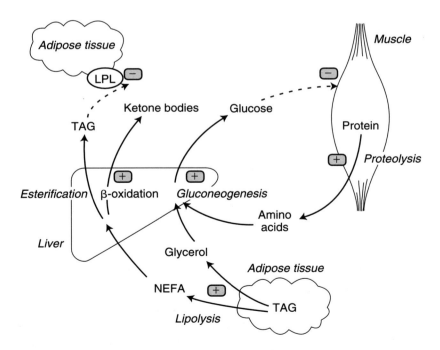

Figure 9.3   The metabolic pattern in untreated IDDM
(+) Indicates pathways accelerated by insulin deficiency; (−) indicates pathways inhibited (partic-ularly glucose uptake by insulin-sensitive tissues such as muscle, and triacylglycerol removal by lipoprotein lipase). Abbreviations used: LPL, lipoprotein lipase; NEFA, non-esterified fatty acids; TAG, triacylglycerol.

> ## Box 9.1 Diagnosis of diabetes mellitus
>
> Diabetes mellitus is defined by an elevation of the plasma (or blood) glucose concentration. It may be diagnosed by a measurement of the plasma glucose concentration after an overnight fast, but usually the disease is more clearly unmasked by observing the response of the plasma glucose concentration after drinking a solution of 75 g glucose, the *oral glucose tolerance test*. The World Health Organization has specified limits for definition of diabetes, and of less severe changes known as *impaired glucose tolerance*:
>
> | | **Typical control values** | **Impaired glucose tolerance** | **Diabetes mellitus** |
> | --- | --- | --- | --- |
> | Fasting | 4.5–5.0 | – | ≥7.8 |
> | 2 h after 75 g glucose | 4.5–6.0 | 7.8–11.0 | ≥11.1 |
>
> Venous plasma glucose concentrations are given in mmol/l; typical non-diabetic control values are shown for comparison.
>
> The figure shows typical results from an oral glucose tolerance test in non-diabetic and NIDDM subjects.
>
>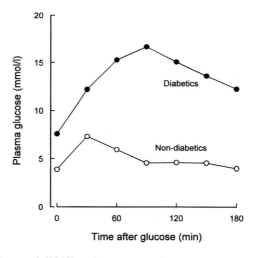
>
> Redrawn from Felber *et al.* (1993) with permission from John Wiley.

ingested becomes exaggerated — the person displays poor *glucose tolerance*. This feature is commonly used for diagnosis of diabetes mellitus (Box 9.1).

The increased glucose concentration of the blood (*hyperglycaemia*) leads to loss of glucose in the urine. Normally glucose is filtered at the glomerulus and re-absorbed in the proximal tubules. But when the blood concentration rises above about 12 mmol/l (the *renal threshold*) re-absorption becomes saturated and glucose spills over into the urine. This would lead to a hyperosmolar urine, so more water is lost through *osmotic diuresis*. Hence the classic sign of increased production of sugary urine. Loss of this extra water leads to thirst, the other classic sign of diabetes mellitus. People who develop IDDM are usually first driven to their doctor by a combination of weight loss, thirst and frequent urination; treatment with insulin rapidly reverses these changes and restores their feeling of health.

The changes in glucose metabolism are usually regarded as the hallmark of IDDM, and treatment is always monitored by the level of glucose in the blood. However, if it were as easy to measure fatty acids in blood as it is to measure glucose, we would think of IDDM mainly as a disorder of fat metabolism. Lack of insulin leads to unrestrained release of non-esterified fatty acids from adipose tissue, and also to lack of activation of adipose tissue lipoprotein lipase. Thus adipocytes fail to take up triacylglycerol from the blood, and there is a dramatic net loss of fat from adipose depots. This, together with the breakdown of protein, leads to the catabolic state and rapidly developing wasted appearance of sufferers who do not receive treatment (see Figure 9.1).

The concentration of non-esterified fatty acids in the plasma in untreated IDDM (normally in the range 0.2–1.0 mmol/l for healthy subjects) may reach 3–4 mmol/l. These high concentrations, together with the lack of insulin (and possible increase in glucagon) lead to increased fatty acid oxidation and ketone body production in the liver (see Figure 9.3). The combined concentration of the ketone bodies 3-hydroxybutyrate and acetoacetate in the blood is normally less than 0.2 mmol/l. In untreated diabetes, their combined concentration may reach 10–20 mmol/l. Remember that these are produced as the corresponding acids, 3-hydroxybutyric acid and acetoacetic acid. Thus the level of acidity of the blood also increases, i.e. the pH falls from the normal value of about 7.4 to perhaps around 7.0. This is a dangerous situation known as *diabetic keto-acidosis*.

In addition, excess non-esterified fatty acids may be diverted into esterification in the liver despite the lack of insulin, and increased very-low-density lipoprotein (VLDL)-triacylglycerol secretion may result. Triacylglycerol clearance from the plasma is much reduced because of lack of activation of adipose tissue lipoprotein lipase (Figure 9.3). Thus hypertriglyceridaemia is another feature of untreated IDDM.

The accumulation of ketone bodies and glucose in the blood, together with dehydration (which is common in the severely affected), leads to an increase in the osmolality of the blood. This, in combination with the increased acidity, causes changes in brain function which lead to unconsciousness — *diabetic coma* or *hyperglycaemic coma*. This will progress to death if not treated. This was the fate of IDDM sufferers before the introduction of insulin treatment. Treatment consists of insulin together with fluid. Deaths from diabetic ketoacidosis are now rare.

The tendency to develop ketoacidosis distinguishes IDDM from NIDDM clinically. Those with NIDDM are not dependent upon insulin in the sense that they will not develop ketoacidosis, apparently under almost any circumstances. It is presumed that the small amount of insulin secretion that remains is sufficient to prevent excess ketone body formation. These people may, however, benefit from treatment with insulin; it may give better regulation of the blood glucose concentration than tablet drugs alone.

9.3.2 Metabolic alterations in NIDDM

The plasma glucose concentration in NIDDM varies according to the severity of the condition; however, if a patient neglects his/her treatment and then attends a diabetic clinic, it would not be uncommon to find a plasma glucose concentration of 20 mmol/l. The plasma glucose concentration is consistently raised throughout the day (Figure 9.4), with an exaggerated response to meals. This highlights the important role of insulin in minimizing the post-prandial 'excursions' in plasma glucose concentration, which is impaired in NIDDM. In addition, plasma non-esterified fatty acid concentrations may be elevated throughout the day (Figure 9.5). This elevation may aggravate a number of features of the condition, by reducing further the ability of insulin to stimulate glucose uptake by skeletal muscle, and promoting hepatic VLDL-triacylglyc-erol secretion.

9.4   Treatment of diabetes mellitus

9.4.1   IDDM

In IDDM, the only satisfactory treatment is to replace the missing insulin. However, this simple statement is not easy to put into practice. Until the last decade, all insulin used by diabetics was extracted from the pancreases of cows and pigs. This had two disadvantages. (i) The supply was finite and there were worries that it would never be sufficient to meet the needs of patients worldwide. (ii) In addition, both bovine and porcine insulin differ slightly in

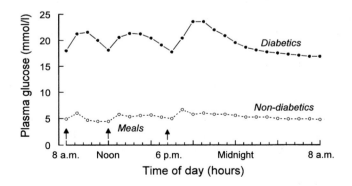

Figure 9.4   Profiles of plasma glucose concentration in non-diabetic subjects and subjects with severe NIDDM over a 24 h period
Non-diabetics were also shown in Figure 5.1. Redrawn from data in Reaven *et al.* (1988) with permission from the American Diabetes Association.

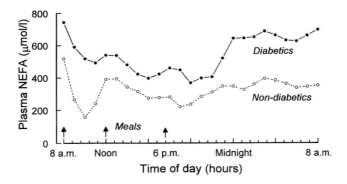

Figure 9.5 **Profiles of plasma non-esterified fatty acid (NEFA) concentration in non-diabetic subjects and subjects with severe NIDDM over a 24 h period**
Plasma glucose concentrations in these subjects are shown in Figure 9.4. Redrawn from data in Reaven *et al.* (1988) with permission from the American Diabetes Association.

amino acid sequence from human insulin, and the extracts were not completely pure. These factors led to the development of *insulin antibodies* in people treated with these preparations. In patients who reacted particularly strongly in this way, the concentration of insulin antibodies became so high (binding the insulin that was given) that enormous doses of insulin had to be used; in fact, this was the original condition known as insulin resistance. Now, a protein identical to human insulin is produced by bacteria in culture using recombinant DNA techniques. The supply is effectively infinite, the preparations are pure and the protein does not cause production of antibodies.

Insulin cannot be given orally because, like any other protein, it would be broken down into its constituent amino acids before absorption from the intestine; therefore, it has to be injected. The number of injections given per day should, ideally, be as few as possible. A major theme of this book has been the way in which metabolism is regulated by constantly changing, subtle alterations in the secretion of insulin. How can this possibly be mimicked by two or three injections each day? The anatomical relationship of the liver and the pancreas has also been stressed in this book. Insulin is secreted into the portal vein and exerts its initial effects on the liver. We cannot inject into the portal vein, and insulin is usually given into the subcutaneous adipose tissue (Figure 9.6). How different will metabolic regulation be if insulin reaches the peripheral circulation in concentrations which can only change slowly and which do not respond directly to changes in the concentration of glucose in the blood? With a suitable combination of injections three times a day, surprisingly normal blood glucose concentrations can be maintained: but never completely normal.

One important reason for the lack of complete normalization is the balancing act that a person with IDDM must perform between too little and too much insulin. Too little and the blood glucose concentration rises unduly and ketoacidosis begins; too much and the blood glucose concentration will

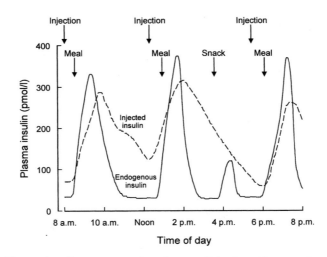

Figure 9.6 Plasma insulin concentrations in non-diabetic subjects and people with IDDM having three injections of insulin during the day
Based on Alberti *et al.* (1990); reproduced with permission from Baillière Tindall.

fall below normal levels. This can happen very quickly, particularly if, for instance, the subject unexpectedly has to miss a meal or take some exercise, having injected his/her normal amount of insulin. If the blood glucose concentration falls below about 2 mmol/l, the brain suffers from a lack of substrate (see Section 3.3) and changes in mood, e.g. irritability and slurred speech, will follow. If the glucose falls further, unconsciousness may occur. This is *hypoglycaemia,* or, if it leads to unconsciousness, *hypoglycaemic coma* or 'insulin reaction'. Because this condition can develop so rapidly, and its consequences can be so severe, most people with diabetes tend to under-treat their condition slightly, keeping their plasma glucose concentration on the higher side of normal. The process of checking their treatment has been made much simpler in recent years by the availability of portable devices to measure the glucose concentration in a drop of blood from a finger-prick.

9.4.2 NIDDM

For those with NIDDM, the balancing act is somewhat easier. Although some will benefit from the use of insulin, many can control their blood glucose concentration reasonably well either by strict adherence to a diet, or by use of drugs.

Dietary measures are largely based on what we know about the processes of digestion, absorption and post-prandial metabolism (see Chapters 2 and 5). The content of simple sugars (mono- and disaccharides) in the food should be low, since these lead to a rapid rise in the concentration of glucose in the blood; a high content of fibre in the diet helps to slow down the rate of absorption of carbohydrate and thus minimize the post-prandial rise in blood glucose concentration. In addition, the calorie intake must be controlled to maintain as low a body weight as possible.

Two classes of drug are available for treatment of NIDDM. (i) The *sulphonylureas* act directly upon the pancreatic β-cells to promote insulin release; in the longer term, they seem to lead also to improved sensitivity to insulin. (ii) The *biguanide* drug metformin acts in a way that is not entirely clear, mainly to improve the sensitivity of the tissues to insulin, i.e. to reduce insulin resistance.

9.5   Longer-term complications of diabetes

People with diabetes may lead very active, normal, long lives. For some, however, life is marred by the development of diabetic complications. These complications seem to be secondary, long-term effects of the disease rather than direct, short-term effects of lack of insulin. However, the distinction is not absolute and it could be argued that they are just as much a feature of the disease as, for instance, ketoacidosis. The complications include vascular disease, both microvascular and macrovascular disease (atherosclerosis); kidney problems (nephropathy); nerve problems (neuropathy); and eye problems (retinopathy and cataract). The development of high blood pressure (hypertension) is also a complication of diabetes.

There has been long-standing debate about whether the progression of complications is related to the degree of *glycaemic control*, i.e. how close to normal the blood glucose concentration is maintained. This simple question has been extraordinarily difficult to answer. Recently a long-term prospective study in the U.S.A. has produced some clear results. Patients with IDDM were randomly allocated to receive either normal insulin treatment or special, intensive insulin treatment which maintained their glucose concentrations closer to normal over a period of 6–7 years. In the group with intensified treatment, the progression of complications was significantly less. Therefore, it is now firmly believed that complications develop because of prolonged elevation of the glucose concentration. However, the down-side was that people in the intensive treatment group suffered many more episodes of hypoglycaemia.

Diseases of the small blood vessels (i.e. the capillaries), the nerves and the kidneys may be inter-related through changes in the *basement membrane*, a structure that surrounds the capillaries in many tissues. In diabetes, this thickens and may restrict permeability. One biochemical mechanism which may underlie these apparently diverse changes is *non-enzymic glycation* of proteins (Figure 9.7). The mechanism by which this changes the function of proteins is not certain, but many proteins may be affected — for instance, changes in collagen structure may result. Since glycation is a non-enzymic process, its progression is dependent mainly upon the prevailing glucose

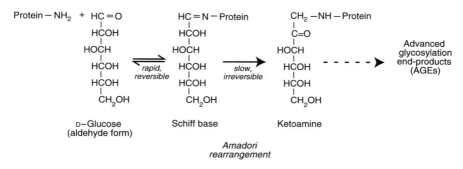

Figure 9.7 Non-enzymic glycation of proteins
A sugar molecule in its straight-chain, aldehyde form reacts non-enzymically with a lysine-NH_2 group in a protein; the resultant Schiff's base is converted with time to an irreversible, ketoamine linkage which may disrupt the functioning of the protein. With further time (perhaps over a matter of years) more changes occur, leading to the so-called *advanced glycosylation end-products* (AGEs), usually brown-coloured. The rate of the first reaction is proportional to the concentration of sugar molecules. Adapted from Alberti *et al.* (1990).

concentration. It probably occurs in everybody over the years, and it is easy to see how it could be a mechanism that relates an increased 'average' glucose concentration over a number of years to the premature development of tissue damage.

Another biochemical change which may relate to the average glucose concentration is the formation of the polyhydric alcohol, sorbitol. The pathway by which this occurs is a normal, physiological one; for instance, it is responsible for the production of fructose which is a normal constituent of seminal fluid. But it occurs at an increased rate when the glucose concentration is elevated. The pathway is outlined in Figure 9.8. It may be responsible for the development of diabetic cataract (opacity of the lens): sorbitol accumulates in the lens, and this may lead to osmotic tissue swelling and damage.

Macrovascular disease means disease of the large vessels, or, essentially, atherosclerosis (see Section 8.4.1). In diabetes, this typically affects arteries in the limbs as well as the coronary arteries. It can lead to impaired blood supply

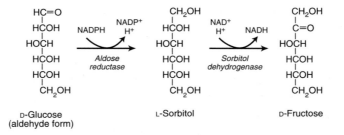

Figure 9.8 The pathway for production and further metabolism of sorbitol
Aldose reductase (EC 1.1.1.21) is present in a number of tissues, including nerve cells and the eye lens. It has a high K_m for glucose; thus the higher the glucose concentration, the greater the rate of conversion to sorbitol.

to a leg, for instance, to the extent that the viability of the leg is threatened. Coronary atherosclerosis is a common finding; in people with diabetes, cardiovascular disease is the most common cause of death.

In untreated or poorly controlled diabetes, alterations in lipid metabolism may give rise to the abnormalities usually associated with atherosclerosis. For instance, lack of insulin leads to failure to activate adipose tissue lipoprotein lipase normally after meals, with the consequences outlined in Section 8.4.3. But in those with apparently well-controlled diabetes, the concentrations of lipoprotein constituents in plasma may be relatively normal. It is probable that more subtle alterations in lipoprotein composition occur, which are not fully understood. For instance, non-enzymic glycation (see Figure 9.7) of the apolipoproteins could affect their ability to interact normally with receptors. In addition, a number of adverse changes have been attributed to chronic (long-standing) elevation of plasma insulin concentration. This will be the situation in many people with diabetes who are treated with insulin or insulin-releasing drugs (sulphonylureas), in the presence of some degree of insulin resistance. Chronic *hyperinsulinaemia* is thought to bring about changes in the arterial wall, particularly promotion of the proliferation of smooth muscle cells, which is an important component of atherosclerosis (see Section 8.4.1). It may also lead to 'inflexibility' of the blood vessels that control the resistance of the peripheral circulation, and thus to inability to regulate blood pressure normally: hypertension may therefore result.

Suggestions for further reading

General features of metabolism in diabetes mellitus

Leslie, R.D.G., ed. (1989) Diabetes. *Br. Med. Bull.* 45

Taylor, R. & Agius, L. (1988) The biochemistry of diabetes. *Biochem. J.* 250, 625–640

McCarthy, M.I., Froguel, P. & Hitman, G.A. (1994) The genetics of non-insulin-dependent diabetes mellitus. *Diabetologia* 37, 959–968

Diabetic complications (including alterations in lipoprotein metabolism)

Howard, B.V. (1987) Lipoprotein metabolism in diabetes mellitus. *J. Lipid Res.* 28, 613–628

Reaven, G.M. & Chen, Y.-D.I. (1988) Role of insulin in regulation of lipoprotein metabolism in diabetes. *Diabetes Metab. Rev.* 4, 639–652

Ruderman, N.B., Williamson, J.R. & Brownlee, M. (1992) Glucose and diabetic vascular disease. *FASEB J.* 6, 2905–2914

10

Energy balance and body weight regulation

10.1 Energy balance

The first law of thermodynamics states that energy can be neither created nor destroyed, although it may be interconverted between different forms. The human body is a device for taking in chemical energy and converting it, by controlled oxidation of fuels, into other forms of chemical energy (e.g. by the synthesis of storage compounds), into mechanical work and into heat. The first law of thermodynamics applies to the human body as to any other isolated system. Therefore, the amount of chemical energy taken in, after correction for any lost as waste products, must equal the total output of heat plus mechanical work plus the chemical energy used in biosynthetic reactions; any chemical energy remaining will be stored. This may be written simply as:

Energy intake (food) = Energy expended (heat, work, biosynthesis)
+ Energy stored

'Energy stored' may include a change in the heat stored, i.e. a change in body temperature, but over any reasonably long period this will be relatively constant.

On an hourly basis, the energy intake and energy expenditure may not match each other at all (see Figure 1.2). Therefore it is necessary to have short-term storage compounds, such as glycogen and triacylglycerol, which can buffer these mismatches. In the longer term — over a period of months or years — the glycogen stores, which have a finite and fairly small capacity (see Table 7.1), cannot buffer mismatches between intake and expenditure. The stores of triacylglycerol in adipose tissue are our long-term buffer. In other words, if energy intake exceeds expenditure consistently, triacylglycerol accumulates in adipose tissue, which accords with common observation.

How precisely do energy intake and expenditure usually match each other over the long term? Many people maintain a relatively constant body weight throughout their adult lives. Suppose that from the age of 25 to the age of 75, a particular individual changes body weight by 10 kg. That's quite a big change, and many people will change much less. We can translate that into a change in energy stores in adipose tissue. Adipose tissue is not all lipid, and its energy density is about 30 MJ/kg. This means that over the person's adult lifetime there has been an imbalance between energy intake and expenditure of 300 MJ per 50 years, which is about 16 kJ (4 kcal) per day. Therefore, many people balance their energy intake and expenditure over their adult life to the extent of about 5 kJ (about 1 kcal) per meal, and indeed many people even more precisely than that. We can look at the precision involved in this example in another way. Most people take in about 10 MJ of food energy each day, or $50 \times 365 \times 10$ MJ (182 500 MJ) over adult life. The imbalance with expenditure might amount to around 300 MJ. This represents an imbalance between intake and expenditure of about 0.2% of the throughput, a pretty impressive figure.

There is no way in which we can judge the energy content of individual meals to this degree of precision, and this sort of reasoning has led some people to believe that there are biological control mechanisms which regulate either energy intake (via changes in appetite) or energy expenditure. However, the existence of such mechanisms other than in a very crude sense (that the larger one's body weight, the more energy one expends) is not proven in humans, although there is good evidence for it in smaller animals. It is important also to remember that there are external cues, such as the tightness of one's belt, which can, perhaps subconsciously, affect one's eating or exercise pattern.

The aim of this chapter is to provide some of the background to what is known about the regulation of energy expenditure (we know very little of appetite regulation), and to show how an understanding of metabolic regulation enables us to take a fairly common-sense look at ideas about body weight regulation.

10.2   Energy expenditure

10.2.1   Measurement of energy expenditure

The measurement of metabolic rate has a long history. Probably Antoine Lavoisier (1743–1794) was the first to study the metabolic rate of a human, his assistant Séguin.

There are two basic approaches. First, we may measure directly the heat liberated by the body. This can be done in a special insulated chamber whose walls contain some device for measurement of heat liberated. Either they contain pipes through which water is circulated; the small difference in temperature between water entering and leaving the system must be measured accurately. Alternatively, the walls contain a large number of thermocouples which respond electrically to the change in temperature. This technique gives a direct measurement of heat liberation, and is known as *direct calorimetry*. It requires sophisticated equipment, and can only be applied in conditions which somewhat restrict the subject.

The alternative approach — used by Lavoisier — is *indirect calorimetry*, whereby energy expenditure is assessed from measurement of the oxidation of fuels, assessed in turn from the whole-body consumption of O_2 and production of CO_2. The basic principles are outlined in Box 10.1. In its simplest form, the subject breathes into a bag, whose contents are later analysed for O_2 and CO_2 concentrations. More commonly nowadays, a clear plastic 'hood' or 'canopy' is placed over the subject's head, air is drawn through this by a pump, all the expired air is collected, and its contents of O_2 and CO_2 measured by on-stream analysers. An indirect calorimeter can also be constructed as a room in which a subject may live a relatively normal, although somewhat constrained, life for several days.

Indirect calorimetry is usually performed over a period which ranges from minutes, breathing into a bag, to a few days in a chamber. Even this is not entirely satisfactory for assessing energy expenditure in people living their normal daily lives. Recently another technique has been introduced, the *double-labelled water* technique. This technique estimates CO_2 production over a period of 2–3 weeks. Energy expenditure can be assessed from CO_2 production alone with reasonable accuracy, although some estimate of the ratio of CO_2 production to O_2 consumption makes the calculation more reliable. To do this, the subject keeps a diary of food intake, and this is used to assess the ratio of CO_2 production to O_2 consumption if all this food is combusted (the *food quotient*, FQ); it is reasonable to assume that the same ratio for the body (the *respiratory quotient*, RQ, or *respiratory exchange ratio*, RER) will approximate the FQ over a period of time. The principle is outlined in Box 10.2. Its advantage is that it allows the measurement of energy expenditure in subjects living normal lives outside the laboratory: the subject comes to the laboratory to receive a glass of labelled water, and then reports back at intervals — say once a week — to provide a sample of urine or saliva.

10.2.2 The components of energy expenditure

We expend energy continuously over each 24 h period. Some of this energy expenditure represents the basic requirements for staying alive: at the cellular level, pumping ions across membranes to maintain normal gradients, turnover of proteins and other cellular constituents; at the organ level, pumping blood around the body, respiration etc. This basic level of metabolic activity is known as the *basal metabolic rate*. It is measured after an overnight fast, at a comfortable temperature, with the subject awake but resting; these conditions give very reproducible measurements. During sleep, the rate of energy expenditure is lower than the basal metabolic rate, but at other times during normal

---

Box 10.1 The principles of indirect calorimetry

The human body takes in the macronutrients carbohydrate, fat and protein. They eventually leave the body as CO_2, H_2O and urea. There is almost no loss of other products (e.g. partial oxidation products such as pyruvic acid or ketone bodies); in other words, the macronutrients are virtually completely oxidized (with the exception of urea formation from protein). The body produces heat and external work from the oxidation of these substances. It is irrelevant that the process of oxidation within the body may not be direct — e.g. glucose may form glycogen, then lactate, then be recycled as glucose before oxidation — or even that glucose may be converted to fat before oxidation. The net heat production will be the same as if the oxidation occurred directly.

The equations for oxidation of the individual fuels are given below,

Glucose

The quantities are shown for 1 mole of glucose.

$$C_6H_{12}O_6 \quad + \quad 6O_2 \quad \longrightarrow \quad 6CO_2 \quad + \quad 6H_2O \quad - \quad \Delta H$$

| 180 g | 6×22.4 litres | 6×22.4 litres | 6×18 g | 2.80 MJ |

where ΔH is the enthalpy change, i.e. heat produced; the negative sign is the convention when heat is liberated.

Note that oxidation of 1 g of glucose liberates

2.80/180 MJ, or 15.6 kJ.

The ratio of CO_2 production to O_2 consumption, the respiratory quotient for this reaction, is 6/6 or 1.00.

Fat

The quantities are shown for 1 mole of a typical triacylglycerol, palmitoyl, stearoyl, oleoyl-glycerol, $C_{55}H_{106}O_6$.

$$2C_{55}H_{106}O_6 \quad + \quad 157O_2 \quad \longrightarrow \quad 110CO_2 \quad + \quad 106H_2O \quad - \quad \Delta H$$

| 2×862 g | 157×22.4 litres | 110×22.4 litres | 106×18 g | 68.0 MJ |

Note that oxidation of 1 g of triacylglycerol liberates 68.0/1724 MJ or 39.4 kJ.

The respiratory quotient for this reaction is 110/157, or 0.70. ☞

---

daily life it is higher. The rate of energy expenditure is increased by physical activity, both by the performance of external work, and by the heat generated in this process. It is also increased after meals. The increase in the rate of energy expenditure after meals used to be called the specific dynamic action of food; more usually now it is referred to as *diet-induced thermogenesis* (DIT);

☞ **Box 10.1 (continued)**

Protein

The quantities are shown for 1 mole of a standard protein.

$$C_{100}H_{159}N_{32}O_{32}S_{0.7} + 104O_2 \longrightarrow 86.6CO_2 + 50.6\,H_2O + \text{other} \quad -\Delta H$$
$$\text{products}$$

$\qquad$ 2257 g $\qquad$ 104 × 22.4 litres $\quad$ 86.6 × 22.4 litres $\quad$ 50.6 × 18 g $\qquad\qquad$ 45.4 MJ

The other products are assumed to be urea (11.7 mol), ammonia (1.3 mol), creatinine (0.43 mol) and sulphuric acid (0.7 mol).

Note that oxidation of 1 g of standard protein liberates 45.4/2257 MJ or 20.1 kJ.

The respiratory quotient for this reaction is 86.6/104, or 0.83.

We may look at this another way, by calculating the heat liberated for each litre of O_2 used:

	Energy equivalent of 1 litre O_2	**Respiratory quotient**
Glucose*	20.8 kJ	1.00
Fat	19.6 kJ	0.71
Protein (forming urea)	19.4 kJ	0.83

---

*Slightly different values will be obtained depending upon whether the substrate is assumed to be pure glucose, or a glucose polymer such as glycogen. The same also applies to fat and protein: different fats and proteins give slightly different values.

Note that the heat produced per litre of O_2 consumed is almost constant. Thus measurement of O_2 consumption alone allows the calculation of energy expenditure (heat production) to a reasonable accuracy. However, the estimate can be improved by also measuring CO_2 production and urinary urea (or total nitrogen) excretion, to allow the appropriate energy values to be used.

These figures may be combined into a formula such as:

$$\text{Energy expenditure (kJ)} = 15.9\,VO_2 + 5.2\,VCO_2 - 4.65\,N$$

where VO_2 represents the volume of O_2 consumed (litres), VCO_2 the volume of CO_2 produced (litres) and N the amount of urinary nitrogen excretion (g), over whatever measurement period is used.

Data taken, in part, from Elia & Livesey (1992).

---

thermogenesis means generation of heat. DIT represents the energy cost of gastrointestinal tract activity, digestion, absorption and the metabolic cost of storing the fuels (e.g. formation of glycogen by the direct pathway from glucose involves the hydrolysis of two high-energy phosphates, one ATP and one UTP, per molecule of glucose).

Box 10.2 Measurement of energy expenditure using double-labelled water

The subject is given water ($^2H_2{}^{18}O$) in which both the oxygen and hydrogen atoms are isotopically labelled with a stable isotope (i.e. not radioactive), so that these atoms can be traced. The oxygen atoms equilibrate with CO_2 through the action of the enzyme carbonic anhydrase (EC 4.2.1.1) in blood. The loss of ^{18}O atoms from the body is related to the rate of expiration of CO_2. However, ^{18}O is also lost in water (in sweat, breath, urine etc.). This is allowed for by monitoring the loss of ^2H. Thus ^{18}O is lost somewhat faster than ^2H, and the difference (averaged over 2–3 weeks) gives a measure of the rate of CO_2 production. As described in the text, this can be used to derive an estimate of energy expenditure. A typical experimental result is shown below.

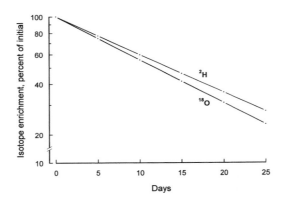

Data for the example are taken from Garrow (1988) with permission from Churchill Livingstone.

The total expenditure of energy over a 24 h period can be broken down into the basal metabolic rate, the energy cost of physical activity and DIT (Figure 10.1). Of course, physical activity varies from person to person. However, the largest component of the 24 h energy expenditure is, for most people, the basal component. The basal metabolic rate is very closely related to the amount of non-fat tissue in the body, the *fat-free mass* or *lean-body mass*[1]. The larger the fat-free mass of an individual, the larger (in general) their basal metabolic rate (Figure 10.2). The basal metabolic rate is also regulated by hormones, primarily by the thyroid hormone, triiodothyronine. During starvation or food deprivation, thyroid hormone concentrations fall and basal metabolic rate decreases (see

---

[1]*Fat-free mass is the total body mass minus the mass of chemical fat; lean-body mass is the total body mass minus the mass of adipose tissue. Although they are not quite the same, they measure the same thing.*

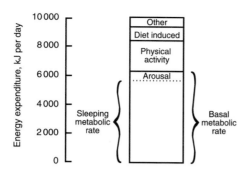

Figure 10.1 Components of energy expenditure

A typical 24 h energy expenditure of 10 000 kJ is shown with its components.

Section 7.3.2.1). The significance of this for weight-reduction programmes will be discussed again later.

10.3 Obesity

10.3.1 Definition of obesity

Obesity may be defined in different ways. It cannot be defined simply from the body weight since a tall, thin person may have the same body weight as a short, plump one. One simple solution is to relate the weight to the height. In 1869, the Belgian astronomer Quetelet observed that, among a large group of individuals, the weight varied approximately in proportion to the square of the height. For people of identical build, the figure given by weight/height^2 will be roughly constant. This ratio is known as the *body mass index* or *Quetelet's index*. It is usually measured in kg/m^2. If the body mass index is greater than the normal, the person is overweight; conversely the person is underweight if the body mass index is lower than the normal. A useful working definition of overweight and obesity is given in Table 10.1.

The increase in body mass in obesity largely represents, as we might expect, an accumulation of fat (Figure 10.3). The fat content of the body may be measured by weighing an individual in air, and then again under water; a

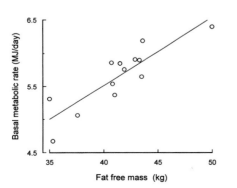

Figure 10.2 Relationship between basal metabolic rate and fat-free mass in lean women

The regression line is shown. Data from Prentice *et al.* (1986).

Table 10.1 A system for grading overweight and obesity

Grade	BMI (kg/m²)	Description
0	20–24.9	Normal
I	25–29.9	Overweight
II	30–40	Obese
III	>40	Severely obese

Based on Garrow (1988).

correction has to be made for the buoyant effect of air in the lungs. This gives a measure of the body density, which can be used to calculate the percentage of fat. More simply, the *skinfold thickness* at different sites on the body can be measured using a calliper to pinch the skin and underlying fat. The skinfolds at defined sites can be related to body fat content using published tables that are based on comparison of these measurements, in large numbers of subjects, with the results from underwater weighing. It is not pure triacylglycerol that accumulates in obesity, but adipose tissue in which there is also non-fat mass — adipose tissue cytoplasm, supporting connective tissue, etc. Thus an obese subject will also have an increased non-fat component (fat-free mass).

10.3.2 How does obesity develop?

If an individual is overweight or obese, that individual must have been through a period when his/her intake of energy was consistently greater than his/her energy expenditure. It does not necessarily follow that this is true now; an obese subject may be in energy balance, with a stable weight. Then we can ask: if energy intake was greater than energy expenditure, did this arise through (i) an elevated rate of energy intake, compared with people of normal and steady body weight, or (ii) a diminished rate of energy expenditure (again, compared with people of normal and steady body weight)? The answer may not be the same for all obese subjects. This question is of interest because if the answer is (ii) — i.e. diminished energy expenditure — it implies that the individual will also have a particularly hard job losing excess calories, because he/she has a 'biologically' low metabolic rate; it also implies

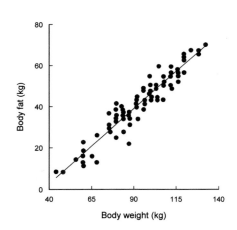

Figure 10.3 Relationship between body fat content and body weight in a series of 104 women
Redrawn from Webster, Hesp & Garrow (1984) with permission from John Libbey & Co.

that we might look, in metabolic terms, for the cause of this oddity of metabolism.

This is a deceptively simple question which has taken many years to answer. The reason for the difficulty in answering it lies in the very precision of energy balance (see Section 10.1). In most people, energy intake and expenditure match each other to within a fraction of a percent over a reasonably long period, but from day to day they may differ considerably. We must also ask what sort of a mismatch we are looking for. Many people who are overweight have become so over a period of many years of gradual accumulation. Take as an example a person of height 1.8 m and body weight 100 kg, i.e. body mass index 30.9 kg/m^2; suppose that he/she increased in weight from 70 kg (body mass index 21.6 kg/m^2) over 10 years. The gain is 30 kg of adipose tissue with an energy density of about 30 MJ/kg (as earlier), i.e. a total integrated mismatch between energy intake and expenditure of 900 MJ, or 90 MJ/year, or about 250 kJ/day. The throughput of energy (i.e. the amount we eat and expend) is about 10 MJ/day, so this is an imbalance of about 2.5%. The task is to measure energy intake and expenditure to a degree of precision that will enable us to say whether one or the other is 2.5% outside normal values, which themselves vary from person to person and from day to day. This is an almost impossible experimental task. What is more, we have to do this not when the person comes to the laboratory complaining that he/she is overweight, but before that, during the phase of weight gain.

The question has been answered quite clearly in a slightly indirect way. The energy expenditure of obese subjects has been measured and compared with that of normal subjects (Table 10.2). On average, obese subjects have higher rates of energy expenditure than subjects of normal weight. Now we see why this is an indirect answer: it is not one of the results we were expecting. At first sight, an increased rate of energy expenditure should result in thinness rather than fatness. But remember that fat itself, i.e. the triacylglycerol in adipose tissue and other tissues, is not metabolically active; energy expenditure occurs in the other components of the body, the fat-free mass. Fat-free mass is also increased in obese people. The rate of energy expenditure is, in fact, closely related to the fat-free mass in people of all body weights, lean and obese (Figure 10.4). Thus obese people have a high rate of energy expenditure because they have accumulated excess fat-free mass along with their excess fat. But, on the other hand, if they are at a stable weight, their rate of energy intake matches their rate of energy expenditure, and is therefore also greater than normal. These are not necessarily measurements made during the period of weight gain; however, it is argued that, if obese people have elevated rates of energy intake and expenditure, it is highly unlikely that their obesity was brought about initially by a decreased rate of energy expenditure.

The message from such studies is clear: for the majority of obese people, the cause of the obesity is not a defect in energy expenditure but a rate of energy intake which is greater than normal. Of course, if energy expenditure is

Table 10.2 Rates of energy expenditure (MJ/day) in subjects measured by indirect calorimetry

	Total metabolic rate	Resting metabolic rate	Sleeping metabolic rate
Lean	8.44	6.12	5.67
Moderately obese	9.60	6.65	6.05
Obese	10.04	7.59	6.22

From Ravussin et al. (1982).

also lower than normal, perhaps because of lack of physical activity, the situation will be made worse. The reasons why some people eat more than others are extremely complex and not well understood, and they are outside the scope of this book.

10.3.3 Health implications of obesity

Obesity is associated with a number of adverse consequences for health, which are outside the scope of this book except in so far as they have identifiable metabolic causes. Some are listed in Table 10.3.

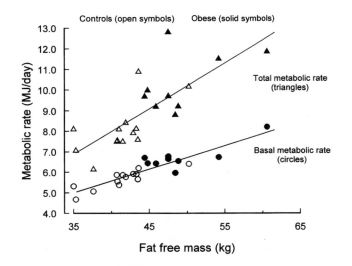

Figure 10.4 Relationship between metabolic rate and fat-free mass (FFM) in lean and obese women
The lean subjects are those shown in Figure 10.2. The graph shows both basal metabolic rate (BMR) (circles), measured in a calorimeter, and total metabolic rate (TMR) (triangles), measured during normal life with double-labelled water (Box 10.2). Open symbols, lean subjects; solid symbols, obese subjects. Note that the obese group have both greater FFM and greater metabolic rate than the lean group. Regression lines for BMR and TMR against FFM are shown. Data from Prentice et al. (1986).

Table 10.3 Health consequences of obesity

	Possible metabolic cause
Problems	
Cardiovascular disease	Elevated LDL-cholesterol, decreased HDL-cholesterol and elevated triacylglycerol concentrations in serum; high blood pressure (see below)
Hypertension (high blood pressure)	May result indirectly from insulin resistance
Non-insulin dependent diabetes mellitus	Insulin resistance
Gallstones	Increased cholesterol flux into bile (possibly related to insulin resistance and high insulin concentrations)
Reduced fertility (males) Polycystic ovary syndrome (females)	Decreased androgens, increased oestrogen production in adipose tissue*
Breast and other cancers	Increased oestrogen production in adipose tissue*
Osteoarthritis in weight-bearing joints	(Not thought to be metabolic)
Accidents and suicides	(Not thought to be metabolic)
Benefits	
Protection against post-menopausal osteoporosis	Increased oestrogen production in adipose tissue*

Based on van Itallie (1985) and Garrow (1991).

*Increased oestrogen production occurs because adipose tissue contains the enzyme *aromatase*, which converts androgens (e.g. testosterone) into oestrogens.

10.3.4 Metabolic changes in obesity

Many of the metabolic changes in obesity seem to stem from the associated insulin resistance. For instance, insulin resistance could, in a susceptible individual, lead to the development of non-insulin dependent diabetes (see Section 9.2.3).

In addition, insulin resistance has effects on lipid metabolism. Some of the major effects of insulin on lipid metabolism in normal subjects are listed in Table 10.4, together with the effects which stem from their disruption in insulin resistance. The typical metabolic picture in obesity is of a tendency to elevation of LDL-cholesterol concentration, a depression of HDL-cholesterol and an elevation of plasma triacylglycerol concentration.

Why does insulin resistance arise in obesity? The answer is not entirely clear. Many changes in insulin action have been shown in animal models of obesity: a decrease in the number of insulin receptors on the cell surface, decreased activity of the insulin receptor tyrosine kinase, and changes in intracellular metabolic pathways which render them less sensitive to insulin. To

Table 10.4 Effects of insulin on lipid metabolism, and the consequences of insulin resistance

Normal effect	Effect of insulin resistance	Secondary effects
Suppression of NEFA release after meals	Continuously elevated NEFA concentrations	Stimulation of hepatic TG synthesis; stimulation of hepatic gluconeogenesis; impairment of glucose utilization in some tissues (especially muscle), thus reinforcing insulin resistance
Activation of LPL after meals	Impaired activation of LPL	Impaired TG clearance; increased transfer of cholesterol from HDL (thus, elevated TG and decreased HDL-cholesterol concentrations)
Stimulation of LDL receptor expression	Increased LDL-cholesterol concentrations*	

Based on Frayn (1993). Abbreviations used: LPL, lipoprotein lipase; NEFA, non-esterified fatty acids; TG, triacylglycerol.

*The increase in LDL-cholesterol concentration is usually not so marked as the other changes in serum lipids.

some extent there is a vicious spiral: for instance, insulin resistance leads to inappropriately elevated non-esterified fatty acid concentrations in the fed state and these impair muscle glucose utilization by the glucose–fatty acid cycle (see Section 5.4.1.2).

Insulin resistance is a function both of the total amount of body fat and of the way in which it is distributed. Different patterns of body fat distribution may be discerned: fat may be concentrated around the abdomen and upper body, or around the hips and lower body. It is predominantly the former pattern which is associated with insulin resistance, and with increased risk of coronary heart disease. Nevertheless, the severely obese usually have plenty of fat in all regions, and insulin resistance to go with it. Upper-body fat distribution reflects accumulation of adipose tissue within the abdomen and subcutaneous fat. Some of this intra-abdominal adipose tissue — associated with the mesentery and omentum which support the small intestine — releases its non-esterified fatty acids directly into the portal vein and thus to the liver. It has been suggested that an increased influx of fatty acids to the liver may have particular metabolic effects, some of which can be judged from Table 10.4.

10.4   Dieting and metabolic regulation

Obesity results from an excess of energy intake over expenditure. If the obese or overweight person wants to lose weight, the solution is simple and unarguable: energy expenditure must exceed intake for a suitable length of time. The only alternative is surgery to remove some excess fat. This message is simple in principle, but extraordinarily difficult to put into practice. We shall consider why it is difficult, and look at dieting from a metabolic viewpoint.

10.4.1   Dieting as a battle against adaptation

It was stressed in Section 7.3 that the body is able to adapt admirably well to starvation. Indeed, it has been important throughout evolution to be able to minimize the impact of a period of partial or total lack of food. We should not, therefore, be surprised that dieting is difficult: it is a fight against mechanisms which have evolved over many millions of years precisely to minimize its effects. In our consideration of starvation, we saw the factors which bring about this protection. As food intake drops, the level of thyroid hormone falls and metabolic rate is lowered. Food intake has to be reduced yet further to drop below the level of energy expenditure. Hunger mechanisms, including the feeling of an empty stomach, lead us to search for food — although the feeling of hunger disappears after a day or so of total starvation, perhaps because ketone body concentrations rise and may suppress appetite. In addition, as weight loss occurs, the lean body mass will drop as well as the fat mass — this in itself will reduce daily energy expenditure (Figure 10.4).

Equally dispiriting for the aspiring dieter is the pattern of weight loss. Over the first 24 hours or so of total starvation — longer if the food deprivation is partial — the liver glycogen store will be reduced almost to nothing. This is a store of around 100 g (Section 7.2.1). Since glycogen is stored in hydrated form, with about three times its own weight of water, 400 g will disappear over a period of a few days, or a week or so with partial food deprivation. Muscle glycogen will also be depleted, again with its stored water, leading to further loss of perhaps 800 g. So more than 1 kg will be lost relatively quickly, leading the dieter to great hopes of a rapid transformation to skeletal proportions. However, the body's strategy is then to derive as much as possible of the necessary energy expenditure from fat, the store of which we have most. Suppose, initially, that almost all the energy expenditure is derived from fat. (This assumption cannot be entirely true, and will be examined in more detail later.) A typical dieter's daily energy expenditure may be around 9 MJ. The energy density of adipose tissue is around 30 MJ/kg. So 1 kg of adipose tissue will disappear every 3–4 days in total starvation; on a diet of 4 MJ/day, weight would be lost at a rate of about 1 kg/week. The contrast is this: when we derive energy mainly from the hydrated glycogen stores, each MJ of energy expenditure represents loss of about 240 g of body weight; when we derive it mainly from fat in adipose tissue, each MJ used represents loss of about 33 g of body weight. Now psychological factors will intervene: weight loss, so promising at first (when it represented mainly water) is now much less than hoped for, and for some there may be a tendency to resign oneself to a life of being overweight, and to resume a 'normal' diet. The situation is not helped if the diet is relaxed for any reason: the first response to a resumption of normal food intake will be the rebuilding of the glycogen stores (with their associated water), so 1 kg or more will go on surprisingly quickly. Thus the body's mechanisms, which have evolved to minimize the effects of a period of food deprivation, lead to difficulties for those who want to over-ride them to maximize the effect of a period of food deprivation.

10.4.2 Quantitative aspects of dieting

A knowledge of metabolism and metabolic regulation enables some common-sense statements about the effects of any particular dietary regimen to be made. For instance, a diet of grapefruit and bacon is likely to be effective only if its total energy content is suitably low, and if it will be sufficiently satisfying to enable the dieter to eat nothing to supplement it for a suitable length of time. An example of this application of metabolic knowledge to quirky diets will be used for illustration. A colleague (who could certainly have benefitted from the loss of some adipose tissue) started one of the proprietary very-low calorie diets which supply about 1.7 MJ/day in the form of soups or bars. Those who try this form of dieting often report favourable results in the short term, and it does seem that such diets can be reasonably satisfying. After two weeks he announced proudly — knowing of my interest in metabolism — "I've lost a stone [about 6 kg] — and it's all fat!". The reader might like to examine this claim. My analysis is given in Box 10.3. From the first principles of metabolism we would expect a weight loss of about this amount; but only about half of it could possibly have represented fat, and there was a considerable loss of lean tissue, potentially harmful if continued for a longer time, but certainly reducing his daily energy expenditure and slowing further weight loss.

10.4.3 Alternatives to rapid dieting

The problem with all special diets is that they cannot be maintained indefinitely. There is a wealth of research on the effects of dieting, with uniformly depressing results when the study is continued beyond the period of the diet. Almost all studies of dieting show that there is weight gain when the diet is stopped, and the long-term results of dieting are, for the most part, thoroughly discouraging. It is not the purpose of this book to recommend diets or exercise regimes, but a few statements can be made, based on sound metabolic principles, about sensible approaches to voluntary regulation of body weight.

An attractive approach would be to alter energy balance by taking a drug. The most obvious intervention to increase energy expenditure would be treatment with thyroid hormone. This has been tried in experimental studies, but it has many adverse effects, including loss of body protein, tremor and increased blood pressure. Alternative approaches are under development, including drugs which may stimulate the production of heat in brown adipose tissue. Their usefulness in adult humans (whose content of brown adipose tissue is at best small) has not yet been proved. Other drugs interfere with appetite, through elevation of 5-hydroxytryptamine (serotonin) levels in the brain. They seem to be somewhat effective in the short term, but in the longer term the problem of weight regain after stopping the drug limits their usefulness. Therefore, we must think in metabolic terms about how to alter energy balance in the required direction.

On the energy intake side, it has been shown many times that when special diets are stopped the dieter tends to resume his or her previous diet — which provided an excessive amount of energy. The long-term solution has to be to change dietary habits. Again, years of research have shown that simply trying to eat less of the same things is desperately unsuccessful. Presumably the body or the brain becomes used to a certain bulk of food, and any less is not satisfying. So the nature of the diet rather than the amount has to be changed. To the metabolically literate, it is obvious that some foods contain more energy than others in the same bulk; like energy stores in the body, fat-rich foods are more energy-rich, whereas carbohydrate-rich foods contain less energy for the amount of bulk — especially hydrated bulk, which is what they will be by the time they reach the stomach. Therefore, the metabolically literate eater consumes a diet relatively high in carbohydrate foods and low in fat-rich foods. By this means, he or she can actually have a very full stomach and yet not ingest excessive amounts of energy, especially if the carbohydrate is largely in unrefined forms (fruit, vegetables, cereals rather than sugar). The trick may be to be aware of which foods contain fat: pastry, biscuits, potato chips and red meat are examples of foods which may be thought of as carbo-hydrate- or protein-rich, but which actually contain a lot of fat. This is not just a theoretical argument; a number of studies have shown that body weight is related to the habitual fat content of the diet, with those on lower-fat diets having, on average, lower body weights.

Another important point about a change in eating habits is that one should think in reasonably long terms. The effect of dieting for a few weeks may be disappointing. Suppose that someone who is at a stable weight, but wants to become slimmer, cuts down on energy intake by about 150 kJ a day, by switching from high-fat foods, such as chips, to lower-fat items, such as baked potatoes. Assuming unchanged energy expenditure, there will be a daily energy deficit of around 150 kJ. As we saw earlier, in the long term this will be met by depletion of the adipose tissue energy stores. Since the energy density of adipose tissue is around 30 MJ/kg, it will take 30 000/150 or 200 days to lose 1 kg of adipose tissue. This may sound depressingly low, but, if this is a true change of habit rather than a temporary diet, then over the next 10 years, around 18 kg will be lost — sufficient for many people to transform

Box 10.3 Weight loss on a very-low-calorie diet

The example is of a moderately overweight person on a 1.4 MJ/day diet (a typical very-low-calorie diet) for 2 weeks. From our understanding of metabolism, how much weight loss would we expect, and what would be its composition?

As usual, the figures are very generalized and should not be taken too literally.

Assume
- Carbohydrate intake = 44 g/day
- Protein intake = 33 g/day
- Fat intake = 3 g/day
- Energy intake = 1.38 MJ/day

(The above are typical for a very-low-calorie diet)
- Daily energy expenditure = 9.8 MJ/day

Let
- Total protein utilization over 2 weeks be P g
- Total fat (triacylglycerol) utilization over 2 weeks be F g

Carbohydrate balance
- The brain needs 120 g of glucose/day, or 1680 g over 2 weeks

- Over a 2 week period, there will be loss of 100 g of liver glycogen and 300 g of muscle glycogen, liberating 400 g carbohydrate

- The diet provides 44×14 g (616 g) of carbohydrate over 2 weeks

- Therefore deficit (to be met from protein and glycerol) = $(1680 - 400 - 616)$ g
$$= 664 \text{ g}$$

- 1 mol (862 g) of a typical triacylglycerol yields 1 mol glycerol, equivalent to 0.5 mol glucose (90 g), i.e. yield $(90/862) \times F$ g of glucose

- It is often assumed that, since not all amino acids can form glucose, about half of any protein loss will be converted to glucose, i.e. yield $P/2$ g of glucose

$$P/2 + (90/862) \times F = 664 \qquad \text{eqn. (1)} \qquad ☞$$

themselves from being slightly on the portly side to rather slim figures. (This is oversimplified because resting energy expenditure will decrease as lean-body mass decreases, but the order of magnitude will be correct.) This is not a miracle cure for those needing to lose weight rapidly, but it is a strategy for those who feel that an upward trend as years go by needs to be transformed to a downward one.

10.4.4 Modification of energy expenditure

The discussion has concentrated on decreasing energy intake. But energy storage is the imbalance between intake and expenditure. So an alternative —

☞ **Box 10.3 (continued)**

Energy balance

- Daily energy deficit (to be made up from bodily stores) = (9.8 − 1.38) MJ or 117900 kJ over 2 weeks
- Energy derived from glycogen (400 g; ~17 kJ/g) = 400 × 17 = 6800 kJ
- Energy derived from fat (F g; ~38 kJ/g) = F × 38 kJ
- Energy derived from protein (P g; ~19 kJ/g) = P × 19 kJ

$$6800 + 38F + 19P = 117900 \qquad\qquad \text{eqn. (2)}$$

Eqns. (1) and (2) may be solved as simultaneous equations to give: $F = 2522$ g and $P = 804$ g

Of these:

3 × 14 g, or 42 g, of fat was supplied by the diet; therefore, net bodily fat loss = 2522 − 42 = 2.48 kg

33 × 14 g, or 462 g, of protein was supplied by the diet; therefore, net bodily protein loss = 804 × 462 = 0.342 kg

[but since lean tissue weight is approximately 20% protein (75% water, 5% other substances) this is equivalent to loss of 5 × 0.342 kg or 1.71 kg of lean body mass].

Summary of bodily losses

- Glycogen and associated water = 1.6 kg
- Fat (triacylglycerol) = 2.5 kg
- Lean body tissue = 1.7 kg
- Total loss = 5.8 kg (as claimed)

Some data for this box were taken from Kreitzman & Howard (1993). The diet composition refers to an earlier version of a proprietary diet: present very-low-calorie diets have somewhat greater energy contents.

---

or additional — means of changing the balance is to increase energy expenditure. The largest component of daily energy expenditure is the basal metabolic rate. Can this be increased? Pharmacological or hormonal measures were discussed above. Otherwise the main regulator of the basal metabolic rate is the lean-body mass: an increase in basal metabolic rate will be achieved naturally if body weight increases, due to the increase in lean-body mass. (Incidentally, we can thus see that obesity is to some extent self-limiting — provided energy intake does not increase continuously, there will come a time at which the elevated energy expenditure matches the energy intake. This was the situation in the stable-weight subjects in the study shown in Figure 10.4.) But since we are discussing reduction in body weight, this is not a useful strategy, unless the proportion of fat to lean tissue is altered — e.g. by exercise training to increase muscle mass relative to fat.

Among the other components of energy expenditure, the one most easily altered is that associated with physical activity. Physical activity has a bad reputation in terms of losing weight. Suppose we summon up the energy for a 3 mile jog. The rate of energy expenditure during gentle jogging is typically 40 kJ/min. It may take about 30 min (nothing too energetic); the energy expenditure is about 1200 kJ. Compare this with sitting at home for 30 min, with an energy expenditure of around 4 kJ/min, or 120 kJ over 30 min. So we have used up an excess of about 1100 kJ — and this may be immediately offset by the snack we feel obliged to eat to make up for our labours. This whole argument is, of course, oversimplified and put forward by those who want an excuse not to exercise! For one thing, the assumptions may be wrong — there is evidence that energy expenditure is elevated for a considerable period of time after a bout of exercise. So the energy deficit may be greater than that assumed above. In addition, the true comparison (with a dietary approach) for one bout of exercise should be foregoing one meal — again, not very impressive on its own. However, if we consider someone of stable body weight, who manages to include three such exercise sessions in his/her normal week, in the longer term the energy deficit per year will be $52 \times 3 \times 1.1$ MJ, or 172 MJ — the equivalent of almost 6 kg of adipose tissue. Over 10 years the person would waste away! (You may like to consider why this would not happen in practice.) Of course, there are many other benefits to health of regular exercise, so for those wishing to regulate their body weight in the longer term a combination of dietary change and increased exercise may be particularly beneficial.

Suggestions for further reading

General reviews on obesity

Bray, G.A. (1990) Obesity: historical development of scientific and cultural ideas. *Int. J. Obesity* **14**, 909–926

Flatt, J.P. (1988) Importance of nutrient balance in body weight regulation. *Diabetes Metab. Rev.* **4**, 571–581. (The views of J.P. Flatt have been very influential. In this review he outlines his views on the importance of the balance of individual macronutrients for the regulation of body weight.)

Health risks of obesity

Flynn, M.A.T. & Gibney, M.J. (1991) Obesity and health: why slim? *Proc. Nutr. Soc.* **50**, 413–432

Garrow, J. (1991) Importance of obesity. *Br. Med. J.* **303**, 704–706

Metabolic associations in obesity, including the distribution of body fat

Brindley, D.N. & Rolland, Y. (1989) Possible connections between stress, diabetes, obesity, hypertension and altered lipoprotein metabolism that may result in atherosclerosis. *Clin. Sci.* **77**, 453–461

Björntorp, P. (1988) Abdominal obesity and the development of non-insulin-dependent diabetes mellitus. *Diabetes Metab. Rev.* **4**, 615–622

Kissebah, A.H. & Peiris, A.N. (1989) Biology of regional body fat distribution: relationship to non-insulin-dependent diabetes mellitus. *Diabetes Metab. Rev.* **5**, 83–109

References

Acheson, K.J., Flatt, J.P. & Jéquier, E. (1982) Glycogen synthesis versus lipogenesis after a 500-g carbohydrate meal. *Metabolism* **31**, 1234–1240

Acheson, K.J., Schutz, Y., Bessard, T., Ravussin, E., Jéquier, E. & Flatt, J.P. (1984) Nutritional influences on lipogenesis and thermogenesis after a carbohydrate meal. *Am. J. Physiol.* **246**, E62–E70

Ainsworth, B.E., Haskell, W.L., Leon, A.S., *et al.* (1992) Compendium of physical activities: classification of energy costs of human physical activities. *Med. Sci. Sports Ex.* **25**, 71–80

Alberti, K.G.M.M., Boucher, B.J., Hitman, G.A. & Taylor, R. (1990) Diabetes mellitus. In *The Metabolic and Molecular Basis of Acquired Disease, vol. 1* (Cohen, R.D., Lewis, B., Alberti, K.G.M.M. & Denman, A.M., eds.), pp. 765–840, Baillière Tindall, London

Arner, P., Kriegholm, E., Engfeldt, P. & Bolinder, J. (1990) Adrenergic regulation of lipolysis *in situ* at rest and during exercise. *J. Clin. Invest.* **85**, 893–898

Åstrand, P.-O. & Rodahl, K. (1977) *Textbook of Work Physiology.* McGraw-Hill, New York

Atkinson, D.E. & Bourke, E. (1987) Metabolic aspects of the regulation of systemic pH. *Am. J. Physiol.* **252**, F947–F956

Bergström, J. & Hultman, E. (1966) Muscle glycogen synthesis after exercise: an enhancing factor localized to the muscle cells in man. *Nature (London)* **210**, 309–310

Bergström, J., Hermansen, E., Hultman, E. & Saltin, B. (1967) Diet, muscle glycogen and physical performance. *Acta Physiol. Scand.* **71**, 140–150

Bergström, J., Fürst, P., Norée, L.-O. & Vinnars, E. (1974) Intracellular free amino acid concentration in human muscle tissue. *J. Appl. Physiol.* **36**, 693–697

Bliss, M. (1983) *The Discovery of Insulin.* Paul Harris, Edinburgh

Bloom, S.R., Vaughan, N.J.A. & Russell, R.C.G. (1974) Vagal control of glucagon release in man. *Lancet* **ii**, 546–549

Brodows, R.G., Pi-Sunyer, F.X. & Campbell, R.G. (1974) Insulin secretion in adrenergic insufficiency in man. *J. Clin. Endocrin. Metab.* **38**, 1103–1108

Brodows, R.G., Pi-Sunyer, F.X. & Campbell, R.G. (1975) Sympathetic control of hepatic glycogenolysis during glucopenia in man. *Metabolism* **24**, 617–624

Brunicardi, F.C., Sun, Y.S., Druck, P., Goulet, R.J., Elahi, D. & Andersen, D.K. (1987) Splanchnic neural regulation of insulin and glucagon secretion in the isolated perfused human pancreas. *Am. J. Surg.* **153**, 34–40

Cannon, W.B. (1915) *Bodily Changes in Pain, Hunger, Fear and Rage.* Appleton, New York

Christensen, H.N. (1982) Interorgan amino acid nutrition. *Physiol. Rev.* **62**, 1193–1233

Coppack, S.W., Fisher, R.M., Gibbons, G.F., *et al.* (1990) Postprandial substrate deposition in human forearm and adipose tissues *in vivo. Clin. Sci.* **79**, 339–348

Cornish-Bowden, A. & Cárdenas, M.L. (1991) Hexokinase and 'glucokinase' in liver metabolism. *Trends Biochem. Sci.* **16**, 281–282

Costill, D.L., Coyle, E., Dalsky, G., Evans, W., Fink, W. & Hoopes, D. (1977) Effects of elevated plasma FFA and insulin on muscle glycogen usage during exercise. *J. Appl. Physiol.* **43**, 695–699

Durrington, P.N. (1989) *Hyperlipidaemia: Diagnosis and Management.* Wright/Butterwoth, London

Dyck, D.J., Putman, C.T., Heigenhauser, G.J.F., Hultman, E. & Spriet, L.L. (1993) Regulation of fat–carbohydrate interaction in skeletal muscle during intense aerobic cycling. *Am. J. Physiol.* **265**, E852–E859

Elia, M. & Livesey, G. (1992) Energy expenditure and fuel selection in biological systems: the theory and practice of calculations based on indirect calorimetry and tracer methods. In *Metabolic Control of*

Eating, Energy Expenditure and the Bioenergetics of Obesity. World Review of Nutrition and Dietetics, vol. 70. (Simopoulos, A.P., ed.), pp. 68–131, Karger, Basel

Felber, J.-P., Acheson, K.J. & Tappy, L. (1993) *From Obesity to Diabetes.* John Wiley, Chichester

Felig, P. (1975) Amino acid metabolism in man. *Annu. Rev. Biochem.* **44**, 933–955

Felig, P., Pozefsky, T., Marliss, E. & Cahill, G.F. (1970) Alanine: key role in gluconeogenesis. *Science* **167**, 1003–1004

Féry, F.D., Attellis, N.P. & Balasse, E.O. (1990) Mechanisms of starvation diabetes: study with double tracer and indirect calorimetry. *Am. J. Physiol.* **259**, E770–E777

Frayn, K.N. (1982) Acute metabolic responses to injury. In *Topical Reviews in Accident Surgery, vol. 2.* (Tubbs, N. & London, P.S., eds.), pp. 47–66, John Wright, Bristol

Frayn, K.N. (1986) Hormonal control of metabolism in trauma and sepsis. *Clin. Endocrinol.* **24**, 577–599

Frayn, K.N. (1991) Out of balance: diabetes mellitus, a disorder of metabolism. *Biol. Sci. Rev.* **3**, 37–41

Frayn, K.N. (1993) Insulin resistance and lipid metabolism. *Curr. Opin. Lipidology* **4**, 197–204

Frayn, K.N., Coppack, S.W., Humphreys, S.M., Clark, M.L. & Evans, R.D. (1993) Periprandial regulation of lipid metabolism in insulin-treated diabetes mellitus. *Metabolism* **42**, 504–510

Gardner, D.F., Kaplan, M.M., Stanley, C.A. & Utiger, R.D. (1979) Effect of tri-iodothyronine replacement on the metabolic and pituitary responses to starvation. *New Engl. J. Med.* **300**, 579–584

Garrow, J.S. (1988) *Obesity and Related Diseases.* Churchill Livingstone, Edinburgh

Garrow, J.S. (1991) Importance of obesity. *Br. Med. J.* **303**, 704–706

Gerich, J., Davis, J., Lorenzi, M., *et al.* (1979) Hormonal mechanisms of recovery from insulin–induced hypoglycemia in man. *Am. J. Physiol.* **236**, E380–E385

Goldspink, D.F. & Kelly, F.J. (1984) Protein turnover and growth in the whole body, liver and kidney of the rat from the foetus to senility. *Biochem. J.* **217**, 507–516

Goldspink, D.F., Lewis, S.E.M. & Kelly, F.J. (1984) Protein synthesis during the developmental growth of the small and large intestine of the rat. *Biochem. J.* **217**, 527–534

Gould, G.W. & Holman, G.D. (1993) The glucose transporter family: structure, function and tissue-specific expression. *Biochem. J.* **295**, 329–341

Griffiths, A.J., Humphreys, S.M., Clark, M.L., Fielding, B.A. & Frayn, K.N. (1994) Immediate metabolic availability of dietary fat in combination with carbohydrate. *Am. J. Clin. Nutr.* **59**, 53–59

Gurr, M.I. (1988) Lipid metabolism in man. *Proc. Nutr. Soc.* **47**, 277–285

Harrison, D.E., Christie, M.R. & Gray, D.W.R. (1985) Properties of isolated human islets of Langerhans: insulin secretion, glucose oxidation and protein phosphorylation. *Diabetologia* **28**, 99–103

Hegsted, D.M., McGandy, R.B., Myers, M.L. & Stare, F.J. (1965) Quantitative effects of dietary fat on serum cholesterol in man. *Am. J. Clin. Nutr.* **17**, 281–295

Henry, C.J.K., Rivers, J.P.W. & Payne, P.R. (1988) Protein and energy metabolism in starvation reconsidered. *Eur. J. Clin. Nutr.* **42**, 543–549

Hitman, G.A. & Niven, M.J. (1989) Genes and diabetes mellitus. *Br. Med. Bull.* **45**, 191–205

Hodgetts, V., Coppack, S.W., Frayn, K.N. & Hockaday, T.D.R. (1991) Factors controlling fat mobilization from human subcutaneous adipose tissue during exercise. *J. Appl. Physiol.* **71**, 445–451

Holloszy, J.O. & Booth, F.W. (1976) Biochemical adaptations to endurance exercise. *Annu. Rev. Physiol.* **38**, 273–291

Hue, L. & Rider, M.H. (1987) Role of fructose 2,6-bisphosphate in the control of glycolysis in mammalian tissues. *Biochem. J.* **245**, 313–324

Humphrey, C.S., Dykes, J.R.W. & Johnston, D. (1975*a*) Effects of truncal, selective, and highly selective vagotomy on glucose tolerance and insulin secretion in patients with duodenal ulcer. II. Comparison of responses to oral and intravenous glucose. *Br. Med. J.* **2**, 114–116

Humphrey, C.S., Dykes, J.R.W. & Johnston, D. (1975*b*) Effects of truncal, selective, and highly selective vagotomy on glucose tolerance and insulin secretion in patients with duodenal ulcer. I. Effect of vagotomy on response to oral glucose. *Br. Med. J.* **2**, 112–114

Hunt, S.M. & Groff, J.L. (1990) *Advanced Nutrition and Human Metabolism.* West Publishing Co, St Paul, MN

Issekutz, B., Bortz, W.M., Miller, H.I. & Paul, P. (1967) Turnover rate of plasma FFA in humans and in dogs. *Metabolism* **16**, 1001–1009

Jackson, A.A. (1989) Optimizing amino acid and protein supply and utitlization in the newborn. *Proc. Nutr. Soc.* **48**, 293–301

Johnson, I.F. (1982) Authenticity and purity of human insulin (recombinant DNA). *Diabetes Care* **5 (Suppl. 2)**, 4–12

Jones, D.A. & Round, J.M. (1990) *Skeletal Muscle in Health and Disease: A Textbook of Muscle Physiology.* Manchester University Press, Manchester

King, R.F.G.J., Almond, D.J., Oxby, C.B., Holmfield, J.H.M. & McMahon, M.J. (1984) Calculation of short-term changes in body fat from measurement of respiratory gas exchange. *Metabolism* **33**, 826–832

Kraus-Friedmann, N. (1984) Hormonal regulation of hepatic gluconeogenesis. *Physiol. Rev.* **64**, 170–259

Kreitzman, S.N. & Howard, A.N. (1993) *The Swansea Trial: Body Composition and Metabolic Studies with a Very-Low-Calorie Diet (VLCD).* Smith-Gordon, London

Leslie, R.D.G., Lazarus, N.R. & Vergani, D. (1989) Aetiology of insulin-dependent diabetes. *Br. Med. Bull.* **45**, 58–72

Lewis, B. (1990) Hyperlipidaemia. In *The Metabolic and Molecular Basis of Acquired Disease, vol. 1.* (Cohen, R.D., Lewis, B., Alberti, K.G.M.M. & Denman, A.M., eds.), pp. 860–920, Baillière Tindall, London

Lewis, S.E.M., Kelly, F.J. & Goldspink, D.F. (1984) Pre- and post-natal growth and protein turnover in smooth muscle, heart and slow- and fast-twitch skeletal muscles of the rat. *Biochem. J.* **217**, 517–526

Mason, A.S. (1960) *Health and Hormones.* Penguin Books, Harmondsworth

Newsholme, E.A. & Challiss, R.A.J. (1992) Metabolic-control-logic: its application to thermogenesis, insulin sensitivity, and obesity. In *Obesity* (Björntorp, P. & Brodoff, B.N., eds.), pp. 145–161, Lippincott, Philadelphia

Newsholme, E.A. & Leech, A.R. (1983) *Biochemistry for the Medical Sciences.* John Wiley, Chichester

Nilsson, L.H. & Hultman, E. (1973) Liver glycogen in man - the effect of total starvation or a carbohydrate-poor diet followed by carbohydrate refeeding. *Scand. J. Clin. Lab. Invest.* **32**, 325–330

Oliver, M.F. & Opie, L.H. (1994) Effects of glucose and fatty acids on myocardial ischaemia and arrhythmias. *Lancet.* **343**, 155–158

Owen, O.E., Tappy, L., Mozzoli, M.A. & Smalley, K.J. (1990) Acute starvation. In *The Metabolic and Molecular Basis of Acquired Disease* (Cohen, R.D., Lewis, B., Alberti, K.G.M.M. & Denman, A.M., eds.), pp. 550–570, Baillière Tindall, London

Pilch, P.F. (1990) Editorial: glucose transporters: what's in a name? *Endocrinology* **126**, 3–5

Pilkis, S.J. & Granner, D.K. (1992) Molecular physiology of the regulation of hepatic gluconeogenesis and glycolysis. *Annu. Rev. Physiol.* **54**, 885–909

Prentice, A.M., Black, A.E., Coward, W.A., et al. (1986) High levels of energy expenditure in obese women. *Br. Med. J.* **292**, 983–987

Randle, P.J., Garland, P.B., Hales, C.N. & Newsholme, E.A. (1963) The glucose fatty-acid cycle. Its role in insulin sensitivity and the metabolic disturbances of diabetes mellitus. *Lancet* **1**, 785–789

Rang, H.P. & Dale, M.M. (1991) *Pharmacology.* Churchill Livingstone, Edinburgh

Ravussin, E., Burnand, B., Schutz, Y. & Jéquier, E. (1982) Twenty-four hour energy expenditure and resting metabolic rate in obese, moderately obese, and control subjects. *Am. J. Clin. Nutr.* **35**, 566–573

Reaven, G.M., Hollenbeck, C., Jeng, C.-Y., Wu, M.S. & Chen, Y.-D.I. (1988) Measurement of plasma glucose, free fatty acid, lactate, and insulin for 24 h in patients with NIDDM. *Diabetes* **37**, 1020–1024

Robertson, R.P. & Porte, D., Jr (1973) Adrenergic modulation of basal insulin secretion in man. *Diabetes* **22**, 1–8

Romijn, J.A., Coyle, E.F., Sidossis, L.S., et al. (1993) Regulation of endogenous fat and carbohydrate metabolism in relation to exercise intensity and duration. *Am. J. Physiol.* **265**, E380–E391

Romijn, J.A., Coyle, E.F., Sidossis, L.S., Zhang, X.-J. & Wolfe, R.R. (1995) Relationship between fatty acid delivery and fatty acid oxidation during strenuous exercise. *J. Appl. Physiol.* **79**, 1939–1945

Ruderman (1975) Muscle amino acid metabolism and gluconeogenesis. *Annu. Rev. Med.* **26**, 245–258

Simons, L.A. (1986) Interrelations of lipids and lipoproteins with coronary artery disease mortality in 19 countries. *Am. J. Cardiol.* **57**, 5G–10G

Snell, K. (1986) The duality of pathways for serine biosynthesis is a fallacy. *Trends Biochem. Sci.* **11**, 241–243

Snell, K. & Fell, D.A. (1990) Metabolic control analysis of mammalian serine metabolism. *Adv. Enz. Reg.* **30**, 13–32

Taylor, R., Price, T.B., Katz, L.D., Shulman, R.G. & Shulman, G.I. (1993) Direct measurement of change in muscle glycogen concentration after a mixed meal in normal subjects. *Am. J. Physiol.* **265**, E224–E229

Thorens, B. (1993) Facilitated glucose transporters in epithelial cells. *Annu. Rev. Physiol.* **55**, 591–608

van Itallie, T.B. (1985) Health implications of overweight and obesity in the United States. *Ann. Intern. Med.* **103**, 983–988

Webster, J.D., Hesp, R. & Garrow, J.S. (1984) The composition of excess weight in obese women estimated by body density, total body water and total body potassium. *Human. Nutr. Clin. Nutr.* **38C**, 299–306

Wright, E.M. (1993) The intestinal Na^+/glucose cotransporter. *Annu. Rev. Physiol.* **55**, 575–589

Subject index

DATE DUE